Faces from the Front examines the British response to the huge number of soldiers who incurred facial injuries during the First World War. These injuries were produced within a short time span, but (for the first time in a major conflict) did not necessarily lead to death due to developments in anaesthesia and improvements in the treatment of infection and blood loss. Casualties were evacuated back to England, where surgeons had an opportunity to develop their skills on a large patient caseload.

Harold Gillies, an ambitious young surgeon, developed a new branch of surgery: plastic surgery of the face. In January 1916, Gillies set up a dedicated ward for patients with facial injuries at the Cambridge Military Hospital in Aldershot, Hampshire. Following the Battle of the Somme and the escalation in the number of casualties with facial injuries, steps were taken to establish a new hospital entirely focused on the treatment of facial injuries at Sidcup in South-East London. The Queen's Hospital treated more than 5,000 patients between its opening in August 1917 and the mid-1920s; its work was mainly funded by charitable donations.

The book uncovers the history of this hospital by analysing a wide range of sources – including numerous photographs and paintings – which detail the experiences of patients and staff. A team of surgeons and other specialised staff were brought together at Sidcup who, like the hospital's patients, came from Britain, New Zealand, Australia, Canada and the US.

The book argues that the development and refinement of new surgical techniques was helped by a multi-disciplinary approach. Detailed patient records – combined with notes, photographs and paintings – were used to evaluate the efficacy of experimental procedures and to educate new surgeons. Treatment often involved multiple operations and took place over long periods of time, and considerable thought was given to the recovery and rehabilitation of patients.

The Queen's Hospital had two important legacies: first, it played a pivotal role in the development of modern medical practice by paving the way for a new surgical specialty – plastic surgery – and by showcasing the benefits of specialist hospitals and multi-disciplinary services; second, the reconstruction of damaged faces had a major impact on the patients themselves.

Drawing on a unique collection of personal and family accounts of the post-war lives of patients treated at Sidcup, the author explores surgical and aesthetic outcomes and the emotional impact of facial reconstruction.

Andrew Bamji studied medicine in London and worked as a consultant physician in rheumatology and rehabilitation at Queen Mary's Hospital, Sidcup from 1983-2011.

As consultant archivist of the hospital from 1989 onwards, Bamji acquired the case files of the British and New Zealand sections who worked at Sidcup during the First World War. These 2,500 files are some of the only surviving clinical records from this conflict and include surgical notes, diagrams, X-rays and watercolours. These records fuelled Bamji's interest in the history of plastic surgery and the work of the Queen's Hospital, Sidcup.

His publications include 'Facial surgery: The patients' experience', in Hugh Cecil and Peter H. Liddle, *Facing Armageddon: The First World War Experienced* (London, Pen & Sword Books, 1996), and 'Facial surgery, rehabilitation and the impact of medical specialisation', in Peter H. Liddle (ed.), *The Widening War: The Central Years of the Great War* (Barnsley: Pen & Sword Books, 2016).

Bamji has lectured to medical and lay audiences in the United Kingdom, the United States, France and New Zealand, and his research has informed many television programmes and exhibitions – including at the Royal College of Surgeons, the National Army Museum and the Tate Gallery.

Faces from the Front

Harold Gillies, The Queen's Hospital, Sidcup
and the Origins of Modern Plastic Surgery

Andrew Bamji

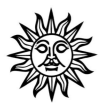 Helion & Company

Helion & Company Limited
26 Willow Road
Solihull
West Midlands
B91 1UE
England
Tel. 0121 705 3393
Fax 0121 711 4075
Email: info@helion.co.uk
Website: www.helion.co.uk
Twitter: @helionbooks
Visit our blog at http://blog.helion.co.uk/

Published by Helion & Company 2017
Designed and typeset by Mach 3 Solutions Ltd (www.mach3solutions.co.uk)
Cover designed by Paul Hewitt, Battlefield Design (www.battlefield-design.co.uk)
Printed by Short Run Press, Exeter, Devon

Front cover: 'Newly Blinded' by Francis Leopold Mond, RFC. (Author's collection)
Rear cover: The interior of the Plastic Theatre, Queen's Hospital, with Gillies seated right
and Rubens Wade standing. (Author's collection)

ISBN 978-1-911512-66-0

British Library Cataloguing-in-Publication Data.
A catalogue record for this book is available from the British Library.

For details of other military history titles published by Helion & Company
Limited, contact the above address, or visit our website: http://www.helion.co.uk

We always welcome receiving book proposals from prospective authors.

Contents

Acknowledgements   vi

Introduction   ix

1   From Injury to Blighty   17

2   The Emergence of a Dedicated Facial Injury Service and the Creation of the
Queen's Hospital   41

3   "A New Art": The Innovative Treatment of Facial Injuries   67

4   A Revolution in Record-Keeping   120

5   Rehabilitation, the Patients' Experience and Public Perceptions   142

6   The Legacy of the Queen's Hospital for Surgeons
and Surgery   161

7   The Post-War Lives of Sidcup's Patients   176

Bibliography   203

Index   210

Acknowledgements

I am grateful to many people who have helped with the research and production of this book, and apologise to any whom I have omitted. I must start by thanking in particular my dear wife Liz, who has put up with my writing and lecturing for several decades with great patience. I am also eternally grateful to Dr Alex Bamji for her invaluable advice – taking me under her wing as a mature, if slow student – and to Dr Chris Phillips for his judicious and meticulous editorial input.

Had it not been for Don Macalister, son of Sandy, none of this book would have been possible, as I would never have found the Sidcup case notes. I owe a debt to my surgical colleagues at Sidcup, Peter Savage and Jeremy Wilson, who decided I was a suitable person to organise the archives after the death of Freddie Herman, and hope I fulfilled their expectations. Valerie Jennings, Charnley librarian, obtained all of my requested reference texts at the drop of a hat and suggested more besides. Her assistant, Sylvia Pateman, typed chunks of text for me, as has Kathryn Wilson when she was my secretary. Stephen Collinson and Helen Moffatt, chief executives of Queen Mary's, gave invaluable practical and financial support. The late Denis McDonnell acted as my unofficial agent for acquiring texts, together with Luc-Daniel Dupire, who provided a number of continental items. Tom Donovan, John Marrin, David Harrison, Graham Nelson and Steve Tilston also watched out for relevant material and passed it our way.

Nick Bamji set up the initial structure of the archive website, without which many important contacts would never have been made. Doreen Hale, Ivy Meader, Brenda Holmes, Jean Holden and the late Pat Howley and Roseann Gibbs were all invaluable in sorting and cataloguing records, as well as maintaining order in the archive at Sidcup. Thereafter, it was a stroke of good fortune to meet Paul Nixon, who arranged digitisation of the entire case note collection and indexed it for the genealogy website FindMyPast; this digital archive has been much used for research.

The late Dr Ralph Millard was very generous both in donating a copy of *The Principles and Art of Plastic Surgery* to Queen Mary's, and for permission to reproduce various extracts from it. Mr Tony Wallace, who was originally responsible for the organisation of the British Association of Plastic Surgeons' Archive, kindly gave me a number of useful papers; my liaison with Brian Morgan and Roger Green, BAPRAS archivists past and present, has been invaluable and I am most grateful to Felix Freshwater, plastic surgeon in Florida, for his advice. It has been a continuing pleasure to collaborate with Dr Simon Chaplin and Dr Sam Alberti, past directors of Museums and Archives, and Louise King and Ruth Neave, all at the Royal College of Surgeons of England. Lyn Macdonald advised on the book's direction when it got out of control, and even did some background research. Susannah Biernoff's interest in the psychology of disfigurement has been most useful, as has the help and encouragement of James Partridge of the national charity Changing Faces. Sophie Delaporte has been invaluable in outlining for me, through her book, the management of facial injury in France; Xavier Riaud, who has written a succinct biographical volume on the war pioneers; through Olivier Roussel, Directeur-Géneral de l'Union des Blessés de la Face et de la Tête, I was introduced to other historians of the French experience – notably Dr Jean-Jacques Ferrandis and Dr François-Xavier Long. Vincent Coupez provided helpful details of German experience and Leo van Bergen introduced me to his own powerful book *Before My Helpless Sight*, which gave me a new perspective on military medical experience. A number of medical historians – including Mick Crumplin and John Richardson – have provided welcome advice.

William Spencer at the National Archives was most helpful in initiating me in the ways of searching Great War records before digitisation, and became interested enough to do some searching himself. The staff of the Imperial War Museum have been particularly helpful – especially Pauline Allwright (Department of Art), Stephen Walton (Department of Documents), and Paul Kemp and Alan Williams (Department of Photographs). Peter Liddle, past curator of the Liddle Collection at the University of Leeds, and his assistant Matthew Richardson supplied some important Sidcup material from their archive, as well as a great deal of encouragement. I have had vital input from Professor Murray Meikle, Colonel Darryl Tong and Sandy Callister on the New Zealand angle. Kerry Neale has researched the Australian section's work and its consequences. The artistic endeavours of Paddy Hartley helped to bring the Sidcup story to a wide audience by driving forward the exhibition 'Faces of Battle' at the National Army Museum in 2007, and his enthusiasm has been infectious. Paul Ferguson of the Royal British Columbia Museum, Canada has found the military files of many of the Canadian patients, which contain some previously unknown medical details, and I am very grateful to him for sharing this information.

In the text, I have acknowledged the many family members and friends who have provided artefacts and personal reminiscences which I have quoted, and there are many more whose correspondence has informed my arguments. I regret that I have not been able to include them all. I would particularly like to thank Jeremy Stevenson, for telling me the story of Norman Wallace; Pamela Campbell, daughter of Sergeant Reg Evans DCM; The Reverend Canon Ian Cohen, for details of his great-uncle Stanley Cohen; John Taylor, historian, for more details of the same; and Dr Hilary Marlow, for his details of the life of Mike Bowen.

As someone who is a physician, rather than a plastic surgeon or a writer, I have benefited from the perspectives of others. Three notable authors have visited the archives, and I have learned from all of them: Juliet Nicholson's book about the aftermath of the war, *The Great Silence*, has been both interesting and helpful, while the novels of Pat Barker and Louisa Young tell what it might have been like at Sidcup – weaving fact and fiction in an utterly credible way.

A number of institutions have provided information, or have helped to bring the Sidcup story to a wider audience. I wish to thank:

Army Medical Service Museum, Aldershot
Auckland War Memorial
Australian War Memorial, Canberra
Blond McIndoe Research Foundation, East Grinstead
Brightsolid Publishing Company
British Association of Plastic, Reconstructive and Aesthetic Surgeons, London
Brotherton Library, University of Leeds
Francis A. Countway Library of Medicine, Boston
Hocken Library, Otago University, Dunedin
Imperial War Museum, London
In Flanders Fields Museum, Ypres
Library and Archives, Ottawa, Canada
Local Studies Centre, London Borough of Bexley

London Metropolitan Archive
Musée du Service de Santé des Armées – École du Val-de-Grâce, Paris
National Archives, Kew
National Army Museum, London
Queen Mary's Hospital, Roehampton
Royal Archives, Windsor
Royal Australasian College of Surgeons, Melbourne
Royal College of Surgeons, London
Science Museum, London
Slade School, University College, London
Tank Museum, Bovingdon, Dorset
Tate Britain, London
University of Birmingham
Wellcome Collection and Library, London

My thanks go specifically to the following:

Ian Lyle, past librarian, Royal College of Surgeons, London, for copies of the Tonks pastels; Colin Smith, archivist, Royal Australasian College of Surgeons, Melbourne, for details of the Australian holding of notes, copies of photographs from Daryl Lindsay's album of the watercolours and the plaster facial casts; Richard Davies, Brotherton Library, University of Leeds, for copies of the essays written in Lady Gough's literacy class; Oliver Everett, late librarian, Windsor Castle, for Queen Mary's diary extract; Sir Brian Mayes, director, Army Medical Services; Shirley Dixon and William Schupbach, Wellcome Institute for the History of Medicine; Tim Wiles, curator, Royal Army Dental Corps Museum, Aldershot; Pete Starling, past curator of the Army Medical Services Museum, Aldershot; Elaine Lewis, librarian, Clinical Teaching Block, University of Birmingham, for a copy of Pickerill's MS thesis; Anne Dale, Dental Museum, Faculty of Dentistry, Toronto; Anna Blackman, archivist, Hocken Library, Dunedin; Emma Chambers, late curator at the Slade School, University College, London; Roy Hopper, librarian, Chislehurst Library; Helen Pugh, archives assistant, British Red Cross Museum, Guildford; staff of the London Metropolitan Archive, for access to the hospital's press cuttings book; Alan Baker, clerk to the trustees, Queen Mary's Roehampton Trust; Margaret Lewis and David Swift, Australian War Memorial; Dr Ian Kelsey Fry; Dr John Taylor, archivist to the Canadian plastic surgeons; Phil Sykes, John Holmes, Michael Tempest and David Eliott – all British plastic surgeons; the late Sir Benjamin Rank and Sir William Manchester; Luis Bermudez (Colombia); Sarah Crellin, for information on Derwent Wood; Mrs Margaret Divers and Mrs Joanna Vernon, Sir Harold Gillies' daughters; Susie Winter, daughter of Sir Harold's son Michael; Julian Lofts; Harvey Brown, biographer of Henry Pickerill; Andrew Wingrove, for details of HMHS *Plassey*; Jason Bate, who has meticulously researched the King George V Hospital, Stamford Street; Deborah Cohen; Mrs Dorothy Martin; Mrs Julia King, for mementoes of her aunt, Sister Emily Bayne; Albert Collins; Dr Robert Goldwyn of Boston, USA, for details of Varastad Kazanjian's records; Mr Lance Bromley; Miss Shelagh Davidson, who donated the original glass negatives of her father Bob; Mrs Barbara Hilton; Janet Harding; Dr John Waldron; Philip Lane, grandson of dental technician Archie Lane; Hazel Basford; Geoffrey Miller, convenor of the WW1 Document Archive; Donald Macalister; Gill Martin; Jim Connor.

Introduction

During the Great War, facial injury became a major focus of medical attention for the first time. Of all the horrific injuries suffered by soldiers during the conflict, facial wounds were the most obvious and had the capacity to cause the most reaction among those who viewed the wounded. This book is about the men who suffered from facial wounds, and the surgeons who repaired them. I examine the injuries men suffered, their evacuation from the battlefield, and the development of a new specialism within surgery. The text discusses surgical techniques and their impact on the injured, looks at the development of multidisciplinary work within the specialism, and tells the post-war stories both of the injured and of those who treated them. The book is based on the work of one centre where, arguably, both the techniques and the principles of modern multidisciplinary surgical management were set out for the first time. It also reviews the fundamental differences between experience in Great Britain and on the continent, and draws upon a combination of medical notes, textbooks, personal accounts and newspaper reports to argue that the First World War represents a turning point in the development of trauma surgery. The work of the surgeons discussed in this book took place at a watershed between the nineteenth and twentieth centuries – enabled by a growing understanding of infection, surgical shock and safe anaesthesia, and facilitated by the prevalence of raw material for experimentation as a result of the scale and pattern of the fighting. In this book, I will show how the development of techniques – reliant upon the concentration of resources, and the careful and accurate recording of the work undertaken – set the scene for the education of the next generation of surgeons. This work places emphasis on one man, Harold Gillies, whose drive and innovative approach were fundamental to these developments.

The book will demonstrate how the vision of one man was translated into a single-site, single-specialty hospital which both concentrated resources and patients, and pioneered the multidisciplinary approach to medical care which remains in place today. In January 1916, Gillies established a small unit for facial injury at the Cambridge Military Hospital, Aldershot, with the support and encouragement of the chief of the Royal Army Medical Corps, Sir Alfred Keogh, and the head of army surgery, Sir William Arbuthnot Lane. When it became apparent that the unit was too small, the Queen's Hospital in Sidcup was commissioned. Gillies took his small team from Aldershot with him, and the 320-bed hospital was formally opened on 18 August 1917.[1] The hospital developed major reconstructive surgical techniques and provided a model for sensitive rehabilitation. The surgical team from the Cambridge Military Hospital was augmented in 1918 by the transfer of contingents from Canada, Australia and New Zealand. The Queen's thus became a centralised hospital dedicated to the repair of faces. The staff list, which excludes the section heads and some other named staff, recorded 115 active medical staff and 18 American surgeons attached for training. Discussions in the Hospital General

---

1   The first patients were transferred in June 1917. The establishment of the hospital and its initial work were recorded in an anonymous report in *The Lancet* on 3 November 1917. A series of articles by Gillies, William Kelsey Fry, John Law Aymard and Geoffrey Seccome Hett followed shortly after.

Committee demonstrate that it is likely an American section would have been established as well had the war continued.[2] However, the Armistice intervened and the patients from the British Empire were slowly dealt with and discharged after the war's end. The Dominions' contingents returned home in 1919 and, after just eight years, Sidcup was closed in 1925.

The work of the surgeons at Sidcup has been largely absent from public memory of the First World War, and deserves a more prominent position than it has hitherto attained. In the past decade, Sidcup's role has begun to re-emerge in popular historical works and novels. *The Great Silence*, Juliet Nicolson's study of the aftermath of the war in Britain, examines the stories of several Sidcup patients and discusses the effects of injury on soldiers' later lives.[3] Pat Barker and Louisa Young have based powerful novels on characters constructed from the men treated at Sidcup, and Conny Braam has created a story of the disfigurement, pain and addiction of a fictional officer whose stay at the hospital resulted in a dependence on cocaine.[4] Howard Brenton's play, 'Doctor Scroggy's War', dramatises a surgical ward at Sidcup and was premiered at London's Globe Theatre in 2014.[5] All the same, academic scholarship on the Queen's Hospital has been restricted to professional journals, and analysis of the events at Sidcup for a lay audience is sparse. Murray Meikle has outlined the work of Sidcup in a book which focused on four surgeons from New Zealand: Gillies; his contemporary at Sidcup, Henry Percy Pickerill; and two of Gillies' later surgical partners, Archibald McIndoe and Rainsford Mowlem.[6] However, Meikle's study does not evaluate the important advances in organisation which were introduced at Sidcup, nor does it examine the effects of injury on the patients. Sophie Delaporte's work has provided important insights into the experience of facial management in France, but without any comparison to work undertaken elsewhere.[7] This book aims to bridge these divides by examining the collaboration between surgeons, dentists and other members of what is now known as a 'multidisciplinary team', and by comparing progress in England with experiences in other countries. The book also looks at the patients themselves, and reflects on the effects that war experience and injury had upon their subsequent lives.

This account of the broken faces of war relies almost entirely upon the records of this one institution. These records, which lay hidden for decades, detail all manner of facial injuries in text, diagrams, photographs and even paintings. Aside from one photograph album from the King George V Hospital in Stamford Street, London; a small collection of dental records from Aldershot and Sidcup, which now reside in the museum at East Grinstead; and a small set of notes in the collection of American surgeon Varastad Kazanjian's papers, which are held in the Countway Library in Boston, no other records survive from the other institutions which attempted to conduct facial surgery during the First World War.

2   A minute from the General Committee for 26 July 1918 notes a letter from Brigadier-General Winter, AEF, which stated that an American presence at Sidcup was no longer reasonable due to 'prevailing conditions'. See Australian War Memorial (AWM), AWM11 1506/8/43 [Australian Imperial Force Administrative Headquarters registry, 'A' (Adjutant-General's Branch) medical (subject) files], The Queen's Hospital, Frognal [Minutes of Meetings of General Committee] (October 1917-August 1918).

3   Juliet Nicolson, *The Great Silence: Britain from the Shadow of the First World War to the Dawn of the Jazz Age* (London: John Murray, 2009).

4   Pat Barker, *Toby's Room* (London: Hamish Hamilton, 2012); Louisa Young, *My Dear, I Wanted To Tell You* (London: HarperCollins, 2011); Louisa Young, *The Heroes' Welcome* (London: HarperCollins, 2014); Conny Braam, *The Cocaine Salesman*, trans. by Jonathan Reeder (London: Haus, 2011).

5   Howard Brenton, *Doctor Scroggy's War* (London: Nick Hern, 2014).

6   Murray C. Meikle, with Andrew Bamji, Bob Marchant and Brian Morgan, *Reconstructing Faces: The Art and Wartime Surgery of Gillies, Pickerill, McIndoe and Mowlem* (Dunedin: Otago University Press, 2013).

7   Sophie Delaporte, *Les Gueules Cassées: Les Blessés de la Face de la Grande Guerre* (Paris: Nöesis, 1996).

Plastic surgery of the face developed into a new specialism during the First World War, but had its roots in antiquity. The term 'plastic surgery' derives from the Greek *plastikos*, which means 'to mould or shape'. Hindu scriptures attest to the practise of nasal reconstruction more than 2,000 years ago. In the West, reconstructive techniques were described by Celsus and Galen, and in the eighth century AD, Emperor Justinian II sought to have his nose repaired after a battlefield injury.[8] The process was developed further during the Renaissance. In his *De Curtorum Chirurgia per Insitionem*, the Italian surgeon Gaspare Tagliacozzi (1545-1599) set out a method for grafting from the arm.[9] These surgeons and their patients encountered numerous problems in the treatment of facial wounds. The difficulties surrounding surgery were partly technical, as patients had to be incredibly stoical to undergo surgery without anaesthesia, and partly related to the cause of deformity. Injury and infection were the major causes of facial disfigurement at this time. Although the principles of tissue repair and scar formation were not understood, it was easier for surgeons to deal with injuries than with deformities caused by infections such as *lupus vulgaris* (cutaneous tuberculosis). Such work was more challenging because the continued spread of the infection could destroy the reconstructed area. The rapid spread of syphilis through Europe from the 1490s onwards also had an impact. Sufferers from the congenital form of the disease had a characteristic sunken nasal bridge, which clearly identified their affliction and brought shame upon them.

As the centuries progressed, plastic surgery continued to develop – and by the nineteenth century, several schools of surgery existed. The Indian tradition had been maintained, and was brought to the West by surgeons such as England's Joseph Carpue (b.1764) and von Graefe from Germany.[10] Von Graefe translated Carpue's *Two Successful Operations for Restoring a Lost Nose*, and was also responsible for the re-introduction of the Italian method. During the Napoleonic Wars, the Edinburgh anatomist Sir Charles Bell observed injuries and surgeries, and several pages of Thomson's *Report of Observations made in British Military Hospitals in Belgium after the Battle of Waterloo* covered the facial casualties sustained by troops in the triumph over Bonaparte's forces.[11] Across the Atlantic, surgeons such as Gurdon Buck and Charles Bell Gibson performed some simple and rather crude operations on soldiers during the American Civil War. In 1891, Denis Keegan claimed to have rediscovered the Indian technique, although his claim was probably based on a book published by Motichand Shah two years previously.[12] A decade later, in France, considerable experimentation culminated in the codification of Charles Nélaton and Louis Ombrédanne, whose two books on rhinoplasty and other reconstructions were published in 1904 and 1907.[13]

---

8   J.P. Remensnyder, M.E. Bigelow and R.M. Goldwyn, 'Justinian II and Carmagnola: a Byzantine rhinoplasty?', *Plastic & Reconstructive Surgery*, 63:1 (1979), pp.19-25.

9   Gaspare Tagliacozzi, *De Curtorum Chirurgia per Insitionem* (Venezia, 1597).

10 M.F. Freshwater, C.D. Su and J.E. Hoopes, 'Joseph Constantine Carpue – first military plastic surgeon', *Military Medicine*, 142:8 (1977), pp.603-606; M.F. Freshwater, 'Joseph Constantine Carpue and the bicentennial of the birth of modern plastic surgery', *Aesthetic Surgery Journal*, 35:6 (2015), pp.748-758; C.F. von Graefe, *Rhinoplastik* (Berlin: Realschulbuchhandlung, 1818).

11 M.K.H. Crumplin and P. Starling, *A Surgical Artist at War: The Paintings and Sketches of Sir Charles Bell, 1809-1815* (Edinburgh: Royal College of Surgeons of Edinburgh, 2005); J. Thomson, *Report of Observations made in British Military Hospitals in Belgium after the Battle of Waterloo with some remarks on Amputation* (London: T. Cadell & W. Davies, 1816).

12 D.F. Keegan, 'Rhinoplasty', *The Lancet*, 137:3521 (1891), pp.419-422; M.F. Freshwater, 'Denis F. Keegan: forgotten pioneer of plastic surgery', *Journal of Plastic, Reconstructive & Aesthetic Surgery*, 65:8 (2012), pp.1,131-1,136; T.M. Shah, *Rhinoplasty: A Short Description of One Hundred Cases* (Soruth: Junagadh Sakari, 1889).

13 C. Nélaton and L. Ombrédanne, *La Rhinoplastie* (Paris: Steinheil, 1904); C. Nélaton and L. Ombrédanne, *Les Autoplasties* (Levres: Joues Oreilles Tronc Membres, 1907).

By the end of the nineteenth century, surgeons operating on the face better understood the technicalities of surgery, but major obstacles to successful reconstruction remained. The first of these was wound infection. The teachings of Ignaz Semmelweis (1818-1865) on the spread of puerperal fever were ignored. Surgeons did not scrub themselves or their clothes, and failed to understand that the mouths and noses on which they tried to operate were full of bacteria. The second was the lack of suitable sedation. The first anaesthetics had appeared in the 1840s and were administered by mask. For facial surgery, a mask covered the very area which the surgeon wanted to repair. The third important issue was the lack of patients, which meant no surgeon was able to gain a great deal of experience in facial surgery. Under such circumstances, it is hardly surprising that surgery of the face was slow to develop. Indeed, some regarded reconstruction as an unattainable goal. Claude Martin wrote in 1889 that "Reconstruction, despite new resources and continuing perfection of procedures, cannot pass certain limits … [The art of] prosthetics still has huge advances to make; it is still necessary to fill out some types of deficit and mask tissue loss."[14] It was easier to cover a defect with a mask than to run the numerous risks which reconstructive surgery entailed.[15] Attempts to restore contour in the face through the use of paraffin wax injections had appalling results. Often the paraffin would migrate, leak, be extruded, or get infected – leaving a worse appearance than before.

Spurred on by the development of new techniques, but somewhat tethered by unease about the prospect of surgery for cosmetic purposes, interest in facial surgery grew in the early years of the twentieth century. However, its practitioners were few and they were isolated. Surgeons such as the American oral surgeon Vilray Blair wrote textbooks which were more comprehensive and less like the lists compiled by Nélaton and Ombrédanne. At the Val-de-Grâce Hospital in Paris, Hippolyte Morestin attracted attention and audiences for his heroic reconstructions.[16] Yet it would take more than the skills of these men and a few syphilitic noses to turn plastic surgery into a formal discipline. The massive casualty load of the First World War offered unparalleled experimental material, and permitted facial surgery to become effective. Previous wars had seen injury, but the photographs of men treated during the American Civil War by Buck and Gibson provide graphic evidence that the results were not good.[17] In any case, it was deemed more important to get men back to the front, and so medical efforts were prioritised towards those who needed less attention and whose return to the battlefield was most likely. Due to the problems outlined above, the victims of facial injury did not fall into that category.

Whilst a cadre of army and naval surgeons existed in most armies before and during the nineteenth century, they were, for the most part, poorly trained and supported. The French had pioneered the concept of casualty triage during Napoleonic times, whereby men were sorted rapidly into three categories: those who could be treated quickly and returned to battle; those who were beyond salvage and were left to die; and those who were in between. These latter cases would be transported from the battlefield and received major intervention. Such men received treatment which was brutally quick – largely because any delay led to intractable infection. Some died because blood-letting was still considered a valuable treatment, and their

14 C. Martin, *De La Prothèse Immédiate, Appliquée à la Résection des Maxillaires: Rhinoplastie sur Appareil Prothétique Permanent; Restauration de la Face, Lèvres, Nez, Langue, Voute et Voile du Palais* (Paris: G. Masson, 1889).

15 M.H. Kaufman, J. McTavish and R. Mitchell, 'The gunner with the silver mask: observations on the management of severe maxillo-facial lesions over the last 160 years', *Journal of the Royal College of Surgeons of Edinburgh*, 42:6 (1997), pp.367-375.

16 J.P. Lalardrie, 'Hippolyte Morestin, 1869-1918', *British Journal of Plastic Surgery*, 25 (1972), pp.39-41.

17 B.P. Bengston and J. Kuz (eds.), *Photographic Atlas of Civil War Injuries: Photographs of Surgical Cases and Specimens* (Grand Rapids, MI: Medical Staff Press, 1996).

surgical shock was thereby worsened. Many received rapid amputations of shattered limbs, and surgeons boasted of how quickly they could remove a leg.

In Britain, medical organisation in the armed forces underwent a minor revolution at the end of the century. Britain's experience in the Crimea had underlined the poor quality of medical staff, as well as the need for satisfactory nursing, and led to a growing clamour for the professionalisation of military medicine. Army doctors had low status and low pay, which resulted in a failure to attract high-quality surgeons. Furthermore, ability, or the lack of it, was irrelevant when it came to promotions, where length of service and patronage were far more influential. It took depressing reports on the medical services in the 'little wars' in the Sudan and Afghanistan to engender change. The Royal Army Medical Corps (RAMC) was established in 1898, and with it a proper career structure, adequate training and decent pay were brought to the army's medical services.[18] However, the new organisation was far from ready at the outbreak of the Boer War, and there was considerable demand for better forward planning. The establishment of the Territorial Force in the interwar period took things further – including medical support on a voluntary basis. Nonetheless, the Director-General of the Army Medical Service, Sir Alfred Keogh, felt this was inadequate and pressed for reorganisation along regular army lines. Keogh had a good working relationship with the Secretary of State for War, Lord Haldane. By 1908, they had created robust plans for field services, as well as for home hospitals based near teaching hospitals, which could be brought into effect at short notice when required.

By 1914, doctors and surgeons had the knowledge and technique to manage what had hitherto been untreatable. The response to infectious diseases had been transformed. Vaccination against the epidemic diseases that had previously decimated armies (such as typhoid) had begun. Wound sepsis was manageable, and anaesthetics permitted technique to triumph over speed. Military medical services were prepared, but not for the war that actually occurred. The First World War was the first in which casualties from trauma were more numerous than those from disease. Previous wars had been wars of movement and manoeuvre, but on the Western Front, machine guns decimated advances across open ground. There had been trenches dug in South Africa, but nothing to compare with the lines of deep, organised trenches and dugouts that stretched by late 1914 from the North Sea to the Swiss border. Even then, the men were not safe: a sniper's bullet could catch anyone who dared to peep over the parapet, whilst the employment of innumerable batteries of heavy artillery – raining down shrapnel and shell fragments – introduced new dimensions to injury. However, whilst men were increasingly exposed to injury, survival was now usual rather than unlikely, and surgeons were able to address the previously untreatable – thus the facial injury patient reached specialist care, only to find that it was often wanting because surgeons were inexperienced and isolated. The stage was set for a sea change in management and outcome, and Gillies and Sidcup provided it.

In the mid-1980s, some members of the modern Queen Mary's Hospital decided to record its history. Freddie Herman, the hospital's pathologist for 30 years prior to his retirement, was appointed as hospital archivist. One of the hospital's medical secretaries, who came from a large family of hospital workers stretching back to before the establishment of the National Health Service (NHS), suggested that the hospital's First World War records had been destroyed. She recalled that her father, who had been on the maintenance staff, had burned large quantities of paper records and photographs, and destroyed a large number of glass negatives in 1928. Queen Mary's only possessed some plans of the old hospital, a booklet dating from 1929, and a

---

18 J.S.G. Blair, *Centenary History of the Royal Army Medical Corps, 1898-1998* (Edinburgh: Scottish Academic Press, 1998).

few photographs. At the end of the war, the detachments from the Dominions had taken their records with them and, in March 1986, Freddie Herman received a letter from Professor Sandy Macalister, who was the professor of Oral Surgery at the University of Otago, Dunedin, New Zealand. Macalister wrote that "some years ago," he had come upon "the complete and original records of the New Zealand personnel treated by Pickerill."[19] He had discovered that they were about to be destroyed by the University, and had removed what he considered to be an important historical record to the safety of his garage.

Macalister had made contact, as he was scheduled to give a lecture on Pickerill's work to the Royal College of Surgeons (RCS) in London, and he wished to augment the clinical content of the records with some background information. Unfortunately, Herman was unable to provide any. However, a large number of the consultant staff attended the lecture and, for the very first time, they saw pictures of the surgery that had been done at Sidcup during the First World War. Sadly, Freddie Herman was not there; he had died of cancer and I had been asked to take on the role of honorary archivist in his stead. After the lecture, I asked Professor Macalister if Pickerill's notes might find a permanent home at Queen Mary's. After two years, Macalister's son Donald, himself a dentist, contacted me to say that his father, who had been incapacitated by a stroke, would be happy for Sidcup to obtain the Pickerill collection. In the meantime, I had purchased several reprint copies of Gillies' 1920 textbook *Plastic Surgery of the Face*.[20]

When two packing cases arrived from New Zealand in spring 1990, what became the 'Gillies Archive' began to take shape. One case contained the notes of 282 Queen's Hospital patients. The large majority recorded gunshot injuries, which were labelled as 'GSW'. A smaller number of injuries were listed as the result of shrapnel or gas shell bursts. The records consisted of typewritten summary notes, drawings of X-rays, mounted photographs (both clinical and of X-rays), and 77 watercolour sketches. Almost all had a grey card folder cover, but most of the records were incomplete. Occasionally, there were two sequential watercolours in a folder. Most of them were unsigned, but four were the work of Daryl Lindsay and a number of others were signed by Herbert Cole – a New Zealand artist who arrived at Sidcup in April 1918. Many of the notes related to British, rather than New Zealand soldiers, which suggests that the New Zealand surgeons helped to manage the overall caseload at the Queen's during the war. The second case contained a life-sized wax model of a head and shoulders, which illustrated some techniques of grafting and reconstruction.[21] Further records – including another 13 watercolours – arrived subsequently after Donald Macalister discovered them in a box in the attic. Additional sections from the New Zealand records were later uncovered in the Hocken Library, Dunedin and collated by Sandy Callister and Murray Meikle. Much of the material contained within these records comprised duplicates of the material previously collected by Professor Macalister. Yet whilst the various files from New Zealand were incomplete, only one set of case notes was missing from the typed list of records that had left Sidcup when the New Zealanders returned home in 1919.

From further research, I discovered that the shipment of the Canadian records to Toronto had required 16 packing cases in 1918. However, aside from the staff's baseball kit, most of the shipment had been lost in transit. Some display photographs and diagrams are now held by John Taylor, the historian of Canadian plastic surgery, and the Canadian facial plaster casts

---

19 Letter from Professor Macalister to Freddie Herman, who was the then honorary consultant archivist at Queen Mary's Hospital. (Author's collection)

20 The reprint had been organised by the British Association of Plastic Surgeons, which is now the British Association of Plastic, Reconstructive and Aesthetic Surgeons (BAPRAS) (London: Gower Medical Publishing, 1983).

21 This model was restored by the moulage artists employed by Madame Tussaud's.

were retained by one of the Canadian surgeons, Fulton Risdon. Unfortunately, Risdon's family had thrown them on a skip after his death.[22] The case notes of the Canadian section, if they still exist, are yet to be discovered. However, the Admissions book of the Canadian section has survived, and from that, it can be calculated that a total of 458 Canadian patients were treated at Sidcup; in addition, the digitisation of Canadian service files has revealed that summary notes were included.[23]

Whilst the Canadian notes were lost, the Australian records survived. The 345 files, which include 68 watercolours and 22 plaster casts, have been preserved by the Royal Australasian College of Surgeons (RACS) in Melbourne.[24] All of the Australian patients treated at Sidcup are documented in these records and, as with the Macalister collection, there were also records of British soldiers. The existence of these British records reinforces how the various national sections at the Queen's Hospital did not operate solely on their own citizens.

In 1992, whilst I was Director of Medical Education at Queen Mary's Hospital, Sidcup, I gave a talk and wrote an article for the journal of the Institute of Medical Illustrators.[25] Two weeks after it was published, I received a telephone call from the photographer at Queen Mary's Hospital, Roehampton. He asked if I knew that there were Sidcup records in his department. I made a visit and discovered two overflowing filing cabinets, which contained the supposedly lost records of the British section at Sidcup. The cabinets contained more than 2,000 sets of notes – documenting the care given to around half of the British section patients treated at the hospital between 1917 and 1925.[26] The records included written and typed notes by surgeons and anaesthetists, as well as diagrams, photographs and X-rays, and notes and proofs for Gillies' 1920 textbook *Plastic Surgery of the Face*.[27] Papers within the files also indicate that Gillies consulted the notes in the preparation of his 1957 work *The Principles and Art of Plastic Surgery*, which was co-authored with Ralph Millard.[28] The notes represent what had survived when Sidcup closed for plastic work in 1925, minus the files of a number of key cases which had been passed to the RCS in 1923. I took them back to Sidcup.

Of the 132 cases discussed in Gillies' first book, 78 sets of case notes survive. Dual sets of records also illustrate that several soldiers were treated by the British section, as well as by the Australian or New Zealand surgical teams. The case notes demonstrate that destruction and mutilation could be, and were, successfully repaired without antibiotics or modern techniques of microsurgery. The discovery of these notes enabled me to see far beyond Gillies' published work. In 1996, I created a website about the facial work at Sidcup, which led to more information (not least, about the patients themselves) being sent to me.[29] The fascinating details that I was sent by many families of Sidcup patients led me to re-evaluate considerations of the psychological effects of facial injury. I also began to compile a large archive of books related to medical and surgical aspects of the war. However, the closure of Sidcup's Postgraduate Centre

22 Risdon family, personal communication.
23 I am grateful to Paul Ferguson for this information.
24 These were a gift from the University of Melbourne.
25 A.N. Bamji, 'The Macalister Archive: records from the Queen's Hospital, Sidcup, 1917-1921', *The Journal of Audiovisual Media in Medicine*, 16:2 (1993), pp.76-84.
26 Thanks to Paul Nixon of www.findmypast.co.uk, there is a complete digital copy of all the records. Through careful research in the National Archives, Paul has located the first names for most of the British case notes where this information had not been recorded.
27 H.D. Gillies, *Plastic Surgery of the Face: Based on Selected Cases of War Injuries of the Face Including Burns* (London: Hodder & Stoughton, 1920).
28 H.D. Gillies and R. Millard, *The Principles and Art of Plastic Surgery* (London: Butterworth & Co., 1957).
29 A.N. Bamji, *The Gillies Archives from Queen Mary's Hospital, Sidcup* <http://www.gilliesarchives.org.uk/> (accessed 15 June 2017).

in 2011 resulted in the dispersal of the archive; most of the clinical material is now held in the RCS. Some of the archive's artefacts are housed within the college, in the offices of the British Association of Plastic, Reconstructive and Aesthetic Surgeons (BAPRAS). The book collection is now held in the Brotherton Library at the University of Leeds, whilst some items went to the Army Medical Services Museum in Aldershot. These objects and documents represent the only surviving full medical records from the First World War – a conflict in which more than 21 million soldiers underwent medical or surgical treatment. As a result of my work with this archive, I have met and discussed my research with students, researchers, authors, playwrights, and television and film producers. All of them have contributed to my understanding of the layman's perceptions of the physical and psychological management of facial injuries, which were a primary motivation behind the decision to write this book.

The book begins with an examination of the battlefield and how the conflict, and military medicine, evolved at the turn of the twentieth century. Next, it discusses injuries and how they were sustained, and follows the casualties of war on their journey from the front line to specialist help. It then considers how a small specialist unit for facial work was set up, and how and why it expanded into a multinational, multidisciplinary establishment known as 'the Queen's Hospital, Sidcup'. The book explores the work of the surgeons at Sidcup, the techniques they developed, and the processes by which they recorded the work and the lives of the soldiers at the hospital. Finally, the book discusses what happened to the surgeons, patients and the specialism itself after the war. It examines the lessons which were learned at Sidcup (many of which would be translated into modern experience), and how the patients themselves lived with the effects of their injuries. Studies of the First World War often focus on the events and the fatalities of the war, or on cultural memory of the conflict. Historians, writers, artists and poets speak of heroic sacrifice. However, few of them give thought to those whose lives were not ended by the conflict, but were changed forever. This book talks of those who were left to grow old, and whom age did weary, and is dedicated to their memory.

1

From Injury to Blighty

This chapter introduces the main causes of facial injuries, with reference to personal first-hand accounts of injury. The pattern of facial injuries had a different profile in each of the fields of conflict: bullet and shell wounds were significant in the context of trench warfare; naval warfare produced burns; and aerial activity led to both injuries and burns. This chapter discusses the survival of facial casualties, the development of casualty evacuation and triage, and the journey made by the soldier from injury to initial treatment, casualty clearing stations, base hospitals and, eventually, to England.

The First World War produced the largest number of facial injuries ever seen in a short time span. An analysis of 48,000 admissions to British army casualty clearing stations showed that face, head and neck wounds comprised nearly 16 percent of the total.[1] The French army Medical Service (the *Service de Santé*) dealt with over 15,000 facial casualties over the course of the war. In previous conflicts, the wherewithal to manage these injuries did not exist. In subsequent conflicts mass confrontations did not occur so frequently, and when they did in places like the Russian Front during the Second World War, survival rates were low. Some injuries were fatal, especially where damage to an artery led to severe blood loss. Others were often compounded by infection.

The high prevalence of facial injuries during the First World War was due to the changed nature of warfare. In the nineteenth century, battles were fought in the open. After an initial flurry of open warfare, for the majority of the First World War the opposing troops dug in and entrenched. The widespread use of machine guns, artillery and tanks expanded the number of ways in which facial injuries could be received beyond those caused by rifle bullets. Moreover, the war was fought on multiple fronts, and the war at sea and in the air generated additional casualties with their own patterns of facial injury. Soldiers went to war in their soft caps until the end of 1915. Thereafter, the newly introduced steel helmet spared many soldiers from death. A large quantity of helmets, dented or split by shrapnel, became battered souvenirs that were kept as talismans. Some men survived with a shattered face rather than died from a shattered skull. Improvements in the treatment of injuries, due in large part to a coordinated system of casualty evacuation, meant that far fewer men died from their injuries than might previously have been the case.

Wounds included simple jaw fractures, wounds of the cheek, damage to or loss of the eyes or nose, complex full-face injuries, and burns. The account of journalist Philip Gibbs, written

---

1   T.J. Mitchell and G.M. Smith, *History of the Great War Based on Official Documents: Medical Services, Casualties and Medical Statistics* (London: His/Her Majesty's Stationery Office, 1931), pp.40-42. Quoted in J. Holmes, 'The Development of Plastic Surgery', in *War Surgery 1914-18*, ed. by T. Scotland and S. Heys (Solihull: Helion & Company, 2014), p.265.

immediately after the war, shows how facial injuries horrified the lay observer. Gibbs recalled how:

> There were other wounded men from whom no laughter came, nor any sound. They were carried on to the train on stretchers, laid down awhile on the wooden platforms, covered with blankets up to their chins … I saw one young Londoner so smashed about the face that only his eyes were uncovered between layers of bandages, and they were glazed with the first film of death. Another had his jaw clean blown away, so the doctor told me … Outside a square brick building … the 'bad' cases were unloaded: men with chunks of steel in their lungs and bowels were vomiting great gobs of blood, men with arms and legs torn from their trunks, men without noses, and their brains throbbing through opened scalps, men without faces.[2]

The number of facial casualties increased during the war, although their numbers followed the broader ebbs and flows of the war. They were at their highest during periods of attack or retreat. The Battle of the Somme in 1916 and the Third Ypres campaign, which began in July 1917 and dragged on until November, both produced a steady flow of casualties. The German offensive of March 1918, and the Battle of Amiens in August 1918, also saw significant spikes in the weekly numbers of facial casualties. The accounts of soldiers, sailors and airmen, and the records of casualties treated at Sidcup reveal the impact of twentieth-century warfare on the faces of the fighters. This chapter examines how the injuries occurred.

The Front Line

The scale of the problem started to reveal itself in 1914 as massed infantry attacks by French and German troops ran into a blizzard of rifle, machine gun, and shellfire. As the Western Front settled into an attritional trench war, bombardment by shrapnel and high-explosive shells became the everyday cause of injury. Attackers faced artillery fire and bullets, but a trench was safe from the latter unless its occupants popped their heads over the parapet to take a look around. Once the steel helmet was established as a regular item of kit the risk of death from brain trauma diminished, and more men with injuries to the unprotected face survived.

The army facial casualties from Britain and the Dominions were not all wounded on the Western Front. Men were injured at Gallipoli, in Serbia, Africa, and even in Dublin during the Easter Rising of 1916. The types of injury can almost be predicted from the dates on which they occurred and the unit in which the casualty served. Infantry casualties during an assault were most often caused by rifle and machine gun bullets, and casualties among artillerymen were largely due to shells used in counter-battery fire. The numbers of casualties fluctuated between busy and quiet times, but the range of the larger guns was sufficient to keep soldiers at risk even when they were well behind the front. Rifles were more accurate, machine guns more prevalent, artillery fire more intense, and the effects of explosives more damaging than ever before. The new technology of modern war produced different patterns of injury from previous conflicts, and as medical management improved the numbers reaching treatment centres steadily increased.

Bullet wounds were a leading cause of facial injury. Rifles in the Great War were mostly fired at close range, and the bullets had not stabilised in flight when they struck their target. Thus they often produced large entry wounds, but then their energy was rapidly dissipated as they

---

2   P. Gibbs, *Now It Can Be Told* (New York: Garden City, 1920), pp.179-180.

rattled around. Some bullets sliced through soft tissue, whilst others struck bone and caused fragmentation of the bony facial structure. Shot side on, a soldier could lose his nose and face, and be blinded.

Gilbert Nobbs of the London Rifle Brigade recalled the moment when he was injured:

> My head at the moment was inclined to the right, for I was shouting at the men. Like a flash I remembered that about fifty yards to the left of me there was a 'German strong point' still occupied by the Germans. A bullet had entered my left temple; it must have come from a sniper in that strong point, for I found some days later that it had emerged through the centre of my right eye. I remember distinctly clutching my head and sinking to the ground, and all the time I was thinking, 'So this is the end – the finish of it all; shot through the head, mine is a fatal wound'.[3]

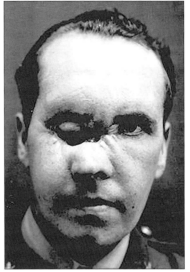

Lieutenant R.G. Tait, 4/5th Battalion, Black Watch, who was wounded on 28 July 1918. Photograph taken on admission to Sidcup, 11 October 1918. (RCS)

Gunshot and shell injuries often caused significant wounds to the eye through fractures, bone loss, and severe disruption to the orbit. Enucleation (removal) of one or both eyes was frequently necessary. As Félix Klein, a French chaplain, wrote in his diary:

> For none of them did I feel greater pity than for a poor reservist hit by a bullet that went through his forehead from right to left, severing the optic nerve and closing his eyes for ever. He does not yet know the extent of his misfortune. 'If only I see clearly again after the dressing!' he keeps on saying; and so far no one has had the courage to crush his last hope – I no more than the others.[4]

The machine gun supplemented the rifle as a major weapon of mass destruction. No man's land was swept by machine gun fire which cut men down in their thousands. When Robert 'Big Bob' Seymour went over the top at Serre with the Sheffield Pals on 1 July 1916, he only got a few yards from his trench before he was hit in the face. He lost most of the left side of his nose. To add insult to injury, the force of the impact spun him round and he took a machine gun bullet in his buttock.[5]

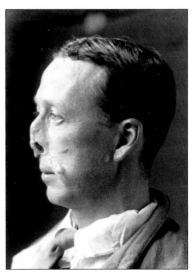

Private Robert Seymour, 12th York and Lancaster Regiment, who was wounded on 1 July 1916. Photograph taken at Aldershot, 26 February 1917. (RCS)

3   G. Nobbs, *English Kamerad! Right of the British Line* (London: Heinemann, 1918), pp.116-117.
4   F. Klein, *Diary of a French Army Chaplain* (London: Andrew Melrose, 1915), pp.169-170.
5   H.D. Gillies and R. Millard, *The Principles and Art of Plastic Surgery* (London: Butterworth & Co., 1957), p.17.

Artillery shells were either shrapnel or high-explosive. Shrapnel shells, which contained large numbers of small shot, were almost universal at the beginning of the war. Like old-fashioned grapeshot they caused widespread devastation among advancing units in the open. However, they did not penetrate deep fortifications, and they did not cut barbed wire. As the war progressed, high-explosive shells were used far more than shrapnel. Their blast effect was substantial, and the irregular, sharp-edged, often red hot shell fragments could cause terrible tearing injuries to the face (See Colour Section, p.iii).

Any part of the face was liable to injury. Private Harold Page, D Company, 8th Norfolk Regiment, enlisted in September 1914 and went over the top near Mametz on 1 July 1916. He and his comrades were, in his own words, "bowled over." As can be seen from the initial photograph of his wound, Page's cheek was torn to pieces by a shell fragment. Lieutenant Smith of the Kent Cyclist Corps, attached to the 1st Battalion, Royal West Kent Regiment, was caught by a machine gun on 27 September 1918. He sustained similar injuries to the lips and jaw.

Accidental injuries also occurred. Alan Nichols, a Bombing Instructor at South Shields who had been wounded in France in 1914, was wounded again in 1917 whilst giving a lecture to trainees on explosives and demolition. As he later wrote:

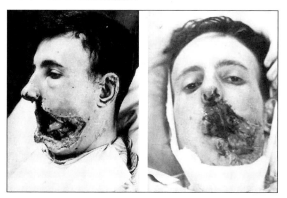
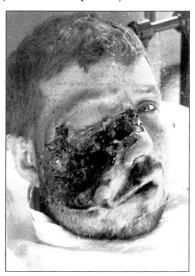

Photograph of Lieutenant Smith, 1st Royal West Kent Regiment. (RCS)

Initial photograph of Private Harold Page, Norfolk Regiment. (RCS)

> After preparing a charge, we proceeded to demolish a barricade adjacent to the hut in which the lecture had taken place. By some mischance, a piece of instantaneous fuse had been inserted instead of time fuse; or perhaps a spark from the fuse may have exploded the primer. It is sufficient to say the explosion occurred instantaneously; and it was fortunate for that particular bombing party that discipline had been observed. At the moment of the explosion the men were lying down at the regulation distance from the barricade, and thus escaped hurt.[6]

Nichols' colleague, Sergeant Sullivan, was less fortunate and died that night. Nichols himself lost both hands and was blinded.

Shell fragments and shrapnel were not the only cause of injury. An explosion could throw up earth and mud. Félix Klein recalled how:

---

6   Alan Nichols, *Sons of Victory: 1914-1918* (privately printed, N.D.), p.7.

two … of the wounded of the day before yesterday had been blinded by the plaster from a high wall along which they were taking shelter, and which had been knocked down by a shell; they have both begun to see a little today. But it's no use deluding oneself; the case of the first is final; he will be for ever in darkness.[7]

On the Somme, sharp flint fragments were as dangerous as shell cases, and around the Ypres salient a shell wound, accompanied by contamination from the bacteria-laden Flanders mud, rapidly developed an infection.

Proximity increased the likelihood of injury among the artillery. Counter-battery fire was more accurate when directed at visible guns so the field artillery, which was closer to the front line, was more vulnerable to incoming shells than the heavy howitzers. Of the Sidcup casualties, 201 came from the Royal Horse and Field Artillery whereas 143 came from the crews of the big guns in the Garrison Artillery.

Indirect injury also occurred among the tank crews. A shell that exploded against a tank shook the occupants severely. They rattled around and struck their faces on the armour plate or any of the sharp projections within the hull. Tiny pieces of metal, or spall, flew about like sharp snowflakes and could cause serious if superficial facial damage. If a shell penetrated the hull it could also cause severe injury, even if it did not explode.

Before the war, military burns injuries were unusual. The technology of modern war resulted in a steady stream of burns victims. Injuries were usually caused by the ignition of petrol after an aeroplane crash, or by cordite, petrol, or explosions of other flammable materials stored at artillery emplacements and ammunition dumps. The increased use of tanks after their introduction in September 1916 also resulted in burns casualties, because their petrol tanks were unprotected and the occupants were sprayed with petrol if an explosion set them alight.

Lieutenant Stanley Cohen, wounded in August 1918, wrote:

> As soon as I realised the tank was on fire I tried to open the escape hatch over my head, but it was jammed … Momentarily I sat still, wondering what next, and recalling an officer who was seen struggling to get through the hatch only to fall back inside. I could see nothing clearly, but my eye caught a light patch in the rear where a door had been opened. I climbed out of my seat and moved towards it. When nearly there I fell to the floor. Apparently the Germans were playing a M.G. on the open door and a bullet went through the left knee.[8]

Cohen's prolonged time in the tank as it burned left him with disfiguring burns of the whole face.

Some facial injuries had unusual causes. Eleven Sidcup patients had wounds which had been inflicted by animals. Army transport in the Great War was largely horse or mule-drawn. Although a number of motor ambulances were available, the majority of the supplies and artillery were brought up by cart. Those responsible for the animals ran some risk of injury not just from shelling but from recalcitrant beasts that were either driven beyond their endurance or frightened by shell bursts. Of the Sidcup patients who were injured by animals, nine had been kicked (one of them also had a shrapnel wound for good measure) and two were bitten. A kick on the jaw could snap it off on both sides below the jaw (temporomandibular) joint. Seven of the 11 were artillerymen, one was from the Royal Army Service Corps (RASC), and two were

---

7   Klein, *Diary*, pp.169-170.
8   Stanley Cohen, personal papers. (Courtesy of The Rev Canon Ian Cohen)

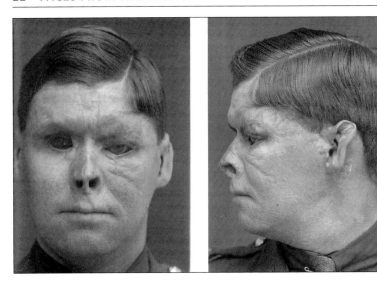

Initial photograph of
Lieutenant Stanley Cohen,
Tank Corps. (RCS)

engineers. Most of the injuries did not have an open wound. Although of little comfort, at least the closed injury was at little risk of infection.

The War at Sea

Fire at sea had been a major fear since the days of wooden warships. Modern dreadnoughts were still at risk because enemy shelling could ignite ammunition and fuel supplies. Cordite, the main propellant of shells, exploded if confined and burned fiercely if not. Private John Harris described how a shell from a German battleship, probably the battlecruiser *König*, led to disaster for HMS *Malaya* at the Battle of Jutland on 31 May 1916.[9] Harris recalled how "one shell dropped amidships, came down through the deck head and exploded. It ignited our ammunition charges throwing every man off his feet. We lay half stunned until the dreaded cry, 'FIRE!!' It was soon roaring like a furnace and we were trapped by watertight doors."[10] The severity of fires at sea was often exacerbated by the practice of storing cordite for secondary armament on deck, and by the disregard of regulations to use flash shutters between magazines and guns in order to increase the rate of fire.

The nature of fires meant that burns particularly affected faces. In many cases seamen suffered flash burns, when only exposed areas were burnt. Wireless telegraphist Frederick Arnold witnessed the first aid given to the burned, and described how "the living badly burned cases were almost encased in wrappings of cotton wool and bandages with just slits for their eyes to see through, in fact, the few 'walking cases' who could wander about the after deck presented a grim, weird and ghoulish sight."[11] A postcard image of a series of wounded men on the deck of a hospital ship shows two such men.

9   A. Gordon, *The Rules of the Game: Jutland and British Naval Command* (London: John Murray, 1996).
10 Private John Harris, Royal Marine Light Infantry. Quoted in Nigel Steel and Peter Hart, *Jutland, 1916: Death in the Grey Wastes* (London: Cassell, 2003), pp.156-157.
11 Wireless telegraphist Frederick Arnold. Quoted in Steel and Hart, *Jutland, 1916*, p.159.

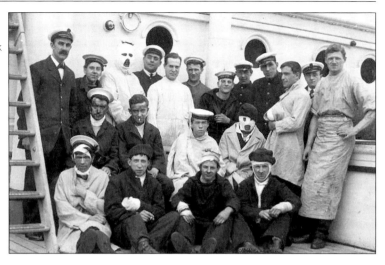

Postcard photograph of injured seamen from the Battle of Jutland on the deck of the hospital ship *Plassey*. (Author's collection)

Ships' surgeons were confronted with the results. Surgeon Lieutenant Lorimer wrote:

> soon after our guns got going we felt a different concussion and soon the ship took a severe list to starboard. I could not help wondering how much damage was done … However, we were soon far too busy to think of anything but our job and a good thing too. The wounded began to come down in great numbers, mostly burns, and very bad burns they were, entailing very extensive dressings and of course morphia.[12]

The consequences were severe, and the burns outside the experience of Lorimer's civilian practice:

> I don't quite understand the immediate cause of death. We talk vaguely of shock, but I don't know that this explains it. A man will walk into the dressing station, or possibly be carried in, with face and hands badly scorched, not deeply burned, nor disfigured. One would call it a burn of the first degree. Very rapidly, almost as one looks, the face swells up, the looser parts of the skin become enormously swollen, the eyes are invisible through the great swelling of the lids, the lips enormous jelly like masses, in the centre of which, a button-like mouth appears. I have an idea that it must be due to the very high temperature of the burning cordite applied for a very short time. It is quite unlike any burns I have ever seen in civil life and would be very easily avoided by wearing asbestos gloves and masks, or similar anti-fire substance. The great cry is water, not much pain, and this is easily subdued by morphia. There is then great and increasing restlessness, breathing rapid and shallow, and final collapse.

Hands and faces, as they were exposed, were most commonly affected. Lorimer's detailed description is harrowing:

---

12 Lieutenant Lorimer. Quoted in Steel and Hart, *Jutland, 1916*, pp.160-161. Unless otherwise stated, all quotations in this passage are taken from this source.

The scorched areas are confined to the exposed parts: face, head, and hands, hair, beard and eyebrows burnt off. The skin of the hands, the whole epidermis including the nails, peels off like a glove. In many cases one has to look twice to be certain that one is cutting off only skin, and not the whole finger. In very few cases does the burning appear to go any deeper than this. And yet they die and die very rapidly. Cases looking quite slight at first become rapidly worse and die in an appallingly short time. It is possible in such circumstances to try many remedies. Stimulants such a spirits and strychnine were useless. We had no time to transfuse. Whether it would have done any good I don't know. I doubt it, the end came so rapidly in many cases. Brandy, hot bottles and drinks with, of course, the dressing of the cases and some operations were the utmost we could do.

Gunners and seamen wore anti-flash gear to protect against the risk of burns, but this was often inadequate. In 1916, Fleet Surgeon Ernest Penfold dealt with the casualties from a shell strike to HMS *Barham*. Many from the gun crews and ammunition parties, over a hundred in all, were very badly burned by cordite fires. Penfold noted that no men were blinded, but that better anti-flash protection would have been useful. Many of the wounds, moreover, were dirty and rapidly became septic, a process which seems to have been hastened by the use of pre-treated dressings.[13]

The War in the Air

Burns were also a prominent form of facial injury which arose from the war in the air. The exposed faces and hands of pilots and observers were vulnerable if an aircraft caught alight. As aeroplane pilots did not have parachutes they had either to try and land a burning plane or bail out and die. The choice was stark. Ralph Lumley, who joined the Royal Flying Corps (RFC), appears to have been an elegant and insouciant young man in his pre-war photograph. On his first solo flight, on 14 July 1916, he crash-landed his B.E.12 and it caught fire. One eye was removed at Tidworth Hospital, while the other was severely damaged. Lumley was transferred to the King Edward VII Hospital in Grosvenor Gardens in January 1917. The hospital had been established by two sisters, Agnes and Fanny Keyser. Agnes Keyser described Lumley in a letter to Sir Reginald Wilson in February 1917. In it, she noted how "His face is burned beyond recognition. One eye removed, the other practically blind. Legs burnt arms burnt thumbs and some fingers amputated. He has very little to live for, poor boy, but we are doing everything possible."[14] In total, 86 airmen were treated at Sidcup, 14 of whom were burns victims.

Other aerial injuries were the result of crashes. Most facial injuries were caused by the sudden deceleration of the craft upon impact with the ground or an object like a tree. Without adequate restraints, pilots hit their faces on the front rim of the cockpit. The surgeons at Sidcup treated 30 members of the RFC and Royal Air Force (RAF) who had sustained facial fractures in crashes. Although parachutes were used by balloonists in the Observation Corps, and were tested in aeroplanes in 1917, both airmen and their commanders were reluctant to adopt them. This reluctance led to a sustained trickle of casualties from crashes until the end of the war. Some planes were shot down by enemy aircraft. Other crashes were caused by inexperience or fatigue. Many men had limited training and arrived at the front barely able to do circuits and bumps, let alone fight aloft. The aircraft themselves were also unreliable and fragile, and even experienced

---

13   E.A. Penfold, 'A battleship in action', *The Journal of the Royal Naval Medical Service*, 3:1 (1917), pp.44-56.
14   RCS: Gillies Archives, Keyser to Wilson, digital copy of letter in Lumley case notes.

pilots like the Canadian Captain C.L. Bath could crash.[15] Although he had fought numerous missions during the war, Bath had a flying accident on 10 March 1918 in which he fractured the base of his skull and broke his nose. Following admission to the Queen's Hospital, Bath suffered an epileptic fit in May 1919, doubtless from an underlying brain injury.

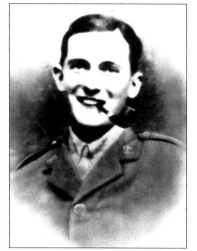

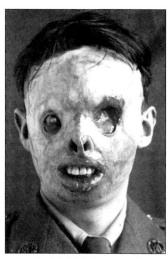

Family photograph of Ralph Lumley in his RFC uniform before injury. (RCS)

Lumley's initial photograph at Sidcup almost a year later. (RCS)

Ordnance wounds were the final significant cause of facial injury in the war in the air. As on the ground, it is likely that many were injured by anti-aircraft artillery fire, or 'Archie', rather than by machine gun bullets in close combat. Twenty-nine Sidcup men from the RFC or RAF were recorded as suffering from such wounds. Regardless of the cause of injury, the next step to be taken by the wounded of all the armed forces was their removal from the battlefield.

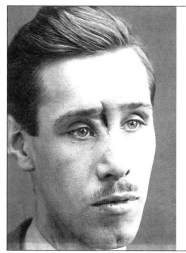
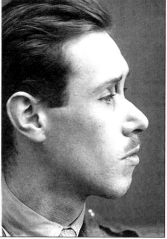

Admission photograph of Captain C.L. Bath, RFC. (RCS)

Casualty Evacuation

All armies in the First World War developed a system of casualty evacuation which involved a triage system connected to the severity of the injury, and a series of treatment settings progressively more distant from the front. This section focuses upon the casualty management of the British armed forces, which was similar in most respects to the systems used by others. The specific management of facial injury needs to be set within the broader context of how the services were organised.[16] First-hand accounts of both the wounded, and those who cared for them, inform the narrative.

---

15 S.F. Wise, *Canadian Airmen and the First World War* (Toronto: University of Toronto Press, 1980), p.387.
16 See Mark Harrison, *The Medical War: British Military Medicine in the First World War* (Oxford: Oxford University Press, 2010); Ian Whitehead, *Doctors in the Great War* (Barnsley: Pen & Sword, 1999).

The British Expeditionary Force comprised only six divisions at first. Based on experience in the Crimea and South Africa, injuries were initially managed at Regimental Aid Posts (RAPs) located at the front line. Certain casualties were subsequently transferred to a Field Ambulance (the term ambulance, as in French, denoted a medical unit rather than the transport itself). At an Advanced Dressing Station (ADS), run by the Field Ambulance, casualties were stabilised prior to a move back to a large base hospital well behind the lines. However, it became rapidly apparent that this system was inadequate. Delays in transport were significant, and the army's senior surgeon in the field, Sir Anthony Bowlby, decided surgery must begin closer to the front line. Bowlby had served in the Boer War, where the concept of the Casualty Clearing Station (CCS) was originated. The CCS was not originally designed to carry out major surgery, but Bowlby recognised that it should act as the main focus for major treatment. If a problem was significant enough, a further transfer to the base hospital was arranged.

A proportion of patients were eventually transferred to Britain if they had a 'Blighty' wound. The term 'Blighty' had been coined in India in reference to England as a corruption of the Urdu *bilayati*, meaning 'British foreigner'. A Blighty wound or illness was one which required highly specialist management or prolonged convalescence. The evacuation process used a wide range of forms of transport: stretchers, ambulances, trains, barges and hospital ships. Treatments included field dressings, vaccinations and surgery. The care of the injured was undertaken by doctors, nurses, orderlies and stretcher-bearers. Many were volunteers, and many were not British. The Quakers, of pacifist persuasions, set up many ambulance units. Numerous American units supported the French armies, and nurses of all nationalities offered their services on all fronts.

The process of triage, which had originally been invented by the French army medical service in the Napoleonic Wars, divided casualties into three broad groups. The first comprised casualties who could be patched and returned to the front. The second included those whose wounds were severe but survivable, and the last group contained those who would inevitably die. Triage was performed at all stages of a casualty's journey back from the front line. Its purpose was to ensure that medical help focused on those who would benefit from it, and that it was not wasted. Those who were expected to die were pragmatically left to their fate, yet mistakes were made in the triage process. George Brooks was injured in the early hours of 12 October 1917. His unit, the 12th Machine Gun Company of the Australian Imperial Force (AIF), was caught by a shell. Brooks was one of 10 casualties. He was taken by two corporals to a clearing post, where the doctor took one look and asked: "Why bring him here? Put him over there." As Brooks observed, "That was where others were dying." Another soldier insisted that Brooks be treated, and he was passed back down the line. Two stops back, at St Omer, "a doctor took one look at me and walked off." Having been triaged as untreatable once again, Brooks "was moved

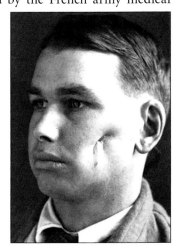

George Brooks on admission to Sidcup. The wound has healed with contracture of the scar. (RCS)

upstairs where I found men were dying." A nursing sister noted that he remained alert and treated his pneumonia. Brooks gradually began to recover. Before he was moved to convalesce, the sister brought the doctor to see him. Brooks later recalled that "he apologised to me for he was sure I was done for, He said: 'Why, your face was as black as ink. I gave you no hope'."[17]

---

17 George Brooks, personal papers; courtesy of the family. The film of Vera Brittain's *Testament of Youth* vividly portrays Vera finding her brother Edward, still alive, in a row of triaged-to-die patients.

From Injury to Initial Treatment (Regimental Aid Post and Advanced Dressing Station)

When a serviceman was injured, he had to get back to a place of relative safety. Disabled by a limb wound, possibly suffering from significant blood loss or following a period of unconsciousness, it was often a difficult process. For members of the infantry, it was not unusual to spend one or two nights out in the open with a serious wound before a stretcher party reached them or they succeeded in crawling back to their lines.

Ernest Wordsworth was injured in the first minutes of the first day of the Somme offensive on 1 July 1916. His story exemplifies the difficulties wounded men faced when attempting to get back to their own lines. He signed up with the York and Lancaster Regiment in Pontefract, and risked the wrath of his master, a butcher, who had already lost two of his staff. He finished his training in May 1916, and was drafted with 90 or so of his colleagues to join the 8th Battalion in France. Wordsworth recalled that Jerry "shot us down as fast as we appeared before him."[18] He was only able to advance around 50 yards before he was shot and lost his left eye. He recalled how he lay "with blood streaming from my face from 7.30 Sat. morning until early Monday morning without assistance of any kind." Wordsworth eventually managed to crawl back to the trenches, and was carried to a dressing station.

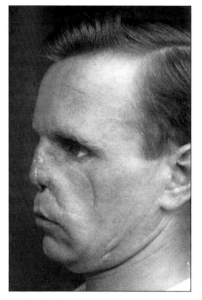

Men carried their own field dressing, which they could apply themselves or get a colleague to do for them. Captain J.K. Wilson provides an example of the former. Wilson's tank crossed the Hindenburg line at Cambrai in 1918. As his tank crested a ridge, the German artillery got the range and the tank was hit twice. "Badly wounded in the face, I succeeded in crawling into a shell hole and plastering my field dressing on the wound, and, although I should not say this in public, fortifying myself with a swig of rum from my water bottle."[19] However, the majority of injuries were initially treated in the front line at an RAP, usually based in a dugout or building in the support trench network. The Regimental Medical Officer was responsible for the RAP, and he would administer morphia and make decisions on patient management. Simple work was undertaken by the stretcher-bearer complement. The bearers, 16 to a regiment at the start of the war but later increased to 32, brought injured men from no man's land or the trenches themselves. The RAP had minimal equipment, only stretchers, blankets, splints and shell dressings, and its exposed position resulted

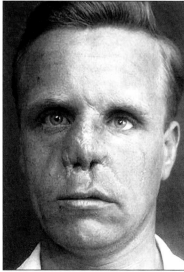

Initial photographs of Private Ernest Wordsworth. (RCS)

---

18 Brotherton Library Special Collections (BLSC): Liddle Collection, LIDDLE/WW1/GA/WOU/34, My Personal Experiences of the Great War, Wordsworth essay.

19 Imperial War Museum (IWM): 12007, Private Papers of Captain J.K. Wilson.

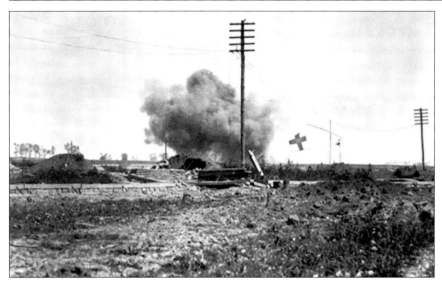

A shell bursting near an ADS (54th Field Ambulance) at Heninel, 27 May 1917. (IWM Q2258)

in the injury or death of many medical officers. The award of a gallantry medal was hardly recompense (See Colour Section, p.iv). The dressings helped to minimise blood loss from an open wound, while correct splinting of a thigh fracture significantly reduced morbidity and mortality, partly because internal blood loss was reduced.

Casualties with significant injuries were then passed back. In the development of a robust system of medical transfer, the RAMC had realised before the war that medical information could get lost during repeated transfers. To combat this, a Field Medical Card was devised, tucked into a waterproof envelope and tied to a button. As a result, the necessary information on the wound and its management stayed with the patient. Each brigade of 4,000 men in the British army had one Field Ambulance in three sections, each of which included a tented unit, the ADS, to which casualties were moved by a stretcher party or cart. A typical ADS was a relatively short distance from the front, and still within range of artillery.

A number of facial casualties recorded their experience of injury and its management. At Neuilly, Félix Klein told of a French officer who:

> wanted to see how the work [of digging trenches] was going on … For ten minutes all was quiet, then the firing began … I was at once hit by a Mauser bullet. It entered, as you can see, below my left eye, went through the nostril and the top of the palate, pierced my right cheek and came out under the ear, breaking the lower jaw bone without touching my teeth.

The blood loss was substantial, and the officer thought he was mortally wounded. However:

> a comrade put on a first dressing, and in spite of the flow of blood from my mouth and nose, I went on foot, leaning on the corporal, along over a mile of trench-branches as far as the dressing-station of our regiment which was installed in a dug-out. The surgeon cleaned the wound, dressed it afresh and telephoned for a wheeled stretcher to take me to the field-hospital.[20]

---

20   Klein, *Diary*, p.185.

David Guild recalled his own injury and evacuation. He:

> was looking over the parapet, not paying much attention, when all of a sudden I got a wallop in the jaw. I found myself sitting in the trench bottom, so I got up, not thinking there was too much wrong, and went on sentry duty again. I had my waterproof sheet wrapped around myself as it was raining. Blood was running down my poncho and I wondered what was wrong. I thought something had knocked my teeth out. I didn't know I had a hole in my cheek. The Sergeant came along … He took one look at me and said, 'Get down to the dressing station!' The medical staff bandaged me up, after a brief stop at Battalion Headquarters. At field ambulance I was trying to smoke as I was reading the funny papers. I don't know why. I couldn't smoke because the air was coming in through the side of my face.[21]

Captain Budd of the 7th London Regiment went over the top on 27 August 1918. He had arrived in France in March 1915, and had survived unscathed for over three years. His Blighty wound was a result of so-called friendly fire. Budd was caught in the creeping artillery barrage that preceded the attack, but which in this case did not advance quite as fast as the infantry were expecting:

> we had not gone far before there seemed to be a lot of bursts too close to be pleasant and [I] concluded that we were moving too fast and had walked into our own shell fire, so I signalled a halt. After a short pause we seemed to draw clear so on we went again, and again, after a short time we bumped into this shell fire, so again I halted. I was discussing the situation with one of my subalterns and had just turned sideways to reply to him when there was a burst just at my feet and I felt something hit my face, which I thought for the moment was a clod of earth. A moment later I felt blood running down over my mouth, and I turned to my batman who was with me and said, 'that blasted shell threw some earth in my face and its made my nose bleed'. He replied, looking at me, 'My God, I should say it has'. He then helped me put on my field dressing and by now I realised that it was more than just a clod that had got me, although it didn't seem much worse than if I had a straight left from a middle-weight. Accompanied by my batman I made my way slowly back to find the aid post, but after we had gone a short way I began to feel rather faint (presumably from loss of blood) and he helped me into a small bit of trench while he went to find a stretcher.[22]

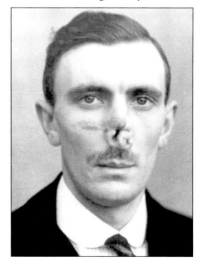

Admission photograph of Captain J.G.H. Budd, which was taken at the Sir John Ellerman Hospital, Regent's Park, London, September 1918. (RCS)

Back at the RAP, Budd "was examined by the doctor, who after glancing at my dressing said, 'You'll do for the

---

21 G. Reid (ed.), *Poor Bloody Murder: Personal Memoirs of the First World War* (Oakville, ON: Mosaic Press, 1980), p.104.
22 BLSC: Liddle Collection, LIDDLE/WW1/WF/REC/01/B43, Budd, JGH, Amateur Soldier.

present, would you like a shot of morphia?' I was not feeling too bad so I refused his kind offer, as I had always had rather a dread of being drugged."

John Bagot Glubb had joined the 7th Field Company, Royal Engineers, in November 1915 at the age of 18. He was wounded, south-east of Arras, on 21 August 1917. In his autobiography, he described the event:

> The road beyond St Martin was in view of the enemy, and it was not yet quite dark. I dismounted and sat on a stone for a short time … Some long range shells whined over, and burst about 120 yards beyond the road … I began to trot at first, but finding shells bursting well over I pulled back to a walk, determined not to run away. Just as I left St Martin, the shelling ceased. Here I met Driver Gowans coming up with a G.S. wagon … As I spoke to Gowans, I think I heard for a second a distant shell whine, then felt a tremendous explosion almost on top of me. For an instant I appeared to rise slowly into the air and then slowly to fall again … Scarcely had I begun to run towards Hénin, when the floodgates in my neck seemed to burst, and the blood poured out in torrents … I was in a kind of dazed panic … I could feel something lying loosely in my left cheek, as though I had a chicken bone in my mouth. It was in reality half my jaw, which had been broken off, teeth and all, and was floating about in my mouth.[23]

Eventually, Glubb reached the aid post. Here:

> I sat on the table in the cellar, while they dressed my wound. The R.A.M.C. orderly put some plug into my neck which stopped the bleeding. They also put a rubber tube in my wound, sticking out of the bandage. They told me there was no ambulance in Hénin and I should have to walk to Boiry-Becquerelle.[24] We accordingly set out, I leaning on the medical orderly's arm. I was not looking forward to the long walk at all, but luckily the orderly remembered that there was some regimental medical officer, who lived in a dugout at the south end of the village … I heard him tell the orderly that it was a good thing they dressed me at once, or I should have been done for.

The initial lack of pain was a common feature of these accounts. That would come later. Morphia was freely available, although many men still suffered. Budd wrote:

> After what seemed an age, but was actually only a few minutes I was slipped into an ambulance and very soon arrived at the Casualty Clearing Station … my dressing was considered satisfactory and was not disturbed, and … I was invited to have a 'shot'. It was the practice to make an 'X' on a man's forehead with indelible pencil when he was given a shot so as to ensure that he didn't get too much by having repeated shots at each stopping place.[25]

The shock of injury resulted in unconsciousness, which sometimes alarmed fellow soldiers. Captain Wilson recalled:

---

23 J.B. Glubb, *Into Battle* (London: Cassell, 1978), p.185. Unless otherwise stated, all quotations in this passage are taken from this source.
24 The distance is about 2.5km, or a 30-minute walk.
25 BLSC: Budd Papers, LIDDLE/WW1/WF/REC/01/B43.

I remember nothing more until finding myself in a field dressing stn well behind the line. Some years after my old friend Wm Bedford of Bere Regis showed me a letter he had received from a tank commander who had seen me on a stretcher on the way back, in which he said 'I have just seen your old friend Jono being carried down on a stretcher. I am afraid you will not see him again'. Which only goes to show that things are not always what they appear to be, and that even a small wound can look pretty ghastly until the mud and the blood have been cleaned away.[26]

An intricate support network developed to facilitate the transport of the wounded soldier from the ADS to the next staging post, the Casualty Clearing Station (CCS). Fleets of motor ambulances plied to and fro. Near the front, they would frequently get bogged down in the mud (See Colour Section, p.iii). Private Page of the Norfolk Regiment, evacuated from the Somme front line by 55 Field Ambulance, got back to the ADS at Carnoy without incident. However, his further evacuation was delayed as the ambulances could not get up the steep hill. When fully loaded, they often had insufficient traction.

Casualty Clearing Station

The CCS functioned as a fully equipped hospital. Initially comprising a staff of 95, each CCS later received three chaplains and seven nursing sisters to add to the workforce. There were two surgical teams which during busy spells could be supplemented by up to four more, sent either from CCSs on a quiet sector or from the base hospitals. When casualties came in the surgeons worked for 16 hours in the day with 8 hours off, but if very busy they worked continuously. Tables were arranged in threes. The first patient would be anaesthetised, the anaesthetist would move to the second table while the surgeons operated, and then on again while an assistant closed the wound of the man on the first table and the surgeon moved to the second. The staff of the CCS embarked on major life-saving surgery, such as amputation, and excision and debridement (cleansing) of wounds. Minor injuries were also treated, and the men returned to duty. Once a patient was assessed as safe to travel, their transfer to a base hospital was arranged.

The merry-go-round took a toll on the staff, and speed often led to errors. Ward accommodation was hutted or tented, and each CCS contained operating theatres, radiography and pathology facilities. Sir Anthony Bowlby's opinion on the problems of delay was underpinned by the high mortality of casualties from blood loss and sepsis. In the first months of the war up to 70 percent of casualties died. Rapid and definitive management reduced this to less than 30 percent by November 1918.

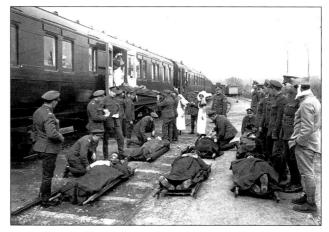

RAMC orderlies loading British and French wounded onto a hospital train at Doullens, 27 April 1918. (IWM Q8752)

---

26 IWM: Wilson Papers, 12007.

In the early days of the war the mainstay of surgical work, the CCS, was kept well back from the front line. However, survival rates of men reaching them were alarmingly low. Conditions taxed the medical staff on and behind the front line.

Regimental officers like Robert Dolby packed their equipment on a two-wheeled cart:

> that carries the medical and surgical panniers. These contain a comprehensive selection of medical and surgical instruments, medicines, condensed milk and beef extract; all as complete as it is compact. Lacking only rubber gloves and sterilisable surgical gowns, there is hardly an operation, of an urgent character, that an adaptable surgeon cannot do in an emergency. Given a house, a stove and a regimental doctor's equipment, his trained N.C.O., and he, will have all the essentials of a temporary hospital.[27]

Richard Clarke recalled the difficulties which faced a staff untrained for their task, and confronted by diseases they had not previously encountered. He had begun his wartime medical career with the 4th Gloucester Regiment in "quiet sectors of the line", and in November 1915 was posted to Number 19 CCS in Doullens. He wrote:

> The surgery, such as it was, was being done by the general practitioner from South Africa and the Edinburgh graduate. As the consulting surgeon hardly ever appeared – and when he did he was as ignorant as we were – the science of war surgery did not get very far in our unit. Looking back on that period in the light of further knowledge, our ignorance was deplorable.[28]

Artilleryman Norman Tennant was "taken by car to the 1st Australian CCS at Blendeque near St Omer where the shell splinter, which had passed through the back of my nose and lodged just below the right eye, was removed."[29]

John Glubb was taken to the main CCS at Ficheux. There he was operated upon and remained for several days. He wrote:

> A good deal of discharge came from my mouth, and I was very miserable, with my pillow always covered with blood and slime. I was later told that I looked very bad, with my mouth dragged down, discharging and filthy … After six days in the C.C.S. we were driven away one morning in a motor ambulance to Boisleux-au-Mont and loaded onto a hospital train.[30]

A network of some three dozen ambulance trains and a number of river barges, often manned by volunteers and conscientious objectors, carried men from the CCSs to the base hospitals on the coast.

On the first four days of the Somme offensive alone, over 33,000 casualties were ferried on trains and barges from the front.[31] James Miles, a member of one of the voluntary units that staffed some of the trains, evoked the grim desolation of a night arrival at a CCS:

27 R.A. Dolby, *A Regimental Surgeon in War and Prison* (London: John Murray, 1917), pp.12-13.
28 R.C. Clarke, 'Evolution of a casualty clearing station on the Western Front', *British Medico-Chirurgical Journal*, 54 (1937), pp.1-20.
29 N.A. Tennant, *A Saturday Night Soldier's War, 1913-1918* (Waddesdon: Kylin Press, 1983).
30 Glubb, *Into Battle*, p.188.
31 For a literary account, see Wilfred Owen's 'Hospital Barge at Cérisy', in *The Complete Poems and Fragments of Wilfred Owen*, ed. by J. Stallworthy (London: Chatto & Windus, 1983).

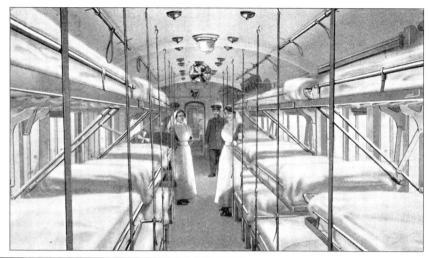

The interior of an ambulance train. (Author's collection)

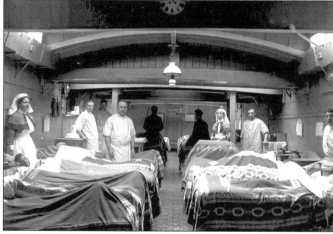

The interior of a hospital barge on the Somme. (IWM Q33443)

up at the far end of the train – a full three hundred yards trudge in ankle-deep mud – the lying-down wards are gradually filling up; more slowly than usual, for the bearers to-night have the gait of men worn out … The long coaches … dazzling white in contrast with the outer darkness, were clean and fresh smelling when the first patient was lifted in through the wide double doors. But now, after half an hour or so, the indefinable, but unmistakable, smell of wounded men straight from the trenches, is making itself felt, and the spotless floor is stained with muddy prints, and running with water where the rain has dropped from the stretchers or scudded in through the open doors.[32]

Miles' recollections underline how the application of proper dressings to replace the filthy field dressings was a long and taxing process. The journey to the hospital was often slow. Men's moods varied: "Some men lie listless and brooding all day, many are cheerful, talkative, and

---

32   M. Tatham and J.E. Miles, *The Friends' Ambulance Unit, 1914-1919: A Record* (London: Swarthmore Press, 1920), pp.137-138.

even nonchalant; some are silent only when sleep or drugs let them forget their agony." As the trains made their way back to the hospitals, "some few … who will never travel further" were unloaded at halts along the route. For them, there was no further requirement for medical treatment, only burial.[33]

Base Hospital

The British army base hospitals were usually on or near the coast, at places like Boulogne, Etaples or Rouen. Some, such as the 3rd British Hospital, were based in large buildings. The Hotel Trianon at Le Tréport, north-east of Dieppe, housed the 3rd British Hospital and later hosted two Canadian hospitals in tents and huts. As the war effort expanded, large hutted encampments were constructed. The increase in casualty numbers as the army grew led to a doubling in the size of the base hospitals during 1915 to 1,000 beds. By 1917, three further hospitals had been constructed, taking the number of available beds to 2,500. The base hospitals treated complicated cases, as well as patients who required prolonged or more specialised treatment. Although base hospitals could do a great deal, as they were well-equipped and fully staffed by specialists, the majority of emergency surgery remained the responsibility of the CCSs.

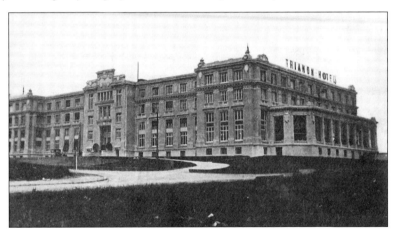

The 3rd General Hospital in the Hotel Trianon, Le Tréport, from a postcard.
(Author's collection)

Casualties arrived daily from the front in hundreds or even thousands. Captain Budd, wounded by friendly fire, described his arrival at the base hospital:

> During the afternoon we were all loaded on to the Ambulance train, and that evening arrived at Rouen … I was put to bed and my first dressing was then removed, which was not too pleasant, and my wound washed and a new dressing put on. I … must confess that I was a bit disappointed to find that I had apparently not got a 'Blighty one'. However, at 6.00.a.m. I was awakened and made to get up and after some breakfast, in company with a number of other stretcher cases I was put on the train again and sent to Le Havre.[34]

---

33 The whole quotation appears anonymously in *A Train Errant: Being the Experiences of a Voluntary Unit in France and an Anthology from their Magazine, 1915-1919* (London: Simson & Co., 1919), pp.91-92.

34 BLSC: Budd Papers, LIDDLE/WW1/WF/REC/01/B43.

Harvey Cushing, an eminent neurosurgeon from Harvard, had organised the second American hospital to be deployed on the Western Front. In his journal, Cushing described the several hundred casualties that arrived at his unit on 25 April 1915. He noted the details of their injuries and indicated one of the major improvements in ballistics management, the localisation of metallic fragments by X-ray. The ever-present risk of infection, despite early management, was also recorded:

> a young lieutenant … who was looking through his field glasses when a Mauser bullet made a direct hit of the lens in front of his right eye, exploding the cylinder and producing an ugly wound not only of his hand but of his right orbital region and cheek. Some metal fragments could be seen by X-ray, driven back into the base of the skull. The eye had been immediately enucleated [removed] by the regimental surgeon, but the whole region had become badly infected – an ugly affair.[35]

Treatment

The initial management of a facial wound focused on survival. Three things threatened survival: blood loss, suffocation, and infection. Facial casualties often experienced a torrential loss of blood because the facial structures are rich in blood vessels. Accounts indicate that soldiers and doctors sometimes took one look at a facial casualty and wrote them off. Disfigurement, coupled with copious blood leakage, often made injuries look much worse than they were. Bleeding was treated with dressings, which applied pressure to the wound, and by stitching wounds. If the bleeding could be stopped survival was likely, provided the wounded man did not choke. The risk of this was compounded both by loss of consciousness, as a man would not cough up the blood as it poured down his throat, and by damage to the muscle attachments of the tongue. If these attachments were compromised by a serious jaw injury then, when a patient was laid flat, he would suffocate as the tongue would fall back into the throat and obstruct the airway. Suffocation could happen during surgery. John Glubb recorded that he "had apparently nearly swallowed my tongue during the operation and, to prevent this, they had pierced my tongue and threaded a wire through it with a wooden rod on the end of it. This was extremely uncomfortable."[36]

Infection management had improved immeasurably since the Crimea. Preventive measures were taken against tetanus. Already common at the beginning of the war, the use of anti-tetanus serum (ATS) became universal. Its application was not a pleasant experience, as David Guild recalled: "The doctor said to me, 'Come on, Jock. It's your turn!' He gave me a shot of tetanus serum which was a darn sight worse than the wound."[37] Although unpleasant, the serum resulted in a rapid diminution of the risk. However, despite these advances, wound infection remained a major and inevitable consequence of a facial injury. The mouth normally contains bacteria. Dental hygiene was generally poor, so pre-existing dental abscesses and gum infection (pyorrhoea) were common. Given the opportunity to enter a wound, these organisms caused local infection that sometimes progressed to septicaemia. Shell wounds were often filthy, as the fragments were accompanied by gobbets of mud, clods of earth or jagged lumps of chalk and flint thrown up by the explosion. The Flanders soil, heavily manured over centuries

---

35   H. Cushing, *From A Surgeon's Journal* (London: Constable & Co., 1935), p.47.
36   Glubb, *Into Battle*, p.188.
37   Reid, (ed.), *Poor Bloody Murder*, p.105.

to maintain its fertility, teemed with noxious bacteria and, in particular, the organism that produced gas gangrene. This infection took hold so fast that it was uncontrollable in the early days of the conflict.

Harvey Cushing wrote of his first encounter with its effects:

> Soon after I joined the casualty clearing station I was introduced for the first time to that dread infection gas gangrene. While I was with the regiment naturally I knew nothing about it, but had noticed that many a man I had evacuated with what was technically called a 'Blighty one' had been reported later as 'died of wounds', and I never knew till afterwards the reason. At that period we had no idea how it should be dealt with.[38]

Delays in the evacuation of casualties also gave infection time to take a grip. Glubb was one of the unfortunate men to succumb in this manner: "I noticed a very evil decaying smell, which I attributed to some foul drains which must be nearby, but when my wound was dressed the stench suddenly became so overpowering that I realised it came from myself."[39]

Base Hospital to Blighty

Men who could take no further part in the war, such as those with amputations or those who needed prolonged treatment and convalescence, were moved to England on one of the hospital ships that ran a shuttle service across the English Channel. Upon arrival at the British ports, ambulance trains transported the men to one of the many military hospitals established across the country. The speed with which military hospitals were built and opened in Britain was impressive, the first Eastern General Hospital in Cambridge admitted its first patients to the newly constructed huts in October 1914.[40]

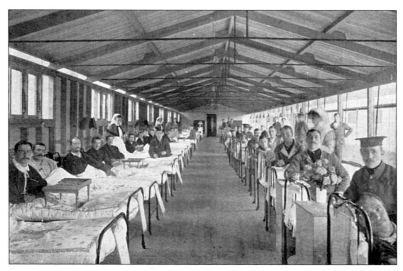

A postcard of a ward at the First Eastern General Hospital, Cambridge. (Author's collection)

---

38 Cushing, *From A Surgeon's Journal*, p.47.
39 Glubb, *Into Battle*, p.189.
40 P. Guillebaud, *From Bats to Beds to Books. The First Eastern General Hospital (Territorial Force) in Cambridge – And What Came Before and After It* (Cambridge: Fern House, 2012).

On the whole, voyages across the English Channel were regular and well-planned. The ships themselves were all shapes and sizes, ranging from small navy tenders through cross-channel steamers, to ocean-going liners. Budd wrote of the sedate nature of the journey:

> we were carried on board the Hospital ship and lay in the saloon on our stretchers with nothing to do all day, until the ship sailed in the evening when there was a certain amount of activity amongst the medical staff, examining our labels and so forth, as it appeared that we were all to be sorted into categories by the type of wound and the places in which our various homes were situated. It was arranged as far as possible that everyone was sent to a Hospital in England as near to his home as could be.[41]

However, a rough crossing was a nightmare for facial casualties. John Glubb recorded his fear of bad weather, as he was terrified he would be seasick. The cots on board were all full and he was put on the floor. The number of patients meant there was little time for proper nursing care: "I was quite a spectacular sight. There were not enough doctors or nurses on board to change anyone's dressings, so whenever mine worked loose, the sister hastily tied another bandage over it."[42] George Brooks recounted how he was given a slate to write on which kept him in good spirits. The English Channel was too rough to cross when he arrived at the coast, but with his tube still in place he was offered bread and soup by an orderly.[43]

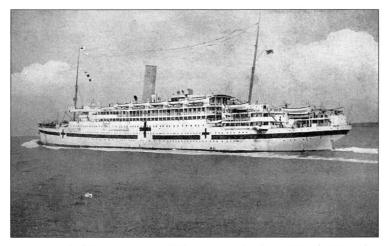

A postcard of HMHS *Asturias*, which was torpedoed on 20 March 1917 and beached at Salcombe, Devon. The author J.R.R. Tolkien had been transported back to England on her in November 1916. (Author's collection)

When patients reached an English hospital, it was not necessarily the end of their medical journey. Although attempts were made to arrange for men to be treated at a hospital near their home, this was not always possible if numbers were large. Furthermore, the medical staff sometimes decided that their unit could not offer the specialist service required. For example, when Ernest Wordsworth was transferred to England, he was treated first at the Brook War Hospital, Woolwich. He was then moved to the 3rd London General, Wandsworth, before he

41 BLSC: Budd Papers, LIDDLE/WW1/WF/REC/01/B43.
42 Glubb, *Into Battle*, p.191.
43 George Brooks, personal papers.

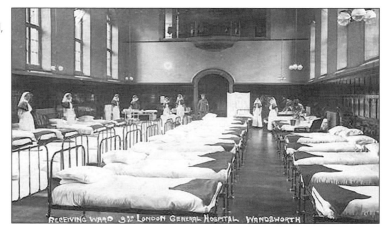

The receiving ward at the 3rd London General Hospital, Wandsworth. (Author's collection)

was transferred to Sidcup in March 1921. It was at the Queen's Hospital that his severe nasal deformity was neatly repaired with a forehead skin flap.

In the Royal Navy, there was a much simpler transfer system. The modern battleship had two medical stations, and immediate first aid packs containing dressings and tourniquets were distributed around the ship. The packs contained special burns dressings soaked in picric acid. The medical stations, or sick bays in the smaller ships, were cramped and limited in what they could do. Accordingly, casualties were trans-shipped direct to a small fleet of hospital ships which came alongside to receive transfers as soon as battle conditions allowed. In the North Sea, the hospital ships docked at Rosyth and men were taken to Edinburgh for further treatment.

The soldiers' experience

Accounts written by soldiers show that many responded to injury with a stoical and fatalistic attitude. As Katherine Luard, a nursing sister who worked at a base hospital on the Western Front, noted, "they all seem to take it as a matter of course; the bad ones who are conscious don't speak, and the better ones are all jolly and smiling, and ready 'to have another smack' … some of the men with their eyes, noses or jaws shattered, are so extraordinarily good and uncomplaining." She highlighted, in particular, "A Reading man, with his face wounded and one eye gone, kept up a running fire of wit and hilarity during his dressing about having himself photographed as a Guy Fawkes."[44] Yet some of the injured never made it into the casualty evacuation system. They were caught in no man's land, taken prisoner, and transferred to detention camps.

Some British soldiers had a difficult experience among their captors. One prisoner of war (POW) described how the sentry in charge of loading men onto a train for transfer to Germany pointed out:

> that one of the *Engländer* had been shot in the face and was badly disfigured; whereupon a German soldier pulled the poor fellow out of the sleeping mass on the floor and sat him upon the seat, the others standing round pointing with their fingers to the poor mutilated face with coarse jeering laughter. The young Irish soldier sat patiently

44 Anon. (K.E. Luard), *Diary of a Nursing Sister on the Western Front* (London: William Blackwood & Sons, 1915), pp.39, 46.

through it all – his blind eye was a running sore, the torn cheek in healing had left a hideously scarred hollow, and the mouth and nose were twisted to one side.[45]

Injured POWs did receive treatment behind enemy lines, but it was rudimentary. When men with facial wounds later returned to Britain they required a great deal of surgical work.

As the war progressed it became evident that delay in primary treatment was a major cause of death for two principal reasons. First, too many men were left to stabilise before transfer. Imperfect understanding of the problem of surgical shock caused by blood loss meant that such men died of blood loss. Second, wounds that were not immediately cleaned and covered got infected, and those covered without cleansing often resulted in the infection being shut in unseen. The initial positions of the emergency treatment centres, the CCSs, were well back from the front line, and transfer from the collecting stations near the front was often slow. It became clear that definitive treatment had to be administered more quickly. The slow realisation of these problems led to the move of the CCSs closer to the front. Furthermore, CCSs were grouped together by function so that, for example, orthopaedic cases might be treated in the same location. Patch and hold was replaced by scoop and run.

By the end of the war the whole process of casualty evacuation could be highly efficient. Medical officer Robert Blackham described an anonymous soldier's journey:

> [He] was wounded in the thigh in the first wave of the attack at 5.0 a.m. He succeeded in dragging himself to a shell-hole, where he was found and dressed by one of the Battalion Stretcher-bearers at 6.0 a.m. In a temporary lull of the enemy's barrage he was removed by the battalion stretcher-bearers to the Regimental Aid Post, where he was dressed by the Medical Officer at 7.0 a.m. He was then carried by R.A.M.C. stretcher-bearers to the first Relay Post, where a change of bearers was effected. The second Relay Post was reached at 9.0 a.m. and the Divisional Collecting Post at 9.30 a.m. At this post he was given a hot cup of tea and afterwards loaded into a Ford Motor Ambulance Car, which took him to the Advanced Dressing Station by 10.0 a.m. At the Advanced Dressing Station his wound was inspected, but the dressing was not changed, an injection of anti-tetanus serum was given, and the Field Medical Card made out. He reached the Main Dressing Station at 10.30 a.m., and, as he was fairly comfortable, he was at once transferred to a Motor Ambulance Convoy Car, and reached the Casualty Clearing Station at 11.0 o'clock. He was placed in an Ambulance train at 2.0 p.m. and reached Boulogne the same night.[46]

The whole process had taken about 16 hours. He had been assessed, dressed, reassessed and given ATS. At the start of the war, the transfer process was five days or more, given the pauses for stabilisation that occurred at both ADS and CCS. Of course, the lengths of time taken for processes to occur were dependent on whether the patient had survived the development of infection or survived the loss of blood.

45 M.V. Hay, *Wounded and a Prisoner of War. By an Exchanged Officer* (Edinburgh: Blackwood, 1916), pp.226-227.
46 R.J. Blackham, *Scalpel, Sword and Stretcher* (London: Sampson, Low, Martin & Co., 1931), p.225.

Conclusion

Injuries sustained during the First World War had a range of effects. Physical pain and psychological distress were often delayed. Many novels appeared in the period between the wars that depicted the tragedy and horrors of trench warfare. The experience of facial injury featured in Ronald Gurner's novel *Pass Guard at Ypres*, a book which encapsulates an injured man's ghastly realisation that his future would be very different.

Following an artillery attack, Private Beard, injured and lying in a shell hole, awaited the stretcher-bearers:

> Bit of a row going on, although from where he was he couldn't see any flashes. Day was a long time coming, but it would be, of course after a night like this. Never known such a night: it didn't seem to matter whether he opened his eyes or shut them he couldn't see a thing. Pity the stretcher bearers were quite so busy; he couldn't help being a bit impatient; after all there was a new arrival waiting for him at home. Bit close, that last one, but a shell never dropped in the same hole twice; he was safe enough, even if he couldn't move and couldn't see a thing.[47]

As he waited patiently, he reflected on the children he would soon see, the youngest but a week old. Finally, with his two friends, he reached medical attention:

> The M.O. still retained something of a bedside manner. He was a stout fellow, done to the world himself after eighteen hours of duty on end; … 'Now' [he said] 'get this bandage off, old son, and let's have a look at you; time to get up, you know.' 'Bit early, ain't it?' Private Beard felt ready for a joke. 'Who wants to get out o' bed at four o'clock?' 'Four o' – what in the world are you talking about? Six o'clock on a bright summer morning, that's what it is, me lad; quite long enough of sleep you've – Hullo, what's up?' 'Six o'clock?' Beard's voice was cracked and ghastly. He put his hand quickly to his forehead. Bettson and Bartlet moved away. There is no need for more than one to be at his side when a man has dreamed for months of his children's faces, and suddenly learns that night has given place to the full blaze of the day, and still he cannot see.[48]

Advances in medical and surgical techniques during the 50 years before the war underpinned the ability of army medical services to deal with injuries that would otherwise have been both untreatable and untreated. Casualty survival during the war increased as a result of better understanding of infection and surgical shock, as well as improvements in the transfer of injured men from front line to definitive management facilities. But the nature of war had changed, and it brought with it a different spectrum of injury. Artillery bombardment exposed men to a blizzard of projectiles which caused widespread damage, and which resulted in facial injury on a scale hitherto unseen. Peacetime navies had no real experience of the actuality of explosions and burns. Aerial warfare had never existed. As a result of better casualty management and evacuation, casualties did not die as they would have done in earlier times. Doctors and surgeons were now confronted with types of injury that were disfiguring, but not fatal. Dealing with these injuries was the challenge. Previous management was limited by ignorance and inexperience, but a major advance was in the offing. The development of specialised treatment for facial injuries would be driven largely by one man: Harold Gillies.

---

47 Ronald Gurner, *Pass Guard at Ypres* (London: J.M. Dent & Sons, 1930), p.133.
48 Gurner, *Pass Guard*, pp.135-136.

2

The Emergence of a Dedicated Facial Injury Service and the Creation of the Queen's Hospital

This chapter examines how a comprehensive response to facial injury was brought about by the large number of casualties and the increased survival of men who received these injuries. The chapter draws attention to the role and methods of Harold Gillies, who established a facial injury service in Britain, and explores why the organisation of treatment was different in Britain and France. Gillies' initial unit at Aldershot was overwhelmed by the number of casualties from the Somme, which led to the development of plans for a larger facility at Sidcup. This facility, the Queen's Hospital, opened in 1917 and became an international unit soon thereafter. The chapter also considers the practical implications of hospital development, given that the new hospital was financed by private donations rather than by the government.

The treatment of a major facial injury, whether caused by bullet or shell, required more than the repair of surface tissues. Wounded men were frequently missing cheekbones, palates, eye sockets and jaws. In these cases, the underlying structures had to be repaired, because if the raw edges of a wound were simply pulled together and stitched, regardless of the amount of tissue loss, the patient was left with a distorted, grimacing mask. There was no tradition of managing such injuries, nor any pool of experienced surgeons upon which the armies could draw. Men who suffered such facial wounds before the First World War either survived with horrible disfigurements, or died. This chapter examines the changes in practice, first in France and later in Britain, which resulted in the establishment of a dedicated service for facial injury care for members of the British and Empire forces, and the genesis of the process by which the outcome of facial wounds was changed from death or disfigurement to reconstruction.

Early Facial Injury Organisation in France and Britain

The French and German armies suffered heavy casualties in the first weeks and months of the war. In France, the significant number of casualties with facial injuries led to the realisation that these patients required better management. The French *Service de Santé* took rapid steps to manage the problems of facial injury, and established a three-tier system which treated men in successive locations: firstly, near the front; secondly, at an intermediate hospital; and, finally, if necessary, at a major centre. Three major centres were initially established. In Paris, Hippolyte Morestin at the Val-de-Grâce Hospital had already performed many operations on patients with facial problems. Morestin was used to performing surgery on cancer victims and had switched effortlessly to trauma work. By the end of 1914, Albéric Pont had established a jaw surgery unit in Lyons. Léon Imbert led treatment in Marseilles, Leon Dufourmentel in Châlons-sur-Marne, Maurice Virenque in Le Mans, Fernand Lemaître in Vichy and Emile-Jules Moure in Bordeaux. These units were far apart and communication between them was almost non-existent. Within each unit, moreover, surgeons worked in isolation from one another and divided patients by site of injury. Morestin's autocratic and patronising attitude extended to a positive refusal to collaborate on facial surgery with his dental colleagues, whom he treated as technicians to be summoned infrequently but peremptorily and then ordered about. His insularity was not unique. Although numerous French surgeons were responsible for treating the more than 15,000 facial casualties that passed through French hospitals during the war, their geographical isolation and professional independence meant that information between the units was rarely shared. Communication was negligible even when geographical constraints were absent. Fred Albee and Varastad Kazanjian, two American surgeons who worked little more than a stone's throw from Paris, in Neuilly-sur-Seine, knew all about Morestin and yet ignored him. The system adopted in France did not facilitate the spread of new techniques in facial injury care, and was not mirrored in the development of the Queen's Hospital.

Albee and Kazanjian operated in the American hospital established at the Lycée Pasteur, Neuilly, in 1914, and began to experiment with bone grafting to the jaw. Albee had worked on bone grafting since 1906, but his pre-war experience was confined to the spine and long bones of the leg. In France, he soon realised that his principles were adaptable to the jaw.

He described how numerous injuries occurred because the troops failed to appreciate:

> the menace of the machine gun. They seemed to think they could pop their heads up over a trench and move quickly enough to dodge the hail of machine-gun bullets. By the time they found out that this was the wrong idea, head-wound cases were filling the hospitals of France … Some of these patients were pitiable to look upon.

He wrote, "The whole side of their face would be blown away."[1] Albee found many who required bone grafts to the jaw among the wounded at Neuilly. The efforts of Albee and Kazanjian, along with those of Jacques Joseph and Johannes Esser on the German side, were largely confined to the patching up of men in a hurry to enable them to return to the front. In 1915 alone, Esser and his team performed around 400 operations.[2]

The United States of America did not enter the war until the spring of 1917, but a number of American doctors and dentists had already rushed to France in order to aid the medical services. The dentists Byron Hayes and William Davenport began work alongside Albee and Kazanjian at Neuilly, and they were joined in July 1915 by James Judd. Accompanied his wife, Judd had made the long trip from Hawaii to volunteer for the American Ambulance. They were stationed initially at Neuilly before moving north-east of Paris to the village of Juilly.

Judd was appalled by the jaw injuries he witnessed, and described them in graphic detail in his post-war account:

> There were some terrible wounds, especially the jaw cases … It does not seem possible that a man could be alive with such wounds. One boy was shot through the shoulder at close range, then the ball tore open his neck and carried away a good part of the lower

---

1   F.H. Albee, *A Surgeon's Fight to Rebuild Men* (London: Robert Hale, 1950), p.108.

2   For a summary of Esser's life and work, see B. Haeseker, *Dr. J.F.S. Esser and his influence on the development of plastic and reconstructive surgery* (Rotterdam: Erasmus Universiteit, 1983). He describes some general rules in the article: 'General rules in simple plastic work on Austrian war wounded soldiers', *Surgery, Gynaecology and Obstetrics*, 24 (1917), pp.737-748.

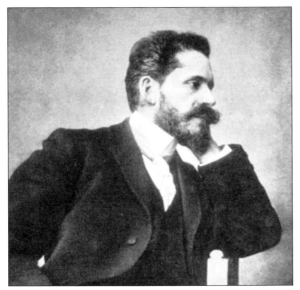
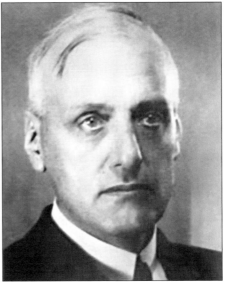

Hippolyte Morestin and Joseph Esser. (Open source images)

jaw, floor of the mouth and tongue. He was a nervous little chap and suffered greatly. He was fed by a tube introduced into his nose, but did not look as if he could survive.[3]

Judd was particularly upset by seeing those blinded by their injury, and recorded that:

often their eyesight has gone beyond hope. It is heart-rending to witness their hope when they recover from the anaesthetic and believe, now that they have been attended to by the American doctor, they will be all right. They get some one to light a cigarette for them, laugh and crack jokes. Later on when the consciousness that they are doomed to everlasting darkness comes to them, they are magnificent.

Such comments illustrate the bond which developed between surgeon and patient, and demonstrate Judd's admiration for the stoicism of the men in his care.

Judd quickly realised that, although there was a certain satisfaction in saving the lives of his patients, early success was no guarantee of longer term survival. Bleeding from major arteries in the head and neck could be torrential. Even if the initial blood loss was stemmed, secondary haemorrhage occurred unseen and without warning when the spread of infection caused the ulceration of a blood vessel.

"One night I was called to the ward hurriedly and by the light of a lantern was appalled to see blood pouring out of a man's mouth," Judd recalled:

The poor fellow was choking and blood poured all over the bed. There was no success in trying to see where the blood came from. A shrapnel ball had struck him in the face alongside of the nose and traversed the neck and the blood poured out of his mouth too fast to sponge it out and see by lantern light the source of the bleeding. A finger in

---

3   J.R. Judd, *With the American Ambulance in France* (Honolulu, HI: Star-Bulletin Press, 1919), pp.48-52. Unless otherwise stated, all quotations in the following passage are taken from this source.

his mouth felt a hole in his hard palate through which the blood poured and the finger was used to plug the hole until the blood could be cleaned out and the wound packed.

Another patient sought help one afternoon. Judd:

> heard a splashing sound and an old chap came staggering in … with blood pouring out from a great hole in his face. He started to bleed as he sat up in bed and, knowing that I was in the dressing room, he came in there after me, leaving a trail of blood behind him. Vigorous packing stopped the hemorrhage [sic] for the time being but later on it was necessary to tie the external carotid artery in his neck … A Chinese bullet fifteen years ago carried away part of his nose and a piece of German shell took away most of what was left and a large piece of his upper jaw. When he was wounded, [he] crawled into a shell hole and packed his wound full of mud to stop the bleeding.

Judd's recollections underline the infancy of reconstructive surgery in France at the beginning of the First World War. His account indicates that the patient's original nasal injury, likely received at the time of the Boxer Rebellion in 1900, was unrepaired at the time the second wound was received.

The European armies did not welcome American support unequivocally. The case of Charles Auguste Valadier provides a notable example. Valadier, a flamboyant French-American who had qualified as a dentist in Philadelphia and practised in Paris, was not actually a doctor. His lack of a medical qualification meant that his services were turned down by the French, whilst the British military medical hierarchy insisted that any operations he undertook had to be supervised by a qualified doctor. Valadier was a wealthy man, and provided much of his own equipment, including a white Rolls-Royce which he had had fitted out as a mobile dental surgery.[4] He initially established a unit for the treatment of jaw wounds in Boulogne, which later moved north to 83 General ('The Dublin') Hospital at Wimereux.[5] It is even alleged that he undertook dental work on the Commander-in-Chief of the British forces in France, Sir Douglas Haig. Cyril Bowdler Henry, a dentist who encountered Valadier, described him as "a charming, jaunty cowboy."[6] Valadier was also a great experimenter, and according to his patients his results were good.

Captain Dougan 'Micky' Chater of the 2nd Gordon Highlanders became Valadier's patient in March 1915. Chater was wounded at Neuve Chapelle on 11 March, during a costly assault for the Highlanders. Five officers, including the colonel, were killed, and a

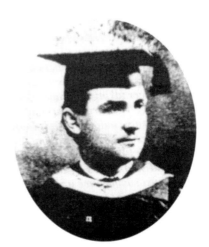

Charles Auguste Valadier.
(Open source image)

4   After the war, Valadier's Rolls-Royce found its way to England and was converted back to a standard saloon. In July 2013, it was sold at auction by Bonhams for £718,000.
5   R.H. Ivy, 'The mysterious A.C. Valadier', *Plastic and Reconstructive Surgery*, 47:4 (1971), pp.365-370; J.E. McAuley, 'Charles Valadier: a forgotten pioneer in the treatment of jaw injuries', *Proceedings of the Royal Society of Medicine*, 67:8 (1974), pp.785-789.
6   Quoted in McAuley, 'Charles Valadier'.

further 10 wounded.[7] What Chater described as his "charming birthday treat charging the German trenches" left him with wounds to the shoulder and arm along with a shattered jaw. He realised his war was over and expected to be sent to England, commenting that "I am not beautiful to look at." Unable to eat solid food he became "frantically hungry." Monica Glazebrook, a family friend, was able to visit Chater and wrote to his mother that, although the medical staff were initially very anxious about him, "he is [now] strong enough to sit up in bed … of course all the lower part of his face is covered but the upper part looked <u>quite</u> himself."[8] Following his surgery, Chater wrote, "I was rather a 'show case' for some time and did not return to England until July. My jaw had been set by Charles Valadier, who was half French and half American and the medical profession considered him a quack as he was not really qualified." Chater was clearly impressed by, and retained an interest in, Valadier's work. An article written by Valadier for the *British Journal of Surgery* the year after Chater's successful procedure had taken place in France was retained by Chater, and was deposited in the Imperial War Museum alongside his wartime letters.[9]

The early British facial casualties from the front joined the mass of other wounded men transported to England for recuperation. Initially, the treatment of facial casualties followed the French pattern. Men were placed indiscriminately in the huge general hospitals that had developed in response to the growing casualty lists, some in

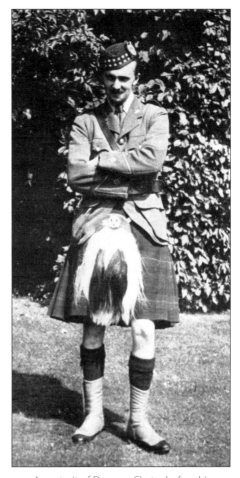

A portrait of Dougan Chater before his departure for France. (Courtesy of the Chater family archive)

existing hospital buildings, some rapidly converted from other uses. A small amount of facial work took place from 1915 at the 3rd London General Hospital in Wandsworth, one of the large clearing hospitals in the capital. Originally sited in the existing buildings of an orphanage, the Royal Victoria Patriotic School, the hospital expanded from 250 beds at the outset to a total of 1,800 beds by February 1917. Treatment was underpinned by the development of a mask unit where the sculptor Francis Derwent Wood made 'Tin Noses' from plaster casts, but the two surgeons at Wandsworth largely confined their work to jaw surgery.[10]

7   MS letter to 'Lionel', 23 March 1915, from the Anglo-American Hospital, Wimereux. (Courtesy of Mr Simon Chater)

8   IWM: 1697-2, Private Papers of Captain A.D. Chater. Unless otherwise stated, all quotations in the following passage are taken from this source. Emphasis in original.

9   A.C. Valadier, 'A few suggestions for the treatment of fractured jaws', *British Journal of Surgery*, 4:13 (1916), pp.64-73.

10 See W. Warwick James and B.W. Fickling, *Injuries of the jaws and face* (London: John Bale & Staples, 1940). This book was based on their Wandsworth experience; in the preface, they note that when they came to

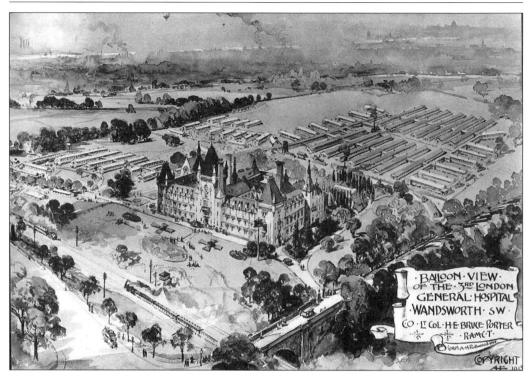

An aerial view of the 3rd London General Hospital, Wandsworth from 'Souvenir of London and the 3rd London'. (Photo Press, 1921)

Elsewhere in London, The King George V Military Hospital on Stamford Street was another hospital which undertook facial work. Converted from a warehouse originally built for the Stationery Office, it possessed 1,650 beds and was funded by subscription. Albert Norman, a doctor who embraced the art of photography, compiled an album of some of the facial cases treated at Stamford Street. The album was assembled for Percival Cole (1878-1948), a dentist who had also qualified as a doctor.[11] A handful of patients from the King George V transferred to the Queen's Hospital when it opened. Two other Red Cross-sponsored hospitals for facial wounds opened in London in 1916, both in private houses. 37 beds were available at 74 Brook Street, and an annexe in a house at 24 Norfolk Street owned by the art dealer Joseph Duveen contained 40 beds. Outside London, a jaw unit was established at Beckett Park Hospital, Leeds. William Maxwell Munby, an ear, nose and throat (ENT) surgeon, ran Beckett Park with the assistance of two dentists, Alan Forty and A.D. Shefford. Of 200 cases discussed in an article

write it, all of the case notes had disappeared.

11   The album is in the Wellcome Library: Royal Army Medical Corps Muniments Collection, CMAC RAMC/760, two albums of photographs of plastic surgery cases at the King George Military Hospital (later Red Cross Hospital), Stamford Street, London, taken by Dr Albert Norman, Honorary Scientific Photographer. See also P.P. Cole, 'Plastic repair in war injuries to the jaw and face', *The Lancet*, 189:4881 (1917), pp.415-418. For a short biography of Cole, see Plarr's 'Lives of the Fellows of the Royal College of Surgeons of England' online <http://livesonline.rcseng.ac.uk/biogs/E003978b.htm> (accessed 10 January 2016).

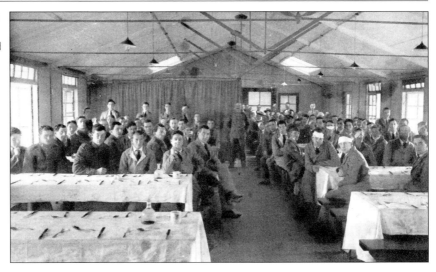

A postcard of the King George V Hospital, Stamford Street. (Author's collection)

written by Munby's team at Beckett Park, 175 patients returned to service.[12] As in France, the work undertaken within these units was small scale, haphazard, and conducted as part of the generality of surgery. However, this would not be the case for the rest of the war.

Harold Gillies and the Birth of Specialist Facial Injury Care

Harold Gillies was 32 years old at the outbreak of the First World War. A New Zealand-born surgeon, Gillies offered his services to the Red Cross and joined a Belgian ambulance unit in February 1915.[13] Prior to the war, Gillies had had an eventful life. He had been sent to preparatory school in England and returned to New Zealand for his secondary education at Wanganui Collegiate School. He was named New Zealand's best young cricketer of the year whilst there, developed the school's golf course, edited the college journal, won several academic prizes, and became a first lieutenant in the school's cadet corps. He then followed two of his brothers to the University of Cambridge, where he studied medicine at Gonville and Caius College. He rowed for the University, and was at number seven in the winning Light Blue boat of 1904. He also attained a golfing blue, and played golf for England in an amateur international. In the early 1930s when a series of famous golfers were immortalised on cigarette cards, Gillies was included alongside the international stars of the day. Restricted in his swing because of a stiff elbow, sustained as a child when fleeing the wrath of a relative he had surprised on the lavatory, Gillies played off a high tee. Initially, he found a beer bottle suitable, but he changed to a wide-bore rubber tube section when the green keepers complained about the broken glass.[14] In addition, Gillies was a keen fly-fisherman, a good violinist, competent pianist and determined practical joker. After Cambridge, he undertook his clinical training at St Bartholomew's

12   See W.M. Munby, A.A. Forty and A.D. Shefford, 'Notes on the principles and results of treatment in 200 cases of injuries to the face and jaws', *British Journal of Surgery*, 6:21 (1918), pp.86-91. Although Munby comments that he and his colleagues intended to analyse more than a thousand cases, no further publication appeared.

13   R. Pound, *Gillies. Surgeon Extraordinary* (London: Michael Joseph, 1964).

14   An illustration of the rubber tee is in D. Vidler, *Rye Golf Club: The First 90 Years* (Rye: Rye Golf Club, 1984).

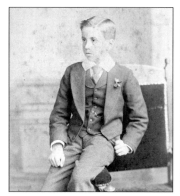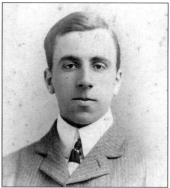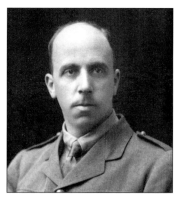

Harold Gillies as a schoolboy; a formal portrait of Gillies while an undergraduate in 1904; Gillies in his first posting with the Red Cross. (BAPRAS Archive)

Hospital in London, where he specialised in otorhinolaryngology (ENT surgery) and worked for Sir John Milsom Rees, Laryngologist to the Royal Household.

The Red Cross sent for Gillies at the end of January 1915. He began by performing general surgery in a Belgian unit at Hoogstadt, near Furnes, but it was not long before he was bored. While passing through Boulogne he met Valadier, who as noted was only allowed to operate under supervision of a qualified surgeon. Gillies took on this role, but became particularly enthused when C.W. 'Bobs' Roberts, an American surgeon and old golfing friend attached to the American Hospital at Neuilly, passed on an article he had received from Germany. Another friend, the Canadian Brehmer Heald who had been a medical student contemporary of Gillies at Cambridge, remarked in passing that it seemed surprising that the British army had not taken any steps to deal with facial injury. This was a turning point. Gillies decided that something had to be done, and that he would do it. In June 1915, he visited Morestin while taking leave in Paris, remarking that Morestin was "rumoured to be performing unbelievable feats."[15] He was allowed to watch Morestin operate on a facial cancer, and decided that facial surgery "was the one job in the world I wanted to do."[16]

After he had met Morestin and Valadier, and observed the treatment of patients in France, Gillies' experience and enthusiasm was translated into action. He reported to the army medical authorities that widespread distribution of patients around many hospitals staffed by generalist surgeons was ineffective, and suggested that special facilities should be developed. Aware of the French surgical diaspora, Gillies felt that inchoate provision in England was unacceptable. Although there was no formal discipline of plastic surgery, and no British surgeons with any experience, Gillies believed that if casualties were pointed in a specific direction, surgeons could learn lessons rapidly and treat casualties more effectively.

Towards the end of 1915, Gillies approached the head of army surgery, Sir William Arbuthnot Lane, to discuss his ideas. Arbuthnot Lane had himself acquired some interest in facial injuries, and was sympathetic to Gillies' views. Furthermore, he had already made a similar move to concentrate the management of amputees at Queen Mary's Hospital, Roehampton, and had sanctioned the development of specialist orthopaedic hospitals following similar lobbying by the surgeon Robert Jones. The concentration of specialists at these hospitals had revolutionised

15   H.D. Gillies and R. Millard, *The Principles and Art of Plastic Surgery* (London: Butterworth & Co., 1957), p.7.
16   Pound, *Gillies*, p.24.

management of amputee treatment and fracture management. Alongside the introduction of the Thomas splint to immobilise thigh fractures, Jones' reorganisation resulted in a marked diminution of both complications and mortality. Gillies' representations eventually reached the Director of Army Medical Services, Sir Alfred Keogh, and in January 1916 Gillies was ordered to report to the Cambridge Military Hospital in Aldershot "for special duty in connection with Plastic Surgery."[17]

The Development of Aldershot's Facial Treatment Capacity

Gillies was convinced that huge numbers of facial injury casualties were on their way, and had a ward cleared at Aldershot in readiness to receive them. While the ward was being equipped he made a quick tour of some French units, but when he made a return visit to Morestin he was rudely turned away. Morestin's unwillingness to collaborate was notorious, to the extent that a contemporary cartoon showed the irascible figure by the door to his operating theatre, on which was a large notice forbidding access. By the time Gillies returned to England, a few patients with facial injuries had begun to arrive in Aldershot. Gillies advised the War Office that in order to facilitate the movement of troops to the new ward, all facial casualties should be directed to Aldershot by means of a special Field Medical Card. The proposal was brusquely dismissed as unworkable, as Gillies recalled: "I was told by the War Office to 'Run away little boy. We are far too busy for that sort of thing'."[18] Nothing if not persistent, Gillies designed a special label to add to the standard card, headed to the Strand, found a printer, and bought a considerable supply of labels himself for £10. He then personally delivered the labels to the War Office with instructions that they should be sent on to the field hospitals. Gillies' proactive approach worked. "It was very amusing," he later recalled, "to find the War House [sic] had found it a very good idea and had copied it."

Within weeks, labelled soldiers began to appear in Aldershot. Among them was Sergeant Reginald Evans of the 1st Battalion, Hertfordshire Regiment. Wounded in February 1916, Evans was initially sent to the 14th Stationary Hospital, Boulogne. Despite his serious injury, Evans remained remarkably cheerful, writing:

> I am getting on quite as well as can be expected and haven't lost my healthy brown looks by any means. I am well looked after here and fed every two hours with a variety of drinks … Fancy I have been nearly 8 weeks in hospital still what's that in a lifetime eh? … Everybody is very good and … I'm not in the least pain at present so you see dear Mother you've no need to worry in the least about your loving son.[19]

Eventually, Evans was shipped across the Channel on 13 April and he was transferred to Aldershot two days later.

Gillies had ensured the supply of patients to his newly established ward and, with the backing of Arbuthnot Lane, he began to recruit his surgical team. He was allotted an assistant, Captain John Law Aymard, who according to Gillies was "a South African practitioner with rather an odd history."[20] Scorning Morestin's attitude to dentists, Gillies arranged for the secondment of two dental surgeons, Alexander (Bill) Fraser and Louis King, and he also acquired the

---

17   Ibid.
18   Gillies, letter to Millard, 12 September 1951. Unless otherwise stated, all quotations in the following passage are taken from this source.
19   Reginald Evans, personal papers. (Courtesy of Pam Campbell)
20   Gillies to Millard, 12 September 1951.

services of an anaesthetist, Captain Rubens Wade.[21] Gillies also developed his own expertise. He studied the extant works on plastic surgery within the library of the RCS in London. We know that Gillies had a copy of Nélaton and Ombrédanne's book *La Rhinoplastie*, published in 1904, but he was unwilling to acknowledge any debt to that text.[22] Indeed, he was reputed to have concealed it hurriedly when another surgeon entered the room where he was consulting it. The identity of the work 'Bobs' Roberts had shown him in France remains unclear. Gillies' biographer, Reginald Pound, claims that Gillies had been shown a book written by the German surgeon August Lindemann, although Gillies' own account suggests that Roberts showed him an article rather than a book. Lindemann was a facial surgeon. Born in 1880, he was eight years Gillies' senior and had contributed to a German textbook edited by Christian Brühn, the first part of which appeared in 1915.[23]

Much of what had been written before 1916 was either about rhinoplasty or did not work in practice. The presentation of the early texts on facial treatment concealed the truth that the results were often dreadful. Denis Keegan's turn-of-the-century account of his work in India was an exception, an honest appraisal in which the author was analytical of his failures.[24] One of the major causes of failure related to the use of unlined skin flaps. The use of tissue flaps, cut and turned, was described at length in *La Rhinoplastie*. However, surgeons did not appreciate that if a flap was used to make a nose, which has skin on the outside and mucous membrane inside, then failure to recreate the inner surface would inevitably result in the collapse of the new nose. The textbooks of the time did not provide this information. Gillies and his team rapidly learned that they had no pool of knowledge from which to identify techniques to apply to patients.[25] As a consequence, the learning curve for the surgeons was a steep one. Gillies also noted that both French and German surgeons had a lack of interest in aesthetic reconstruction. "There was indeed," he continued, "too much truth in the French gibe that 'before' the patient was horrible and 'after' ridiculous."[26]

The new ward required more than just good surgeons. Gillies realised that drawings of actual operations were necessary in order to use his patients as an educational resource. To improve his draughtsmanship, Gillies joined the Press Art School – a correspondence course outfit founded by the artist Percy Bradshaw. However, after showing some of his efforts to another golfing friend, Bernard Darwin, Gillies learned that there was already an outstanding artist at Aldershot. Henry Tonks, who had trained as a surgeon but did not have much enthusiasm for the profession, had drifted into art and become a teacher at the Slade School. Tonks

---

21 For a full account of Wade's life, see D.J. Wilkinson, 'Who was Dr. Reubens Wade?', *Proceedings of the Fourth International Symposium on the History of Anaesthesia*, ed. by J. Schulte am Esch and M. Goerig (Lübeck: Verlag Dräger Druck, 1999), pp.113-116.

22 C. Nélaton and L. Ombrédanne, *La Rhinoplastie* (Paris: Steinheil, 1904).

23 Pound, *Gillies*, p.23. Gillies relates this story in *The Principles and Art of Plastic Surgery*, but his 1951 letter to Ralph Millard is less than clear. Indeed, later in the letter he mentions an apocryphal story which he is happy to have repeated for its effect. The only record for a book authored by Lindemann is for a work first published in 1939: A. Lindemann, *Leitfaden der Chirurgie und Orthopädie des Mundes und der Kiefer* (*Manual of surgical and orthopaedic management of mouth and jaws*) (Leipzig: Verlag von Hermann Meusser, 1939). If Roberts had produced a book rather than an article, it is likely to have been by C. Brühn, *Die Gegenwärtigen Behandlungswege der Kieferschussverletzungen. Ergebnisse aus dem Düsseldorfer Lazarett für Kieferverletzte (Kgl Reservelazarett)* (*Management of Gunshot Injuries of the Jaw, Based on the Experience of the Jaw Hospital in Düsseldorf*) (Wiesbaden: Verlag von J.F. Bergmann, 1915-1917). This contained an extensive section by Lindemann and is mentioned in Pound's biography.

24 D.F. Keegan, *Rhinoplastic Operations with a Description of Recent Improvements in the Indian Method* (London: Baillière, Tindall & Cox, 1900).

25 I am grateful to Felix Freshwater for this analysis.

26 Gillies and Millard, *Principles and Art*, p.10.

was 52 when the war began, and was already a major figure in the art world. In patriotic vein despite his advancing years, he had applied for a commission as an RAMC lieutenant and been posted to Aldershot.

He reflected in a letter to his friend Nelson Ward that:

> I have joined the British Army, and in so doing have entirely deprived myself of all freedom of action. I may remain here two days more or nearly twelve months, I may have something to do or nothing. A wisdom far above anything we can grasp has taken me in hand, and I have got to do what I am told, a lesson I only learn at 53. So you see I cannot dine with you, because by an ingenious arrangement we sign our names between six and seven, which just nips any jaunts to London.[27]

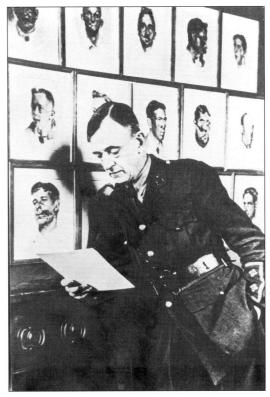

Henry Tonks at Sidcup with his pastels.
(Author's collection)

Tonks was working as the adjutant's secretary at the time of Gillies' request that he be attached to the plastic surgery unit. His new role was to observe Gillies in the operating theatre and make lightning sketches, which he elaborated later by annotating the drawings and making portraits of the men on the ward. These pastels and drawings were the basis of Gillies' early reconstructions, and the source of Gillies' appreciation of the need both to restore function and to produce a result that was aesthetically acceptable. Tonks pointed out that the latter, if achieved, ensured the former.

Tonks, at last, had "something to do," writing that:

> I am doing a number of pastel heads of wounded soldiers who had had their faces knocked about. A very good surgeon called Gillies who is also nearly a champion golf player is undertaking what is known as the plastic surgery necessary. It is a chamber of horrors, but I am quite content to draw them as it is excellent practice. One poor fellow has the D.C.M., a large part of his mouth has been blown away, he is extraordinary modest and contented. I hope Gillies will make a good job of him. You bring up flaps from wherever is convenient.[28]
>
> I may be going abroad. I put down my name when I was not satisfied with my work here; now I might just as well stop, as I am a faint use … One [pastel] I did the other day of a young fellow with rather a classical face was exactly like a living damaged Greek head as his nose had been cut clean off. Another I have just finished with an enormous hole in his cheek through which you can see the tongue working, rather

27   Quoted in J. Hone, *The Life of Henry Tonks* (London: Heinemann, 1939), p.126.
28   Glasgow University Library (GUL): MacColl Papers, MS MacColl T201, Tonks to MacColl, 21 April 1916.

reminds me of Philip IV as the obstruction to the lymphatics has made the face very blobby.[29]

The "poor fellow" with the DCM referred to in Tonks' letter was Reginald Evans. The "young fellow" was Private A.H. Palmer of the Royal Kent Regiment (See Colour Section, p.v). Palmer had enlisted underage by using the name of his brother Edward who had died at birth in 1895.

The Battle of the Somme Overwhelms Aldershot

Gillies' prediction that the new form of warfare would result in a great deal of face work for his team proved accurate. The casualties of Neuve Chapelle and Loos in 1915 were nothing compared to the numbers of men wounded in the colossal battles of 1916 onwards. On 1 July 1916, the Allies launched their offensive on the Somme. Despite a preliminary bombardment by the British artillery of unprecedented ferocity, the German wire across no man's land was not sufficiently cut, the deep enemy dugouts were not destroyed, and the advance on 1 July was slow enough along much of the front for the enemy to emerge from their shelters and man their machine guns. The result was the single bloodiest day in British military history. The assault of 1 July alone resulted in the loss of almost 60,000 killed, wounded or taken prisoner.

A significant number of facial casualties were among those wounded by the German machine gunners. Every conceivable type of facial injury appeared as a result of the Somme. Arbuthnot Lane, the Commandant at Aldershot, allocated Gillies an extra 200 beds, but Gillies recorded, perhaps with some exaggeration, that 2,000 patients arrived. Although he worked flat out all day, invented techniques as he went along, and pushed patients into convalescent beds as fast as he could, Gillies and his little team could not cope with the continued influx of men. He despaired of the size of the task, and wrote of "Men without half their faces; men burned and maimed to the condition of animals. Day after day, the tragic, grotesque procession disembarked from the hospital ships and made its way towards us."[30] The facilities at Aldershot were not sufficient to deal with the demands of industrial warfare. Gillies' team required a dedicated hospital rather than a dedicated unit. Consequently, Gillies sought to ameliorate the problem through the development of a large convalescent facility which would free up the limited number of surgical beds.

Arbuthnot Lane discussed this possibility with some of his acquaintances and one, Lady Rodney, offered her house at Great Alresford, in Hampshire. Lady Rodney's offer added a further 50 beds to the overall complement. Waverley Abbey, another Georgian mansion near Farnham in Surrey, was also pressed into service for convalescent patients. However, the growing number of casualties made it apparent that simply providing more convalescent beds was not enough. As the post-war *Report of the Joint War Committee of the British Red Cross and Order of St John* recorded: "It was not possible to enlarge the Cambridge Hospital, nor, indeed, were the surroundings suitable, in any case, for patients of the type in question. Quiet, good air and ample space, we understand, are amongst the essential conditions for securing success."[31] Facial reconstruction was not a one-step procedure. Each operation required time for healing before the next step could be performed, and Gillies knew that haste was unacceptable. Each

---

29 GUL: MacColl Papers, MS MacColl T212, Tonks to MacColl, 28 June 1916.

30 Quoted in Pound, *Gillies*, p.33. A photograph album survives from the Aldershot convalescent unit at Waverley Abbey.

31 *Report of the Joint War Committee of the British Red Cross and Order of St John on Voluntary Aid rendered to the Sick and Wounded at Home and Abroad and to British Prisoners of War, 1914-1919* (London: His/Her Majesty's Stationery Office, 1921), p.260.

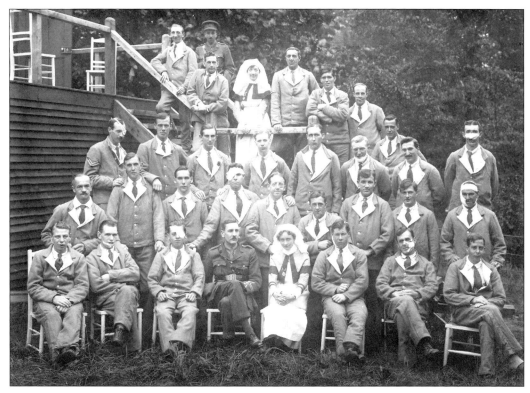

Gillies at Aldershot with some of his patients. (Author's collection)

new patient required frequent re-admittance for surgery that could only be performed in stages. Gillies badgered the Aldershot authorities ceaselessly, and finally appealed above their heads to the Red Cross. Ultimately, "a committee … was formed which had such social and political prestige that the War Office finally gave us permission to move to new and larger premises."[32] The committee, chaired by Viscount Chilston, began to hunt for an alternative site. Charles Kenderdine, one of the trustees of the amputee centre at Queen Mary's Hospital at Roehampton, thought that a new hospital dedicated to the management of facial injuries could be organised on the same lines, and be of the same scale, as Queen Mary's.[33] A well-connected London land agent, Kenderdine also believed that the proposed small increase in bed numbers from Lady Rodney's offer was insufficient, and "advised a far more ambitious scheme."[34] In addition, Kenderdine had a potential site for the hospital in mind, the estate of Frognal House in Sidcup. As he was the estate's own agent, his knowledge of its availability was hardly surprising.

Frognal House, the seat of the Earls Sydney, had been put up for sale following the death of its owner, Robert Marsham-Townshend, in December 1914. Marsham's eldest son, Hugh, inherited the estate and had prepared an auction catalogue containing the house itself, the adjacent estate of Scadbury, a number of other properties and businesses, and a great deal

32 Gillies and Millard, *Principles and Art*, p.30.
33 Kenderdine's involvement came about through his acquaintance with Lady Rodney and Lord Clarendon, who had been involved in attempts to establish a convalescent unit for Gillies near Aldershot.
34 This information is drawn from a commemorative booklet. BLSC: Bamji Collection, QUE, The Queen's Hospital, 1917-1929: The Queen Mary's Hospital, 1929-1967: Sidcup: Kent, p.4.

of land. From Monday 7 June 1915, the contents of Frognal House were disposed of in a huge sale. Starting with the family portraits by Kneller, Gainsborough, Romney, Zoffany, Kauffmann and others, continuing through the Second Viscount Sydney's extensive correspondence with William Pitt, and down to the last cart in the stables, the contents of Frognal House were disposed of over the course of 11 days. The estate itself, some 1,740 acres, was offered as a whole or in lots. But Lot 10, the mansion and its grounds, did not sell. Kenderdine thought that it might be a suitable location upon which to build the required facial

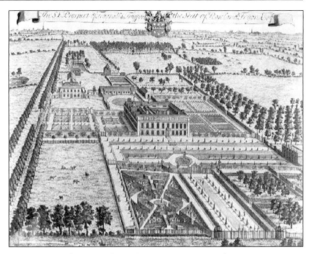

Frognal House, from Dr Harris, *History of Kent*, 1719. (Author's collection)

injury hospital. He became the treasurer of a committee charged to raise money by public appeal, and threw his enormous energy into the cause. The Joint War Committee chipped in, as did Sir Heath Harrison, the shipping magnate and High Sheriff of Hampshire, who offered an instant and enormous contribution of £10,000 to get things going.[35] The Queen also provided funds, not to mention her name, to encourage further donations. In short order, a lease was taken out on Frognal House and its immediate surrounding land.

The house was converted to provide nursing accommodation, administrative space, and a mess for convalescent officers. A hutted hospital was built in the grounds to the south-east. The first part, or Central Hospital, was designed by Mr D.C. Maynard of the partnership Hayward & Maynard. The unique arrangement of the wards suggests that Gillies had substantial input in the design process. Sidcup's wards were arranged in a semicircle around the specially designed plastic and septic operating theatres, unlike most of the new military hospitals which had been laid out on a grid pattern with the wards in long rows.

Full facilities were provided for medical illustration, X-ray, and for the dental technicians. An appeal in the London *Evening Standard* raised money for recreational facilities, including a cinema. A canteen was funded by the Y.M.C.A., and in addition to the standard wards some convalescent accommodation for officers was built to house those awaiting their next operation. A chapel was also provided, thanks to a donation of £200 from the Church of England Missionary Society and the Soldiers and Sailors Institute.

The aims of the Queen's Hospital were supported both by the army's senior medical establishment and its wealthy and aristocratic donors. Some of the latter served on the hospital's management committee and acted to keep it firmly in the public eye. The hospital's cuttings book, which contains nearly 90 folio pages full of newspaper articles and pictures dating from January 1917 onwards, documents the committee's approach. The cuttings book is dominated

---

35 Harrison was noted for his generosity. His obituary in the *Liverpool College Magazine* in 1934 said: "Kind hearted and generous to a degree, he held always before him the Christian ideal of Charity, and used his great wealth in the way which wealth is meant to be used, in helping his fellow men. He was a true benefactor: anything tending towards good had his sympathy and help. Of Sir Heath Harrison it may truly be said that he faithfully performed the whole duty of men. He left the world a better place than he found it."

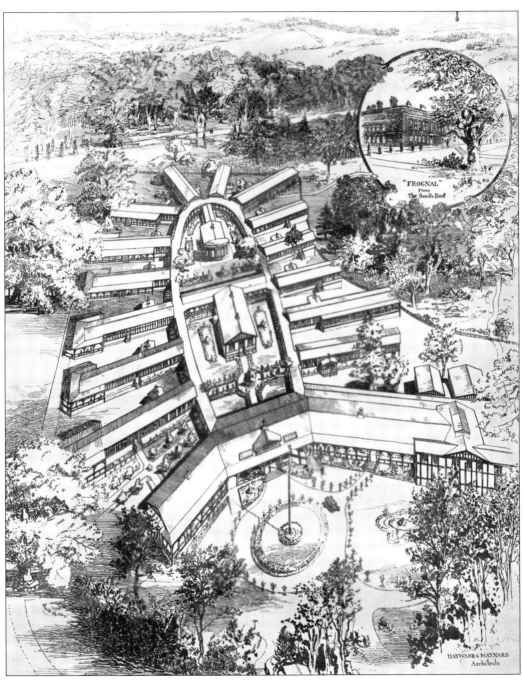

An architect's drawing of the Queen's Hospital. (Author's collection)

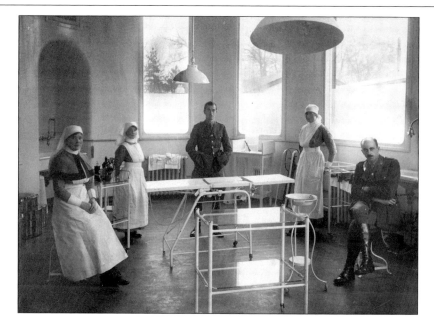

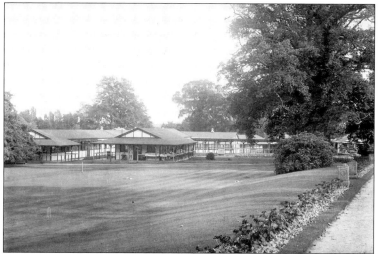

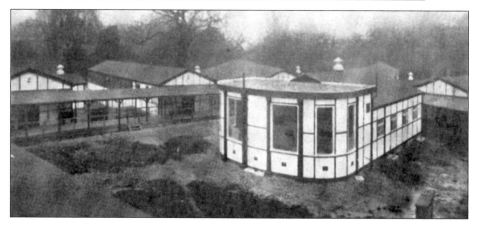

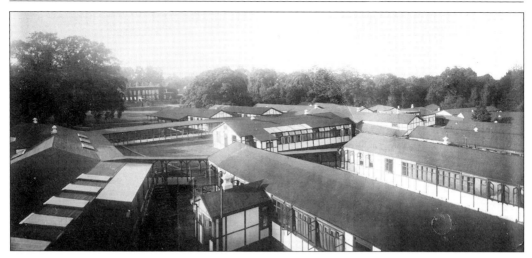

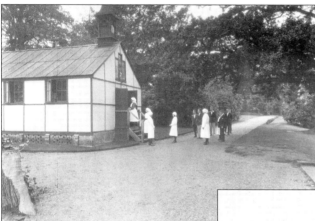

Views of the Queen's Hospital: the interior of the Plastic Theatre, with Gillies seated right and Rubens Wade standing; the wards from Frognal House lawn; the Plastic Theatre; the general view looking north; the hospital chapel; the walkway between wards; the dental workshop. (Author's collection)

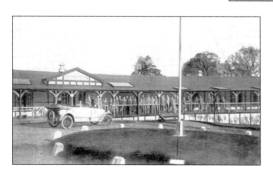

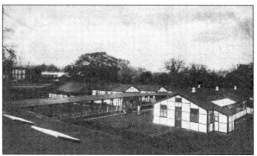

by the widespread media coverage of the development and construction of the hospital, and by a corresponding number of exhortations to potential contributors.[36] Similar appeals appeared in a number of newspapers across England, and the publicity was clearly designed to raise money.

The cuttings also underlined another important aspect of the hospital's function. Repeated explanations of how the hospital would rehabilitate the disabled men, so that they could survive and gain employment after their discharge, were provided:

> Extensive gardens and a farm of 100 acres are attached to the house, where they, with a view to their future employment, will be instructed in outdoor occupations, such as gardening, market-gardening, dairy work, poultry-keeping, forestry, etc. In addition, workshops will be provided for practical instruction in estate carpentry and other handicrafts, and work in connection with electricity, agricultural machinery and motor traction … no effort must be spared to give these men – many of them lads – a fresh interest and a new start in life … and make them realise they are not useless wrecks … [T]hese gallant lads, as they recover, will have an opportunity of learning a trade or gaining experience in outdoor occupations.[37]

Alongside the pitying words for the disfigured men who were to be treated there, the newspaper coverage made clear the need for continued funding of the hospital. As the Joint War Committee reflected after the war, the costs involved in running the Queen's Hospital were substantial:

> It has been pointed out that a hospital of this nature has to contend with very heavy expenses. At the Queen's Hospital the majority of patients were living on 'tube' feeds or upon a diet of fresh milk and eggs, at a period when both these foods were scarce and very costly. The cost of all building materials was abnormally high, and tended constantly to increase … The operating theatres … were equipped with every modern appliance … [and this] necessitated a constant outlay … in order to keep pace with the discoveries made and the improvements suggested.[38]

The daily requirement of 200 gallons of milk was provided by various local sources including the cows of Scadbury Park Farm, which was part of the hospital estate and even featured on a hospital postcard. In December 1917, there were problems with supply and the Secretary, Sir Charles Kenderdine himself, was sent off to a local cattle auction to try and purchase an additional six or seven cows. Unfortunately, according to the hospital Minute Book, "none of the cows were sufficiently good to warrant the Committee making any purchase."[39] Fortunately, a local contractor called Fisher was able to maintain sufficient supply and the crisis passed.

---

36   London Metropolitan Archives (LMA): Westminster Hospital Group, H02/QM/Y/01/005, The Queen's Hospital, Sidcup, Kent: newspaper cuttings.

37   LMA: H02/QM/Y/01/005, cutting from the *Rotherham Advertiser*, January 1917. On the same page are similar articles from the *Daily Telegraph*, *Morning Post*, *Surrey Comet* and the *Darlington North Star*.

38   *Report by the Joint War Committee and the Joint War Finance Committee of the British Red Cross Society and the Order of St. John of Jerusalem in England on voluntary aid rendered to the sick and wounded at home and abroad and to British prisoners of war, 1914-1919* (London: His/Her Majesty's Stationery Office, 1921), p.261.

39   AWM: AWM11 1506/8/43, Queen's Hospital Minute Book.

The hospital's accounts evidence the ongoing running costs of Sidcup. The average messing cost was just over 2s. 6d. for the hutments in May 1918 ("1 Officer = 3 Men Patients"). At Parkwood, a convalescent home near Swanley in Kent where the egg and milk requirements were somewhat lower, it was 1s. 9d. The messing cost at Sidcup is equivalent to nearly £6 per head per day in twenty-first century prices, considerably more than current daily expenditure on food in the National Health Service. Nor did the end of the fighting bring about relief from the financial pressure. By 1922 the hospital was in deficit, and reduced to subtle appeals to the Dominions for financial assistance. As none of their own men were still at Sidcup by this point, they politely declined to help.

The Development and Expansion of the Queen's Hospital

Patients were moved from Aldershot to Sidcup from June 1917, and the new hospital was officially opened on 18 August. Queen Mary visited the site in November, and graciously agreed that it might be known as the Queen's Hospital. The Queen wrote in her diary:

> Tuesday 13th November 1917. Very foggy day. Went at 1.30 to Sidcup in Kent to see the Queen's Hospital for facial cases at Frognal … Charming place and grounds. Fine afternoon. Met by Ld. Clarendon, Ld. Chilston, Mr Kenderdine, Ly. Rodney, Ly. Gough, Mrs Corbett, Sir Arbuthnot Lane, Major Gillies etc. and visited the 12 wards, theatre, recreation room etc. Saw some marvellous results of the treatment. Very interesting visit.[40]

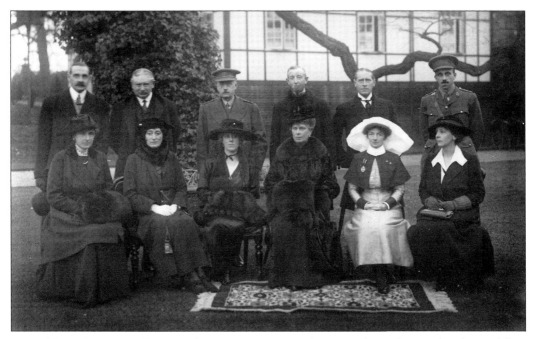

A publicity photograph of the visit of Queen Mary, 13 November 1917. Left to right, seated: Lady Ampthill, Mrs Bertram Corbett, Lady Rodway, Her Majesty, Ethel Barber (matron), Lady Gough. Standing: the Earl of Clarendon, Viscount Chilston, Lieutenant-Colonel Colvin (commandant), Sir Edward Wallington (the Queen's private secretary), Mr Charles Kenderdine, Major H.D. Gillies. (BAPRAS Archive)

---

40 Royal Archives, Windsor: Diary of Queen Mary. (Courtesy of HM The Queen)

The Prince of Wales also visited and, apparently against advice, decided to view wards which housed the worst cases. He reputedly emerged white and shaken. Queen Alexandra and other members of the Royal family also came to Sidcup, and their visits were recorded in group photographs which appeared in the press reports.

At the outset the hospital contained 320 beds, but Gillies had even grander designs. By the beginning of 1918, the hospital had developed a momentum of its own. The sustained publicity campaign had raised awareness of the hospital across the country, and the concept of a single dedicated maxillofacial hospital became attractive, even fashionable. Arbuthnot Lane was among those who saw the potential of the Sidcup facility. His backing may not have been entirely altruistic, as the success of Sidcup was certain to reflect well upon him. Yet regardless of his motivations, Arbuthnot Lane encouraged Gillies to lobby for more facilities in order to make Sidcup "the biggest and most important hospital for jaws and plastic work in the world."[41]

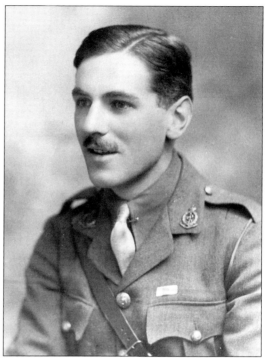

William Kelsey Fry when medical officer of the 1st Battalion, Royal Welch Fusiliers. (Courtesy of Dr Ian Kelsey Fry)

To help plan and develop the hospital, Gillies was aided by an ally with significant wartime experience. William Kelsey Fry had qualified in medicine, then taken a dental degree, and was running a lucrative practice in London when war broke out. A 25-year-old in 1914, Fry volunteered as a regimental medical officer and served with the Royal Welch Fusiliers. His life at the front was full of incident. He continued working after receiving a bullet wound; a photograph of him with his team of orderlies and stretcher-bearers shows him with his left arm in a sling. In May 1915 he was awarded the regiment's first Military Cross, for crawling out into no man's land with his sergeant to try and rescue one of the regiment's lieutenants, the grandson of William Gladstone. Although they succeeded, Gladstone died of his wounds and Fry and Sergeant Woods accompanied the body home. Fry hoped that the coffin would not be opened as the wounds were severe and disfiguring. According to family folklore the poet Siegfried Sassoon, a fellow officer whom Fry thought was quite mad, was so jealous of Fry's MC that he decided to undertake a daring exploit so he could get one too. When he did, Fry removed his own medal ribbon and pinned it on Sassoon.[42]

At the front, Fry saw why so many jaw casualties succumbed when they might have been saved. Gillies described one such case in his post-war writing:

> A young man who had his jaw blown apart during a night raid staggered back to the dugout soaked in blood. In the light of a torch stuck in the mud Captain Fry made a

---

41 Arbuthnot Lane to Gillies, 6 September 1917. Quoted in Pound, *Gillies*, p.42.
42 Ian Kelsey Fry, personal communication.

quick examination and then the two of them marched down along the trench toward the dressing station. Fry walked in front of him so the wounded officer could lean against him, keeping the head forward to allow blood and bits of jaw to fall free of the airway. They arrived without mishap except that Fry's back was covered with blood. The medical orderly was informed about the patient, and as the lieutenant's condition seemed quite good, Fry started back up the line. He had not gone fifty yards along the trench when a message caught up with him that the lieutenant was dead. He had been laid on his back on a stretcher and had died immediately of respiratory obstruction.[43]

Fry's own frontline service also ended in tragedy. At the end of August 1916, when his RAP was hit by a shell and his detachment wiped out, Fry was the only survivor. Sent home with shellshock, he spent a period of convalescence at Parkwood. During his recovery, Fry was walking through the colonnade at Guy's Hospital when he encountered Arbuthnot Lane. As a result of their meeting, Fry went to join Gillies at Sidcup. Like Gillies, and all of the other surgeons who arrived at the Queen's, Fry had no prior experience of facial reconstruction.

Gillies took responsibility for handling the soft tissue work, and allocated the hard tissues to Fry. Between them, the two men learned the procedures and, sometimes accompanied by Tonks, stayed up into the small hours to discuss the details of the cases with which they were confronted. In addition to Fry, Gillies also gained the services of Gilbert Chubb, who had been resident house surgeon to the Hospital for Diseases of the Throat before joining the RAMC in 1914. Gillies' successor as Valadier's supervisor at Wimereux, Captain Frederick Cleminson, an ENT surgeon trained at the Middlesex Hospital, was also later appointed to the Sidcup staff, as were George Lawson Whale and Captain L.A. King who had also been at Aldershot. Lawson Whale had been Chief Assistant in the Ear department of St Bartholomew's Hospital, had worked at the Val-de-Grâce Hospital in Paris, and translated Martinier and Lemerle's textbook on face and jaw injuries into English.[44] In civilian life, King was a dentist from Northampton. Both he and Lawson Whale had contributed articles to journals with Valadier. Gillies was also lucky to have Henry Johnston posted to Sidcup. A genial Irishman, Johnston had been a surgeon in Newcastle before the war and had developed an interest in radiology which resulted in his having designed and built his own equipment. At Sidcup, Johnston developed the infant radiology service. X-rays were used for the localisation of bullet and shell fragments and clearly outlined bony damage in the face, which allowed for analysis of fracture and bone graft fixation.

In pursuit of their ideal to create the biggest and best jaw hospital in the world, Gillies and Arbuthnot Lane organised the transfer of Dominion units which had been established elsewhere. Carl Waldron and Fulton Risdon from Toronto arrived with the Canadian contingent. Waldron had tried to gain a commission in the Canadian Army Medical Corps but, because there were some 400 doctors ahead of him in the queue, had failed to do so. Consequently, he had paid his own passage to England with a letter of recommendation from the respected Canadian physician Sir William Osler. Commissioned in London in December 1915, Waldron was delegated to organise a Canadian facial unit at Folkestone, and it was this unit that transferred to Sidcup.[45] Risdon had qualified as a dentist in 1907, and obtained his medical degree seven years later. As a result of his dental background, he specialised in jaw work and

43 Gillies and Millard, *Principles and Art*, p.23.

44 P. Martinier and G. Lemerle, *Injuries of the Face and Jaw and their Repair; and the Treatment of Fractured Jaws*, trans. by G. Lawson Whale (London: Baillière, Tindall & Cox, 1917).

45 Norman Rowe, personal communication, 1986.

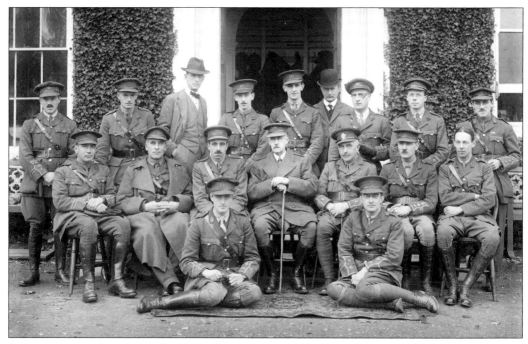

The British section at the Queen's Hospital, August 1917. (BAPRAS Archive)

contributed to the development of bone grafting. Gillies and Arbuthnot Lane trod a fine line by procuring Waldron and Risdon; only four miles away, in Orpington, the huge Canadian Ontario hospital had its own jaw unit.

The senior surgeon appointed to the Australian section at Sidcup was Henry Simpson Newland. Unlike Gillies, Newland had some acute surgical experience. He had previously been the senior surgeon at the 3rd Australian CCS, based near Poperinghe, and held the rank of colonel. The artist Daryl Lindsay had met him in France, as he later recalled:

> He was pointed out to me with great pride by one of his theatre orderlies, an old friend of mine, now a very prominent business man in Melbourne. I learned from the orderly that the unit had just come back from the front, and that during the Bullecourt stunt the Colonel had taken all the major cases and operations for the first two days with practically no sleep at all. My memory of him then was of a spare, wiry-looking man with a serious face and lips drawn close together in concentration as he passed us on the duckboards.

At Sidcup, Newland was a hard but learned taskmaster, who underneath his austere exterior was rather shy: "the hospital staff was rather in awe of the Colonel. He was a disciplinarian and kept everybody on their toes. He never spared himself and expected everybody to keep up with him … I realized that behind the blue-grey eyes was a man of wide knowledge and scholarship with a great understanding of humanity."[46] Newland was senior to Gillies by virtue of both age and rank, not to mention frontline experience. However, within the hospital amity prevailed, and Newland proved quite content for Gillies to continue as Chief Medical Officer.

---

46   D. Lindsay, 'Five men', *Medical Journal of Australia*, 18 January 1958, p.62.

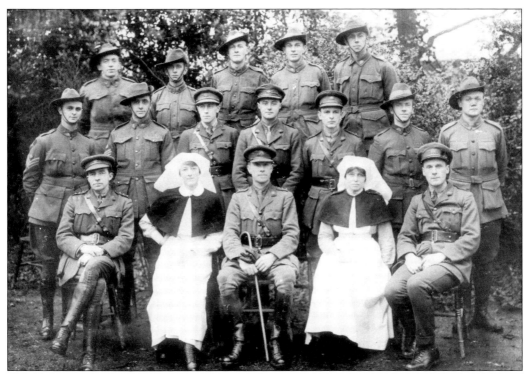

Henry Newland and the Australian team at Sidcup. (RACS Archive, Melbourne)

The New Zealand section was led by Henry Percy Pickerill. Originally a dentist, Pickerill had taken his medical degree at Birmingham University and emigrated to Dunedin. He had developed several techniques for lip reconstruction. Pickerill was less than pleased to be told that his department at the 2nd New Zealand Hospital at Walton-on-Thames was to be transferred to Sidcup, and dug in his heels until Queen Mary herself intervened. Despite a separate operating theatre being built for the New Zealanders, relations between them and their hosts continued to be strained throughout the war.

Alongside the surgeons drawn from within the British Empire were a number of surgeons from America, whose posting to Sidcup anticipated a likely flood of American soldiers once the United States entered the war. Among them were George Dorrance, Ferris Smith, and Vilray Blair from St Louis, Missouri. Blair, who had published the first edition of his textbook *Surgery of the Face and Jaws* in 1912, was present purely in an observational capacity, while the others are recorded in the notes as having operated at the hospital.

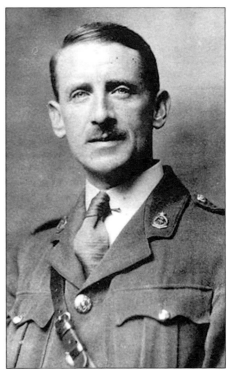

Henry Pickerill, who was the head of the New Zealand section. (Author's collection)

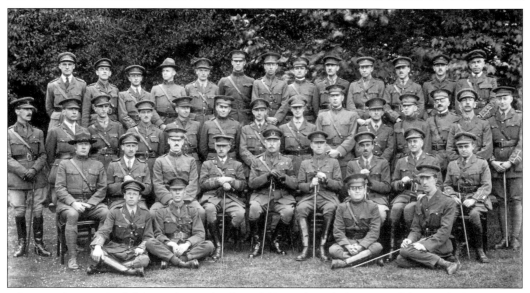

A group photograph of all the sections at the Queen's Hospital – including some of the attached American surgeons. (BAPRAS Archive)

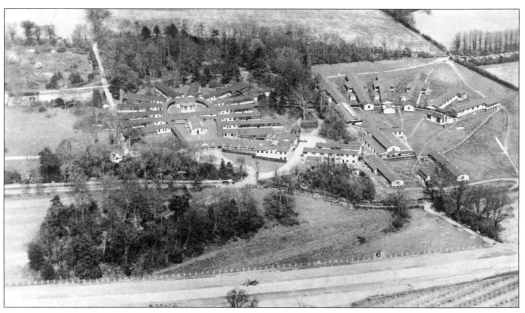

A postcard showing an aerial view of the Queen's Hospital, with the Lower Hospital on the right. (Author's collection)

Following the arrival of the Canadian, Australian and New Zealand sections, the number of beds in the new hospital was once again woefully inadequate in number. New surgeons demanded the establishment of new beds, so the original hospital was increased in size by the addition of the Lower Hospital. Built in concrete, the new construction brought the total number of beds close to 700.

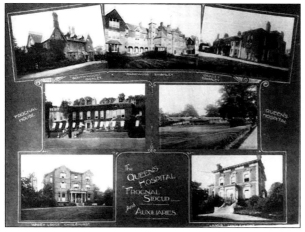

The convalescent hospitals attached to the Queen's Hospital. (Author's collection)

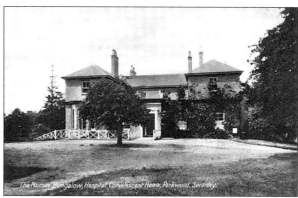

A postcard of Parkwood Convalescent Hospital. (Author's collection)

Known later by its inmates as 'The Jungle', even this addition was not enough to cope with the pressures of frequent admission and re-admission, so the surrounding area was scoured for suitable convalescent accommodation. The need for convalescent beds led to the requisitioning of a number of local private houses. As Gillies wrote:

> No plastic unit is any good unless it has an equal number of convalescent beds. We went in search of them. Then someone told us of Parkwood, a mental hospital up on Swanley Hill. Kelsey Fry and I drove off immediately, and on the front porch of a large, lovely home found two sweet old ladies rocking in the sun. It turned out they were graduate nurses of Bart's Hospital, and as they bewailed loudly that they had no patients, we promised them 100 on the morrow ... By merely picking up a phone we could send one patient off for convalescence and call another back for further surgery.[47]

Gillies' plan was approved after a further visit by the hospital's General Committee. A whole series of hospitals and private houses, from Chislehurst to Swanley, were pressed into service. By the final year of the war, over a thousand beds were available.

Eventually, nearly every soldier who had sustained a major facial injury at the front came through Sidcup. By November 1918, the delay between injury and admission was sometimes as

---

47 Gillies and Millard, *Principles and Art*, p.31.

little as a week, although the Queen's Hospital continued to act as a secondary referral centre for patients originally treated elsewhere. Meanwhile, the newspapers continued to seek funds for the hospital, and donations were reported in vivid detail. In June 1918, the *Daily Sketch* advertised the Frognal Fund under the headline: "Tax on Good Looks: One way of helping men who have lost theirs."

The corresponding article included a bordered section of text reporting that:

> On the recent anniversary of her birthday the Queen received from the Maharao of Kotah the offer of £6,600 to be devoted to such purposes connected with the war as her Majesty might decide. The Queen has accepted the generous gift, and has decided to devote it to the Queen's Hospital for Sailors and Soldiers suffering from facial and jaw injuries, at Frognal.[48]

Similar articles continued to appear until 1925, ensuring that the hospital remained in the public consciousness even after the fighting had stopped. Two years and four months had elapsed between Gillies' initial posting to France and the opening of the first hospital dedicated to the management of facial injury. Slowly but surely a new specialism, plastic surgery, had established itself as an important branch of surgery.

Conclusion

The French army's response to the increasing number of facial casualties that appeared from the end of 1914 was to establish a number of separate units. This provision diminished the likelihood of cooperation between surgeons at different units, whose work remained based on inadequate texts. The arrival of Harold Gillies in France and his exposure to the problem, coupled with his persistence and anticipation of the likely increase in facial casualties amongst British soldiers, led to an acceptance by the military hierarchy of the advantages to be gained from the establishment of a single-site, specialist unit. Public support for Gillies' vision was drummed up by a media campaign, assisted by the personal contacts of the prime movers with their wealthy friends. Gillies' success in developing a unit at Aldershot, and then the Queen's Hospital at Sidcup, illustrates that his views on patient management, though on occasion unorthodox, were accepted and indeed embraced by the army. Nonetheless, it is important to remember that the funding of the hospital was entirely unofficial. By concentrating interested specialists in one place, Gillies ensured that the isolation of surgeons in small dispersed units did not happen in Britain as it had done in France. He created the setting for a revolution in the management of facial injury in the areas of technique, record-keeping and rehabilitation.

---

48 *Daily Sketch*, June 1918.

3

"A New Art":
The Innovative Treatment of Facial Injuries

This chapter examines the causes and patterns of facial injury during the First World War, including wounds to the jaws, noses, lips, cheeks, eyes, and the area surrounding the eyes. It analyses the effects of developments in wartime surgery upon injuries and their treatment, and provides a number of case studies from the Sidcup records to demonstrate how industrial warfare at sea, in the air, and on land stimulated developments in burns surgery. Drawing upon the patients' written records, photographs and other notes generated by the surgical team at Sidcup, this chapter explores how lessons were learned from failed surgery, how experimental surgery was performed, and how surgical challenges were overcome in what Harold Gillies described as the 'New Art' of plastic surgery.

Many records of work at Aldershot and the Queen's Hospital have been lost or destroyed, so it is impossible to determine the exact number of men who passed through the facial surgery service in the Great War. Some of the extant statistics deal with men, some with numbers of operations, and some reports include both. Table 3.1 presents known patient information, drawing on two reports of work compiled in England, the almost complete case records of the New Zealand and Australian sections, and the Admissions book for the Canadian section which, unlike the records themselves, has survived.[1] As the sections did not treat men from their own countries exclusively, a degree of overlap and duplication in the files must be acknowledged. The exact number of patients treated by Gillies and his team cannot be ascertained, but it can be estimated that around 5,000 men received treatment for facial injuries at Aldershot and Sidcup between 1916 and 1925.

A large proportion of facial injury patients had relatively straightforward injuries. Many cases were dealt with by units elsewhere, such as at the jaw injury department in Leeds or Sir Frank Colyer's unit at Croydon. Sidcup became the destination for the most severe and complex injuries, and for those which had proven impossible to treat successfully elsewhere. The system of collaboration allowed the surgeons of the Queen's Hospital to quickly learn from their mistakes and to refine their techniques. Experience led to the development both of new techniques and of new principles to guide the specialty. Gillies published two textbooks which provide a permanent record of the work undertaken by the team at Sidcup. Many of the cases in this chapter featured in Gillies' first post-war text, *Plastic Surgery of the Face*.[2] Others

---

1 In 2016, Paul Ferguson (Royal British Columbia Museum, Victoria) discovered that summary notes still existed in service files held at the Library and Archives Canada (RG 150, Accession 1992-93/166). Many of these files have now been digitised.

2 H.D. Gillies, *Plastic Surgery of the Face: Based on Selected Cases of War Injuries of the Face Including Burns* (London: Hodder & Stoughton, 1920).

Table 3.1 Patients Treated for Facial Injuries at Aldershot and Sidcup

Section	Officers	Other Ranks	Notes
British	546	4,380	2,327 surviving files or firm attributions. Section notes include 65 Australian patients, 55 Canadians, 12 South Africans, 1 American, 1 Chinese, 1 Indian, 1 Japanese, 1 Nigerian, 1 Russian and 1 Serb
Australian	19	601	345 files at RACS
Canadian	30	475	388 Other Ranks from Admissions book
New Zealand	24	184	294 files recorded; 148 of British men
UK readmissions	243	1,517	

derive from Henry Percy Pickerill's Master of Science thesis, later published as *Facial Surgery*.[3] Although some of the procedures which Gillies and his colleagues developed have been side-lined to some extent by modern surgeons, the scope of their work demonstrates why the servicemen who they treated can be considered the pioneer patients of modern facial surgery. Given the conditions of the time, the results were often impressive. All the same, it should be remembered that while the work aimed to provide a good cosmetic appearance, it also sought to achieve an acceptable functional result.

Many of the surgeons who went to the Queen's Hospital to learn and work were credited by Gillies with the invention, or refinement, of different surgical techniques. However, their involvement was often limited to the short period that the Queen's Hospital was open, and most, apart from the Americans and Canadians, returned to their original specialties following the Armistice.

Gillies' vision, like that of Sir William Arbuthnot Lane, was to develop a service that would make surgical advances. As the disparate group of ENT surgeons, oral surgeons, and dentists settled in to their new hospital, that vision was realised. The enormous throughput and the diversity of staff engendered constant dialogue and disagreement among the medical practitioners. As Gillies put it:

> Clinics were held for open discussion of immediate problems and for presentation of difficult cases. Out of many a heated meeting floated a symphony of accents, the Canadian North Irish brogue, the New Zealand Fiji twang, the Australian cockney, a Midwestern Drawl, a Philadelphia bark and a New York Oxford accent. It made it more difficult to hide a bad case than to get a good one, and consequently our standards rose.[4]

Alongside illustrating the cosmopolitan nature of the surgical team, Gillies' phraseology underpins the truism that some of the best learning experiences arise from mistakes. George Dorrance echoed Gillies' view, and noted that the division into sections "stimulated a healthy rivalry which

---

3   H.P. Pickerill, 'Facial Surgery' (unpublished Masters Dissertation, University of Birmingham, 1923); *Facial Surgery* (Edinburgh: E. & S. Livingstone, 1924).

4   H.D. Gillies and R. Millard, *The Principles and Art of Plastic Surgery* (London: Butterworth & Co., 1957), p.31.

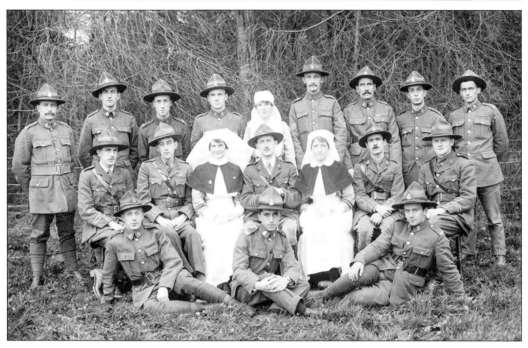

The New Zealand section. Seated left to right: Captain Turner, Tommy Rhind, Sister McBeth, Henry Percy Pickerill, Sister Finlayson, Captain Marshall, Captain Seed. (Courtesy of Gillian Martin)

assisted materially in the excellent results obtained."[5] There were peaks and troughs of activity, but collaboration and discussion were sustained throughout. These concepts were not widely valued at this time, as the insular system adopted by the French demonstrated. A painting of the main Plastic Theatre at Sidcup shows two operations going on at the same time (See Colour Section, p.v). Today, such a practice would be frowned upon because of the risk of cross-contamination, but the rigorous antiseptic and aseptic management of patients meant that the risks were outweighed by the benefits of having access to an immediate second opinion.

Gillies was the only surgeon to make a definitive record of surgical life and times at Sidcup. The views of a young New Zealand surgeon, Tommy Rhind, who had served on the front before moving to Sidcup, have been shared by his daughter. Gillies considered his patients as equals, and treated them in a jocular fashion. Rhind did not agree with Gillies' approach to the wounded. Rhind's daughter recorded that her father "felt that what he considered the overuse of humour, was not always appropriate and though appreciated by some, many other staff and patients were at a loss to find anything amusing or encouraging about their predicament. Some comments were considered to be inappropriate and unhelpful."[6] Rhind also considered that Gillies' major achievements were administrative rather than surgical, and recalled that he did not like "getting his hands dirty," an observation completely at odds with the case records, and a view which may have been shaped by the initial reluctance of the New Zealand section to move to Sidcup and their work in a separate operating theatre.

---

5   G.M. Dorrance, 'Observations on the work at Queen's Hospital in England', *The Dental Summary*, 39 (1919), pp.865-867.
6   Gillian Martin, personal communication, July 2007.

Sites of Injury

Wounds caused by the penetration of bullets and shell fragments posed differing problems according to the site of injury and what caused it. Bullet wounds were frequently clean, although a bullet which struck bone caused fractures or fragmentation of the jaw or cheek. A wound through the orbit regularly damaged the eye itself. If infection or damage was not immediately dealt with by removal of the eye, patients were susceptible to blindness as a result of a curious phenomenon, known as sympathetic ophthalmia, in which the unaffected eye developed an inflammation (uveitis). Major tissue loss was relatively uncommon, and bony injuries were dealt with largely through stabilisation of the fracture. Shell wounds were, in many cases, more difficult to deal with. The whirling splinters from a shell burst were accompanied by razor-edged pieces of flint on the Somme, or by gobbets of Flanders mud thrown up by the explosion (See Colour Section, p.vi). The irregular and often large fragments caused huge tearing injuries and the loss of both hard and soft tissue.

The fields of Flanders were very fertile, largely because for centuries they had been heavily manured by farmers. As a result, infection was almost inevitable. Antiseptic measures were essential, as persistent infection resulted in the erosion of vital structures and torrential haemorrhages were a frequent occurrence when a major blood vessel in the face or neck became eroded. In addition, infections delayed or prevented the healing process, and often resulted in ugly scars. Although the success of surgery despite the complete absence of antibiotics

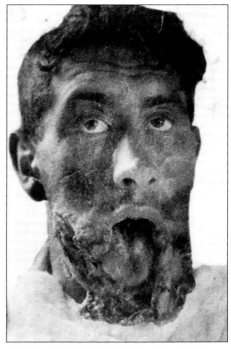

Lieutenant F.G. Adams, Hampshire Regiment. Photograph in case file taken in France; his tongue has become stuck to the raw tissue. (RCS)

may seem surprising, as the war progressed it became more and more apparent to surgeons that primary cleansing had to be accompanied by rapid triage and transfer of patients. As a result of rapid transfer, secondary complications diminished and the survival rates of wounded men improved.[7] Nevertheless, it also soon became apparent that primary closure of large wounds was a mistake. "Pieces," wrote Gillies, "were missing from the puzzle."[8] Attempts to stretch normal tissue beyond its capacity resulted in serious distortions which were exacerbated as the patients' healing scars began to contract.

Contracture was also a major issue for burns patients. As well as the aesthetic impact of a full facial burn, as the skin tightened men became unable to open their mouths or close their eyes. Both caused secretion issues which added to the patients' problems. Men who could not close their mouths suffered as a result of the mild acidity of their own saliva, which dribbled persistently across the intact tissue and led to soreness and ulceration of the intact skin. The drawing-down of the lower lids with turning outward of the normal mucous surface (ectropion) led the patient's eyes to water

---

7   T. Scotland and S. Heys, (eds.), *War Surgery 1914-18* (Solihull: Helion & Company, 2012).
8   Gillies and Millard, *Principles and Art*, p.13.

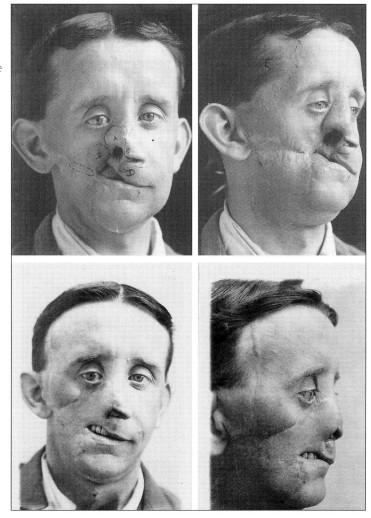

Private Hartley, on admission to Sidcup. The primary closure of the wound, despite tissue loss, has resulted in considerable distortion of the cheek and mouth. (RCS)

uncontrollably. However, as the tears no longer lubricated the eye surface, the cornea became dry and ulcerated.

There was longstanding experience of surgery to the nose, although its limitations were significant due to infection and the failure of surgeons to understand issues of scar healing and the need to line flaps. The management of other facial injuries was almost non-existent. Earlier surgeons left contracted scars well alone, and they had no experience whatsoever of facial burns. Gillies wrote that the work was "confused in its principles, and though overflowing with diagrams and mathematical formulae, was rendered unconvincing by lack of systematical [sic] photographic recording."[9] The remedy required the concentration of surgeons and patients, which did not occur anywhere until Gillies established his unit at Aldershot in 1916. There was no such concentration anywhere else during the whole of the First World War, the primary reason why the work done at Aldershot and Sidcup formed the basis for subsequent surgical developments.

---

9   Gillies and Millard, *Principles and Art*, p.10.

Jaws

Injuries to the lower jaw (mandible) were common, and their management was more complicated if combined with fragmentation and loss of bone. It was difficult to repair and restore function in these cases. A simple fracture could be stabilised with a splint, but if a portion of the jaw was missing any attempt to realign the remainder only succeeded for as long as the supporting splint remained in place. Cartilage and bone grafts restored a relatively normal jaw architecture, but the splint had to be retained until the graft had united. Immobilisation of the lower jaw created major feeding problems, which were sometimes made worse by concurrent injury to the jaw joint (temporomandibular joint). In these cases, the patient was left unable to open his mouth at all if the jaw joint became stuck. In occasional cases, this process occurred even without injury, as a consequence of prolonged immobilisation. Therefore, the provision of a liquid diet during the initial stages, and attempts to re-open the oral aperture through the use of an expanding splint were both necessary components of the surgical process. Yet there were further complications which surgeons had to take into account. First, in cases where injury to the hard palate had occurred there was a possibility that liquid feed could pass up into the nose. Second, there was the likelihood of dental loss. Many of the men had poor dentition; some had lost all their teeth before their injury occurred, and others lost them in the process of being

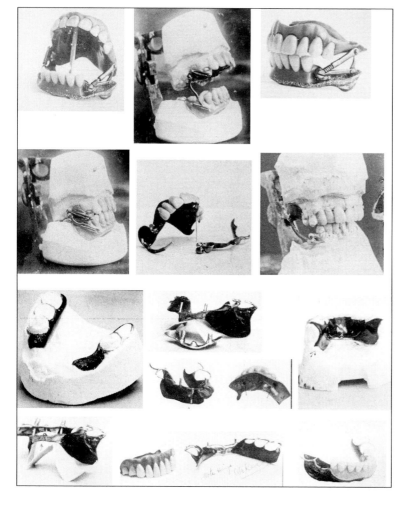

Dental splints made and photographed by the technician Archie Lane. (Antony Wallace Archive (AWA) and the BAPRAS Archive)

injured. Issues with dentition compounded the difficulty of splinting, as traditional methods relied upon cap splints applied over the existing teeth which were then aligned and screwed together with the jaws correctly opposed. Without teeth, external splints were required. A number of splints were devised at Sidcup, and were probably influenced by German textbooks on orthodontics.

Unlike splinting, bone and cartilage grafts were an unknown quantity. Many grafts failed, either through simple non-union or because the graft ends were resorbed. Great care had to be taken not to disturb the alignment of the broken segment, and the tube diet was increasingly complicated if there was any concomitant damage to the upper jaw and palate. In the acute stage of management great care had to be taken to avoid the spread of infection, which appeared to be worse among patients whose fractures were fixed with wire. Almost every jaw wound was effectively open and, as the normal mouth harbours a multitude of bacteria, almost every wound became infected at some stage.

The results of early bone grafts were uniformly poor. Bone grafts in the jaw only became routinely successful after proper splinting had developed. Gillies acknowledged his debt to Gilbert Chubb for advances in this field. Splints became ever more complex, and ensured that the fractures were maintained in a good position both to the broken bone and to the other jaw. As a consequence, malalignment of the bite became less of an issue. Refinement, using a hole-and-peg technique and mortice and tenon fashioning as pioneered by Fred Albee at Neuilly, led to better stability. In addition, Pickerill developed the living bone screw in which, rather than use a simple peg, he cut threads with screw dies and taps so that tibial grafts held more firmly. Despite these developments there were still failures. However, not all failures could be ascribed to deficiencies in the surgical process. One set of notes records the failure of a graft because the patient was allowed to remove his splint in order to have Christmas dinner.

The cases of Ashworth, Gardiner and Kensington exemplify the complexities which surrounded the jaw wounds treated at Sidcup. Walter Ashworth, 18th West Yorkshire Regiment (Bradford Pals) worked for a leading tailor in Bradford before the war. His regiment formed part of the second wave of the attack on Serre on the first day of the Battle of the Somme, 1 July 1916. The regiment had not even advanced across the frontline trenches before it came under fire. Ashworth was wounded and evacuated to Aldershot, where he arrived on 5 July. Later, he was transferred to Sidcup to complete his treatment. Tonks drew two pastels of Ashworth (See Colour Section, p.vi). The first showed him awaiting the orderly washout round, kidney dish below his chin, when the wound was irrigated with sterile water or Dakin's solution (hypochlorite). The second pastel showed Ashworth after the soft tissue had been repaired. Union of the jaw was finally achieved after splinting and two operations. However, at the time of discharge his repair was less than perfect, and Ashworth faced significant problems when he attempted to return to his old job.

Private Gardiner, a New Zealander of the 7th Canterbury Infantry Regiment, and 2nd Lieutenant Kensington of the 1st Battalion, Rifle Brigade, were also wounded on 1 July 1916. In Gardiner's case, there was significant loss of bone in the jaw. Gillies initially used a 2.5-inch-long rib graft, fixed at one end with a bony peg and at the other as a crude mortice and tenon joint (See Colour Section, p.vii). The structure immediately looked unsound and failed shortly after the procedure. Kensington's wound was badly infected, and recurrent severe bleeding forced Gillies to tie off the external carotid artery in his neck. An initial attempt to oppose the broken ends of Kensington's jaw failed, as did an attempted rib graft. Ultimately, it was a suggestion made by Albee that worked; a bone graft from the ilium in the pelvis, shaped into a peg and slotted into a drilled hole in the anterior fragment. Kensington's final operation took place almost two years after his injury, and he was eventually discharged to duty in October 1918.

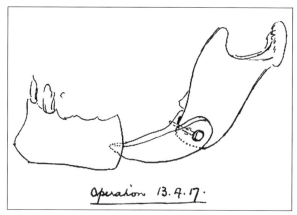

Private Gardiner, 7th Canterbury Infantry Regiment. Diagram by Tonks of the (unstable) bone graft to the jaw. (RCS)

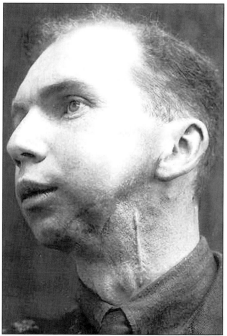

2nd Lieutenant Kensington. Final appearance. There is a large neck scar and the contour of the jaw is distorted because of tissue loss from earlier infection. (RCS)

Private Williams of the 3rd Nigerians is the only African soldier for whom notes survive. Williams' records exist in the form of a single annotated card, a pastel by Tonks in the Slade School collection, and a photograph in one of the dental technician Archie Lane's albums which is absent from the case file (See Colour Section, p.vii). Wounded on 7 September 1917, Williams was transferred to Sidcup from the 1st London General on 4 December of that year. In true army tradition, he was nicknamed 'Snowball'. The whole of his lower lip, jaw, and the floor of his mouth had been lost, and he had a persistent infection in the mouth. Williams suffered from three attacks of pneumonia in nine months and, owing to his poor general state of health, he was fitted with a dental appliance. The photograph in Lane's album attests to the cosmetic success of the splint. Williams' notes end: "To return later for operation," but there is no indication that he did. Gillies referred to Williams' case in *The Principles and Art of Plastic Surgery*. "'Snowball' … was being sent home to Nigeria on convalescent leave. Fear widened the whites of his eyes and he begged first to have his deformity repaired, else his chief and tribe were certain to kill him on arrival."[10] Whether in the end he did return to Africa is not known.

---

10 Gillies and Millard, *Principles and Art*, p.320.

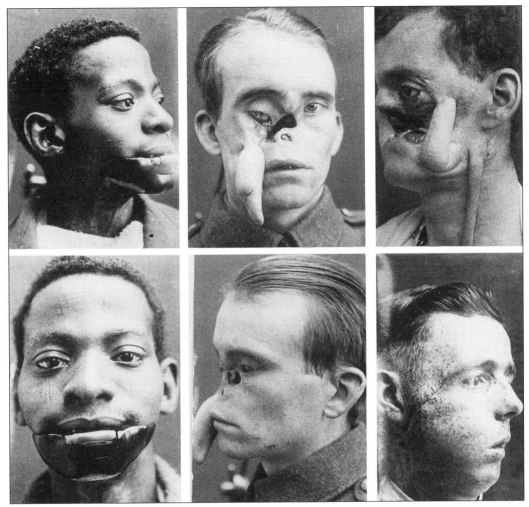

A page from Lane's album. Top and bottom left: Private Williams, 3rd Nigerian Regiment, with the dental appliance in place. (RCS and AWA, and the BAPRAS Archive)

Noses

Although evidence suggests that the reconstruction of the nose had been the subject of successful procedures since antiquity, the existing texts on rhinoplasty at the outbreak of the First World War were completely inadequate given the severity and variety of injuries which required treatment. The dreadful appearance of men who had lost their noses is evident from the existing photographs of the men and in the 23 plaster casts which survive in Melbourne (See Colour Section, p.vii). Gillies adopted a pattern book approach to the task of replacing the appendages and was proud of his results. He and his colleagues showed their patients an album of different shaped noses and invited them to choose one. Some, like Joseph Pickard from Alnwick, cared little about the process.

Pickard recorded his war experience for the IWM, in which he described what happened after he had been sent to Sidcup to have his nose restored:

Joseph Pickard, 5th Northumberland Fusiliers. Admission photographs, 26 July 1919; final appearance, 6 May 1921. (RCS)

I travelled down there, and was there for two years altogether … First of all, they take photographs – I've got them as well – and I had to go to a small hut, and was smothered with plaster of Paris … they take a mask, and when that comes out, that shows every little blemish. And gradually they build up, and I had various operations like a rib graft … the first lot went wrong. It curved – must have been improperly cured, you see! And [Tommy] Kilner said 'What are we doing? It shouldn't go like that.' And I said 'Well, you put it in!' … [Kilner] says 'Come up the office', so I went up the office, he takes the mask from off the wall … and he says 'Now, what do you want? A Wellington nose or a Roman nose?' and I says 'I don't care what it is as long as I get one!'[11]

---

11 IWM: 8946, Joseph Pickard (IWM interview).

Others were less laid back than Pickard. Bob Seymour was injured at the start of the Somme offensive and arrived at Aldershot where he was shown the album of different shaped noses by Gillies. Seymour chose a Roman profile, and Gillies used a local flap which he termed the Bishop's Mitre to affect the repair. Local repair was speedy, and therefore the procedure of choice when there was a rush of new casualties such as in July 1916. Despite the relatively swift procedure, Seymour was pleased enough with Gillies' results that he became his secretary and remained so for over 30 years.

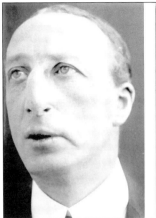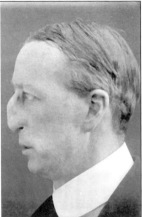

Private Seymour, 12th York & Lancaster Regiment. Initial photograph and final appearance. (RCS)

Seymour was one of the first 'nose jobs'. The large numbers of casualties which continued to arrive led Gillies and his colleagues to a better understanding what worked and what did not. Soft tissue reconstruction did not produce a satisfactory result without support. If the bridge of the nose and its cartilaginous support were damaged, then any repair simply collapsed. The same thing happened if the nasal cartilage was destroyed by infection. Lieutenant Frederick Stacey of the Royal Naval Division was one patient who suffered from the latter complication. Stacey was wounded on 8 April 1918 and arrived at Sidcup four days later. Photographs of the primary repair show a very reasonable appearance. However, within days the nose became infected and a large hole appeared in the side of it.

Gillies was always concerned when he perceived that the blood supply along a proposed flap was precarious. In Stacey's case, Gillies planned the transposition flap with great care. He used a plaster cast to make a paper template, and deliberately altered the origin of the flap so that it included the large artery (the temporal artery) within it. Once the nasal repair was complete, he used part of the residual flap to fill in a defect in Stacey's cheek. In the preparations for his 1957 book, Gillies noted that he thought the Stacey procedure was the first recorded use of an arterial flap. He was mistaken, however, as Theodore Dunham had used the technique some 20 years earlier.[12]

Other examples serve to illustrate the variety of nasal injuries which arrived in front of Gillies and his team. For some, such as William Spreckley who had lost his nose entirely, the procedures were relatively straightforward. Gillies decided to turn a forehead flap and, following an example in Charles Nélaton and Louis Ombrédanne's textbook, implanted a shaped piece of cartilage to create both the nasal bridge and the alae. It was a successful procedure, unlike many of those which relied on heterografts to hold the nasal contour. One patient, whilst treated as a POW in Germany, had a piece of chicken bone inserted. No less bizarre was the case of Sergeant White, who received a graft of a whole toe to fill the gap, skin, bone and all. Replacement of the toe with a forehead flap, which featured a proper cartilage graft, produced a much-improved result for White.

---

12 T. Dunham, 'Method for obtaining a skin-flap from the scalp and a permanent buried vascular pedicle for covering defects of the face', *Annals of Surgery*, 17:6 (1893), pp.677-679.

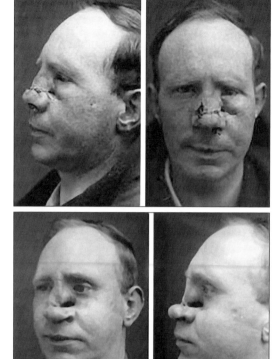

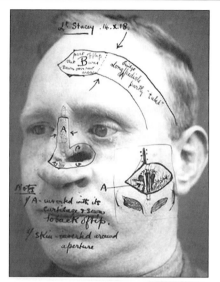

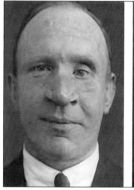

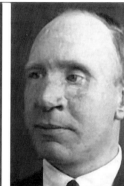

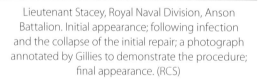

Lieutenant Stacey, Royal Naval Division, Anson Battalion. Initial appearance; following infection and the collapse of the initial repair; a photograph annotated by Gillies to demonstrate the procedure; final appearance. (RCS)

The injury to Leonard Tringham of the 12th Middlesex Regiment was one of the more substantial to be dealt with at the Queen's Hospital (See Colour Section, p.viii). Tringham arrived at Sidcup after failed surgery in Birmingham. He had lost his right eye, cheek, and most of his nose on 8 August 1917. The attempted rotation flap had two problems: first, it was not supported by a cartilage bridge, and had therefore collapsed inwards; and second, it had been taken from within the hairline on Tringham's forehead. The operation site had been carefully shaved, so once moved the hair grew back luxuriantly on the nasal tip. Gillies also noted that it was important, if possible, to restore the lining of the nose, since this had not been carried out in Birmingham. In his 1920 text, Gillies made several comments on the subject.[13] At Sidcup, the surgeons restarted the process by restoring the failed flap to its original position. Pickerill then brought up a flap with a tubed base from the chest wall, lined with a second flap, and took a portion of rib to create the new bridge. After several adjustments, over the course of 21 operations between November 1918 and May 1923, the appearance was vastly improved.

---

13   Gillies, *Plastic Surgery*, p.228.

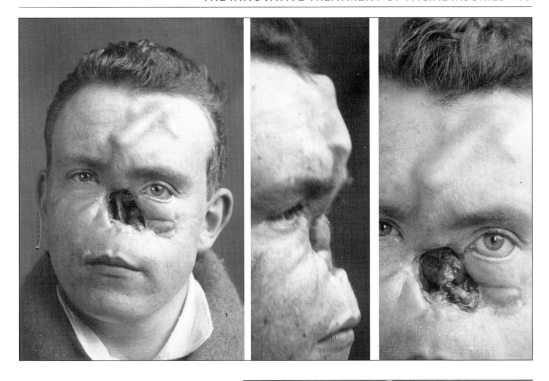

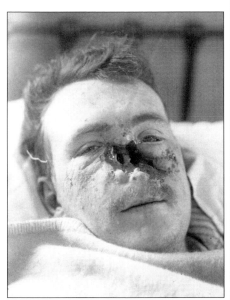

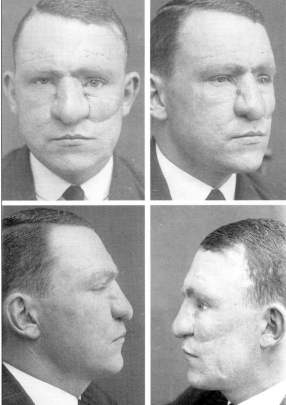

William Spreckley. Initial appearance; a photograph showing the cartilage graft placed under the forehead flap; final appearance. (RCS)

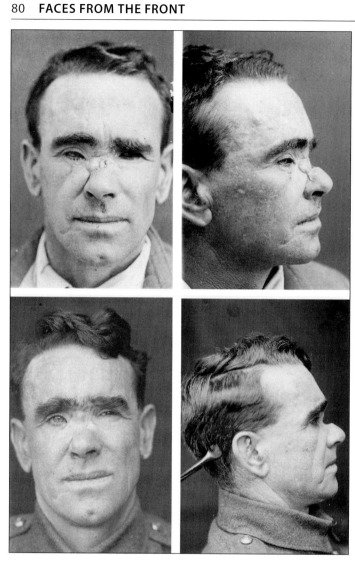

Sergeant John White, New Zealand Field Artillery. Initial appearance (note the bump on the right side of the nose, which is the grafted toe); final appearance. (RCS)

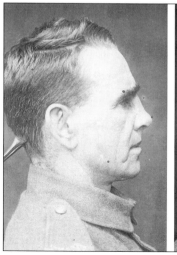
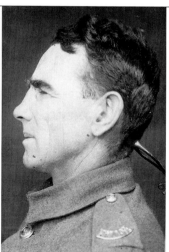
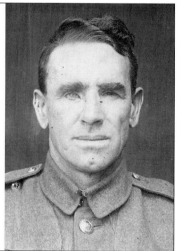

William Thomas, who had originally enlisted in the Royal Engineers but transferred to the 1st Cheshire Regiment, presented with a devastating nasal injury. Thomas' wound, received on 23 October 1918, left him with nothing in the centre of his face at all. The watercolour created by Daryl Lindsay graphically illustrates his appearance, and demonstrates that Thomas required repair and reconstruction of the cheek and upper lip in addition to that of his nose (See Colour Section, p.viii). Gillies and his colleagues agonised over how to support a new nose when so much had been lost, and settled on the use of a prosthesis which could act as a former, but made in three pieces so that it could be removed through the mouth. With a palatal prosthesis and dentures, the end appearance was far from normal but an undoubted improvement upon the gaping hole with which Thomas had started. It had taken 19 operations over almost six years.

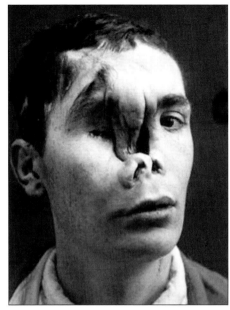

Private Len Tringham. Photograph showing the failed forehead flap with a hairy tip. (RCS)

The nasal injuries treated by Gillies and his team were not only caused by enemy action. Occasionally, a nose was lost to some form of friendly fire. Horace Sewell, of the Irish Horse, received one such unfortunate injury in 1914 when his nose was stove in by a horse's kick. His original deformity was not that severe, but was enough to prompt trouble during his convalescence at Walton-on-the-Naze, Essex. The matron there was requested by local residents to keep the inmates inside as it "gave them the shivers to see us out walking."[14] Sewell developed cutaneous tuberculosis (lupus vulgaris) and his deformity was considerably worse by the time the infection had been eradicated by cautery. Admitted to Sidcup in late 1919, he contracted diphtheria and did not have his first operation until May 1920. Nevertheless, the end result was excellent and Sewell was very pleased.

In 1963, he recalled in a letter to Gillies' biographer the discussion he had had with Gillies over the type of nose which would look best:

> He made various sketches of me, full face and in profile, with different shaped noses. 'I'm not fussy, Sir', I told him, when he asked me to choose. He decided that I should have a Roman nose, as my face was rather round. I underwent well over twenty operations, covering four and a half years. I have never regretted it. We who are left today have been able to go about all this time and not feel any embarrassment. As far as I am concerned, my nose is as good today as when he grafted it on.[15]

---

14 Horace Sewell, letter to Pound, 17 March 1963. Quoted in R. Pound, *Gillies: Surgeon Extraordinary* (London: Michael Joseph, 1964), p.52.

15 Pound, *Gillies*, p.58. The case notes record Bedford Russell as the surgeon who performed the initial procedure.

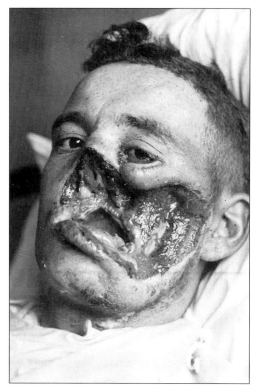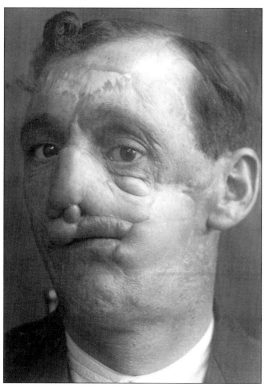

Private William Thomas, 1st Cheshire Regiment. Photograph on the day of admission, 6 November 1918; final appearance, 16 June 1924. Opposite: Intermediate stage, 16 October 1920; prosthesis former inserted, 4 May 1921; double pedicle to create nose, 20 September 1922. (RCS)

Although his post-war text indicated the importance he attached to the acknowledgement of surgical failures, Gillies was equally happy to publicise some of his successes. Reginald Pound recorded that Gillies was so proud of the nose job he performed on Rifleman Maggs, wounded on 10 August 1918 near Arras, that he took his patient to a meeting of the British Medical Association. "At the end of the meeting," Pound wrote, Maggs:

> was called to an ante-room where Gillies was waiting with a group of medical colleagues. As Maggs entered, he was greeted by Gillies in a foreign tongue. Not understanding, Maggs blushed. 'Look, look!' Gillies called out to his fellow surgeons. He had proved that there was circulation in the nose and the surrounding tissue. Guardsman Maggs' nose has functioned satisfactorily ever since.[16]

As the photographs demonstrate, the cosmetic appearance of Maggs' nose was remarkably good.

Nasal work appears to have been Gillies' favourite both during and after the war. The only surviving page proofs for *Plastic Surgery of the Face*, relate to nasal surgery. They were also the subject of an anecdote recalled by Pound in his biography of Gillies. When the proofs began to

16 Pound, *Gillies*, p.57.

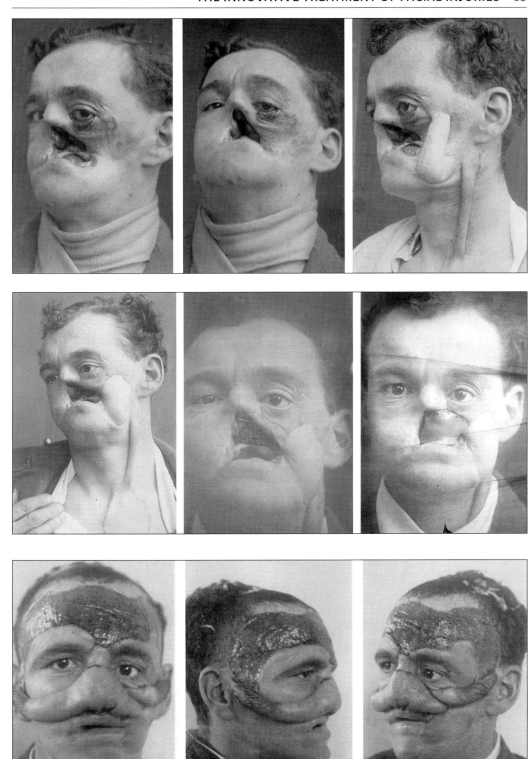

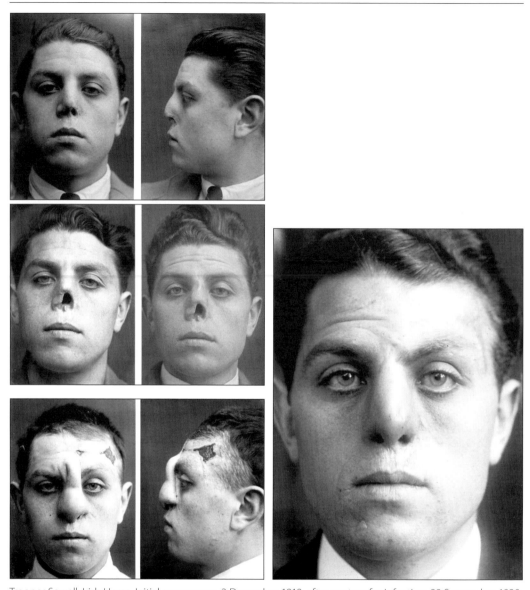

Trooper Sewell, Irish Horse. Initial appearance, 2 December 1919; after cautery for infection, 28 September 1920; forehead rhinoplasty, 10 March 1921; final appearance, 13 November 1923. (RCS)

return from the publishers, Gillies took a batch of them on a fishing weekend in Derbyshire. The daughter of the innkeeper at Gillies' lodging was, according to Pound, a "comely lass with a fearsome nose." Gillies left the page proofs dealing with nasal reconstruction on his dressing room table, in the assumption that the girl would see them when she dusted his bedroom. Sure enough, shortly after his return to London, Gillies received a request from the local doctor to accept the girl as a patient. In full recognition of his lifelong affinity for riverside pursuits, Gillies wrote, "the trout rose, was hooked and returned to the water with an undersized nose."[17]

---

17 Pound, *Gillies*, p.61.

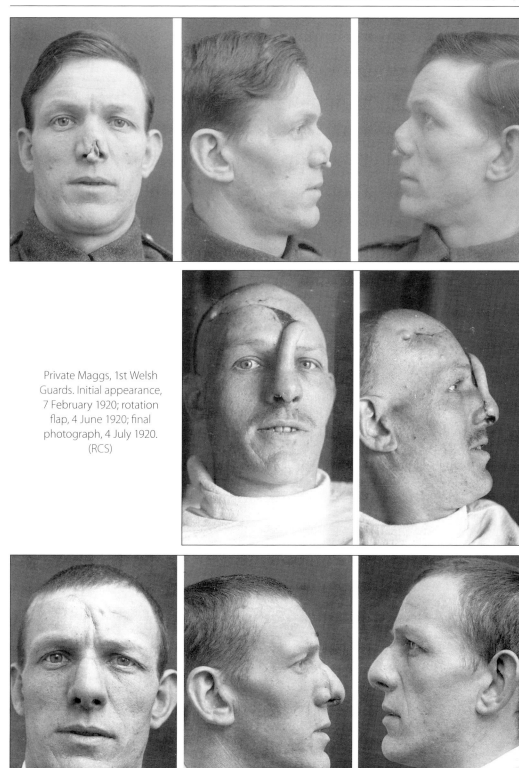

Private Maggs, 1st Welsh Guards. Initial appearance, 7 February 1920; rotation flap, 4 June 1920; final photograph, 4 July 1920. (RCS)

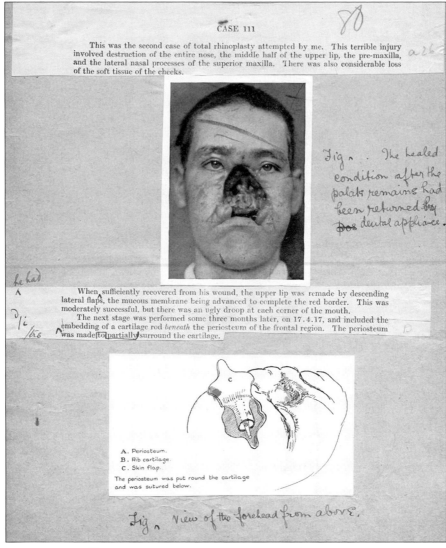

A 'paste-up' page proof for the chapter on noses in *Plastic Surgery of the Face*. The annotations are Gillies' suggestions for picture captions. (RCS)

Lips

Surgeons had attempted the closure of hare-lip prior to the war, but such defects were small in comparison to the tissue loss sustained from the tearing effect of a shell fragment. Furthermore, the defects presented as effectively clean and healed wounds, so surgeons were not confronted with large, irregular, infected wounds with major tissue loss. As with wounds in other parts of the face the temptation for front-line surgeons was to sew wounds shut, but the results were appalling. Closing an open wound reduced the likelihood of subsequent infection, but deformity resulted when tissue was stretched too far and scars contracted. In addition, as Pickerill noted, "the results were not satisfactory simply because the element of tension was introduced with consequent loss of function and therefore of appearance over a much larger area that the original lesion."[18] The lips themselves had contours which, if lost, produced an odd appearance, and if there was skin loss associated with loss of underlying muscle and bone, resulting in the inability of a man to close his lips, then saliva would dribble unchecked from the open mouth, causing significant irritation. Failure to recreate the fold between lip and the gums (the buccal and labial sulci) meant that the provision of dentures was almost impossible.[19] Consequently, the facial specialists had to devise ways of restoring structure, with at least an attempt to make a new lip, in order to provide function.

Private George Stone, of the Newfoundland Regiment, lost most of his upper lip on 1 July 1916. A watchman on Bell Island in civilian life, Stone was one of the more than 650 men from the regiment who became casualties within minutes of zero hour on the opening day of the Somme. He was admitted to Aldershot on 16 July, but was not operated upon until 9 October due to an infection. Henry Tonks' pastel of Stone clearly illustrates the loss of almost the whole of the upper lip, as well as a large scar across Stone's right cheek (See Colour Section, p.viii). Unfortunately, Stone scarred easily, and suffered recurrent adhesions of the reconstructed lip to the jaw. Advancement flaps replaced the lost tissue, but Stone remained a patient at Aldershot and Sidcup for two years. Finally, he tired of the repeated interventions and insisted upon being sent home. Gillies was unhappy, as he thought that more could have been done, but Stone was adamant. He left Sidcup for the final time at the end of August 1918.[20]

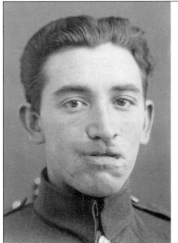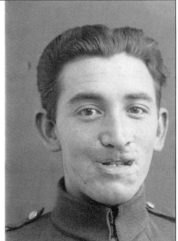

Private Stone. Final appearance. (RCS)

Frank Whipp did not even reach Sidcup until after the Armistice had come into effect. Whipp, from the Borders Regiment, had been taken prisoner on 23 March 1918 at the start of what turned out to be the final major German attack on the Western Front. He was initially treated in Germany to poor effect. The scar on his upper lip had contracted and left a permanent sneer. Gillies undid the repair, and moved the tissue around so that the normal contour was restored.

---

18 Pickerill, 'Facial Surgery', p.16.
19 H.P. Pickerill, 'Intraoral skin grafting: the establishment of the buccal sulcus', *Proceeding of the Royal Society of Medicine, Section of Odontology*, 12 (1919), pp.17-22 (p.18).
20 Stone emigrated from Bell Island to Montreal and subsequently moved to California, where he died at the age of 81. He remained unable to open his jaw fully and never ate solid food again. Information from Jim Connor, Memorial University, Newfoundland.

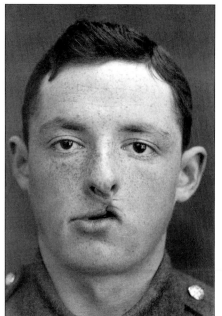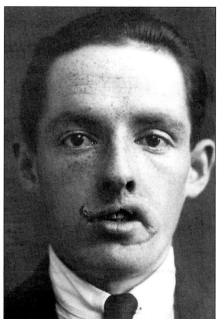

Private Frank Whipp. Initial appearance and final appearance. (RCS)

Pickerill was inventive in his approach to lip surgery. Percy Green, a telegraph messenger from Hackney who had lost both upper and lower lips to a shell shard, benefited from an ingenious idea thought out by the New Zealander. Len Tringham had provided a good example of what happened when hair appeared in the wrong place. Green, on the other hand, demonstrated that hair could be made to appear in the right place and hide the surgical scars all in one. Pickerill took a large forehead flap from within Green's hairline and brought it down to recreate the missing upper lip and provide a ready-made moustache. The lower lip was recreated with an adjacent, hairless flap. Six sequential watercolours made of Green highlight the surgical process and reveal that Green was a redhead (See Colour Section, p.ix).

Wounds of the Cheek

As with the jaws, noses and lips, men returned from the front or arrived at Sidcup from other hospitals with a variety of wounds to the cheek. Where the raw edges of the wounds had been pulled together and stitched, as was standard practice on the continent, the result had been distorted contours which got worse as the wound healed and contracted. Gillies realised that the treatment of such injuries required a complete revision. His first step was to restore normal tissue to normal position, usually by cutting through the healed scars and then interposing new tissue from elsewhere in the form of a flap or tubed flap. Even then an extensive injury was not necessarily amenable to complete restoration. A deep injury frequently damaged the underlying facial nerve, leaving the patient with a persistent facial palsy. Gillies experimented with muscle transpositions, but these were largely unsuccessful. A skin graft with a substantial section of underlying fat was also employed. Pickerill devised a double tube flap. For this, a first graft was taken from the hairless part of the neck and laid surface inward to create a new surface to the inside of the mouth. Then, a second flap of hair-bearing skin was used to create

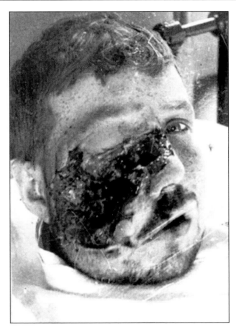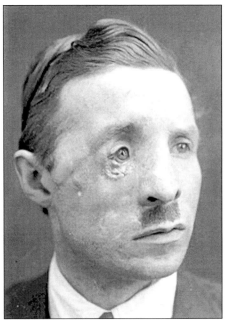

Private Harold Page, Norfolk Regiment. Operative diagram; final appearance, 1 July 1917. (RCS)

the outer side of the cheek.[21] While all of these methods worked reasonably well, a normal cheek contour proved almost impossible to achieve if the zygomatic arch had been lost.

The injury to Private Harold Page, Norfolk Regiment, was repaired by a series of flaps. Page arrived at Aldershot just five days after the regiment's disastrous attack on the first day of the Battle of the Somme. The initial entry in his case file states that Page had "a large lacerated wound involving practically the whole of the right face and right eye. Much necrosing tissue and blood clot about. Right eye has pus in anterior chamber. Right facial paralysis complete." As so often happened with injuries of his type, the eye had been penetrated and became infected. It was removed four days later. A year later, Page was still in hospital.[22]

The next case illustrates the drawbacks involved in attempting primary closure of a large wound with significant tissue loss. The solution Gillies proposed was to open the scars, allow the tissue to fall back into its normal place, and then begin reconstruction using tissue from elsewhere. Sidney Beldam, a sergeant in the Machine Gun Corps, was one of those treated with this method, and provided a detailed case study for Gillies' *Plastic Surgery to the Face*.[23] Beldam was wounded in November 1917, and transferred to Sidcup in March the following year when the wound across his cheek, nose, and upper lip had healed. The contracture in the scar had pulled the lip into a sneer. Gillies opened the scar, swung a new nose down from the forehead, and used a fat flap to try and recreate the cheek contour. The four pages devoted to Beldam's surgery illustrate the satisfactory nose and lip, and reasonable cheek contour which Gillies produced. Beldam remained under Gillies' watchful eye after the procedure had been completed because he became Gillies' chauffeur.

21 Pickerill, 'Facial Surgery', pp.42-44.
22 For a full account of the life and service of Harold Page, see Robert Burkett, Andrew England and Richard Rayner, 'Private Harold Page: a Norfolk man', *Stand To!*, 106 (2016), pp.117-124.
23 Gillies, *Plastic Surgery*, pp.240-243.

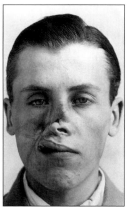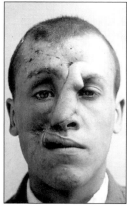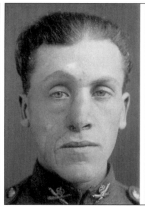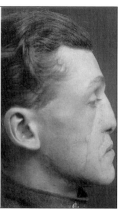

Private Beldam, Machine Gun Corps. Initial appearance, 11 June 1918; after forehead rhinoplasty, 9 July 1918; final appearance, 26 September 1920. (RCS)

Wounds Around the Eyes: 'A Presentable Blind Man'

A large number of soldiers who lost their sight passed through Sidcup (See Colour Section, p.x). Corporal Arthur Cima, a 21-year-old Australian from the 17th AIF, was one of them. Cima was a stereotypical Digger, brash, keen, and disdainful of army discipline. He had signed up in May 1916 in Newcastle, New South Wales, but was of English stock. His widowed mother resided in Tottenham, London. Cima was, at first, somewhat unreliable, with two failures to appear on parade and one absent without leave on his record within six months. By the end of 1916 he had accumulated a total of 21 days' detention, 26 days of Field Punishment No. 2, and lost over a month's pay. However, he was also a brave soldier, and was awarded the Military Medal in late 1917. On 4 July 1918, he was struck by an explosive bullet at Villers Bretonneux. The bullet entered under his lower jaw and traversed the face. Initially Cima was treated in Birmingham, but was transferred to Sidcup on 8 October 1918. He underwent 18 operations in all, but despite the extensive surgery the end result was not attractive.

Private Moss lost both eyes, both cheekbones, half his nose and most of the palate, leaving him with one of the most horrifying appearances of any wounded soldier. The importance of his case to the surgical team is underlined by the duplication of Moss' records, his notes, Tonks' pastels, and the photographs in Archie Lane's albums. Unsurprisingly, his case was included in Gillies' book as well.

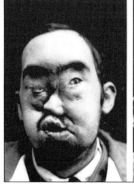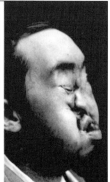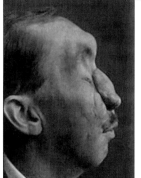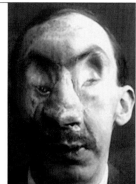

Arthur William Cima, 13th Battalion, AIF. On admission, 16 October 1918; final photograph, 9 August 1921. (RCS)

Gillies commented:

> What has been pushed in can be pushed out again. The soft tissues were first freed
> from the bone and an adjustable splint, designed by Fry, was affixed between face and
> skeleton. This procedure prompted Tonks' comment, 'Beauty is only skin deep'. Fitted
> with an external prosthesis, at last he was presentable enough to become a blind man."
> At this point Gillies succumbed to a rare burst of emotion, adding, *Are these wars
> really necessary?"*[24]

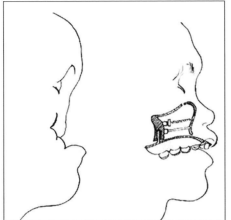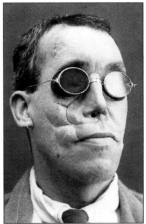

Rifleman Moss. Tonks' diagram showing the adjustable splint, 27 March 1917;
final appearance with mask, 21 February 1918. (RCS)

Men who had become blind as a result of their wounds were often remarkably, in some cases
even unbearably, cheerful. Gillies referred to the "unquenchable optimism" of his patients,
whilst Ward Muir wrote of the unceasing flow of cheerful conversation from a patient called
Briggs who he escorted home from Wandsworth to Yorkshire.[25] The Blinded Soldiers' and
Sailors' Care Committee commenced work at the beginning of 1915, and in the following
February its Chairman, Arthur Pearson, wrote a passionate piece about the importance of St
Dunstan's, the centre for the blind first established in Regent's Park, London:

> Sympathetic folk foretold that the gathering together of a large number of men
> suddenly deprived of sight in the prime of their youth and strength would mean the
> creation of a centre where gloom, dejection and unspeakable sadness reigned supreme.
>
> These prophecies have, I am happy to say, been entirely falsified. The thing which
> invariably strikes the visitor as being most noticeable about the men at St Dunstan's
> is their cheeriness, their brightness, and their apparent disregard of the fact that they
> are anything but normal.
>
> The 'handicap spirit', as it may be called, pervades the classrooms and workshops.
> That horrible word 'affliction', and all the gloomy ideas to which it gives rise, are
> forbidden entry.

---

24 Gillies and Millard, *Principles and Art*, p.27. Emphasis in original.
25 W. Muir, *Observations of an Orderly* (London: Simpkin, Marshall, Hamilton & Kent, 1917), pp.235-249.

'If', wrote the other day a well-known worker among the blind in the North of England, 'Private — is a fair sample of your St Dunstan's men, I must warmly congratulate you. He came to see me this morning, looking a different man from the crushed and sad fellow I had seen before he went. He looked in robust health, and was full of smiles and happiness. He and his wife and children are comfortably off with his pension and the earnings from the mats and bags he makes at home, and at present he has more orders than he can fill.

I am proud to say that Private — is a fair sample of St Dunstan's output.[26]

Pearson's account is certainly rosy, but resonates with Gillies' description of unquenchable optimism and exemplifies rehabilitation at its best. Cima, Moss and another five Sidcup patients were transferred to St Dunstan's, which provided the platform from which one man rose from humble railway clerk to barrister, as we shall see. Yet there was a darker side. Henriette Rémi, a nurse at the Val-de-Grâce Hospital in Paris, wrote a series of vignettes on facial injury in a little book entitled *Hommes Sans Visage*. Her story of Lazé offers the counterpoint to Muir's depiction of Briggs' homecoming. Laze's arrival home was a traumatic one, as his small son ran from him screaming, "That's not my Daddy!" Lazé descended into an irrecoverable gloom and ultimately committed suicide.[27] The deformities of those who had been blinded may have been more bearable to the wounded because they could not see themselves, which led to their cheerful disposition around the surgeons. However, Lazé's case emphasizes how important it was for the surgeons to ensure that appearance was not subordinated entirely to function for those who could not see the results of their surgeries. Likewise, it underpins the despair engendered by the negativity of many of the French surgeons, as Sophie Delaporte has found.[28]

Eye injuries presented a number of challenges which the surgeons struggled to solve adequately. In the first instance, Pickerill noted that a glass eye produced an unnatural stare because the eye did not move. One case file details an experiment which he undertook to remedy this issue. As the eye was removed, Pickerill inserted a cartilage ball. The eye muscles attached themselves to the cartilage ball, which then moved as the gaze did. However, it is likely that the technique was not widely adopted as the advantage of movement was offset by the disadvantage of appearance.

The Sidcup surgeons were also unable to find a satisfactory solution when the eye socket itself was damaged. Whilst the loss of the eye alone was remedied in a cosmetic sense by the provision of an artificial eye, the retention of the new eyeball was dependent on the existence of a satisfactory socket. However, if the bony ring of the orbit was disrupted by the loss of the lower part (the zygomatic arch), the eye socket both widened and dropped. Despite the best efforts of all surgeons, it proved extremely difficult to restore the defect with a bone graft. All too often the eye ended up sitting much lower on the injured side than the uninjured one. A related problem existed when the orbit was damaged but the eye was not. In these cases, the eye's position, and the compromise of its movements, resulted in persistent and untreatable double vision. Lieutenant Elderton, Bedford Regiment, was described by Gillies as a patient of "considerable interest." Elderton had lost his maxilla and eye, which resulted in a major deformity. Gillies attempted, with partial success, to restore the cheek contour with a temporal flap. However, his record of Elderton's procedure in *Plastic Surgery of the Face* notes that final

---

26 A Pearson, Letter to the *National Review*, February 1916.
27 H. Rémi, *Hommes sans Visage* (Lausanne: Editions Spès, 1942). A translation by the author is included as an appendix.
28 S. Delaporte, *Gueules Cassées. Les Blessés de la face de la Grande Guerre* (Paris: Éditions Noesis, 1996).

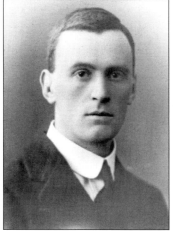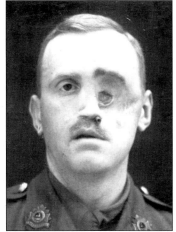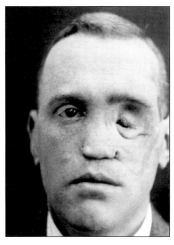

Lieutenant T.H. Elderton, 3rd Battalion, Bedford Regiment. Photograph taken before the war; on admission, 10 February 1918; final appearance, 17 January 1919. (RCS)

treatment had been "deferred for two or three years" at Elderton's request. The case file stops at the same point. Elderton never returned.

When reconstruction was unwanted by a patient who had endured enough surgery, or if it was impossible, gaping defects were concealed by a mask. The experience of Private Scott, a New Zealander, offers an example of the process. Scott provided a pre-war portrait for the mask-maker to work from. The effect was aided by the attachment of a pair of spectacles which helped to conceal the artifice. However, as Ward Muir recorded, it was a time-consuming process. The face was first painted with oil and the hair with Vaseline to stop the plaster from sticking. Then the wet quick-setting plaster of Paris was applied with small pieces of tissue paper over the closed eyes or empty socket. If necessary, straws were inserted into the nostrils. The technician had to judge when the plaster had set, and then lifted the mould from the face. A positive cast was then made of this negative, upon which the sculptor modelled the features to be restored with Plasticine, opened the closed eye, and then built up the correct contours for the missing part.[29]

Metal masks, known as 'Tin Faces', were made from the casts (See Colour Section, p.x). The masks were fashioned in the Dental Workshop. Both Archie Lane's album from Sidcup and the Official History's chapter on facial injury show a multitude of masks, some applied with gum arabic and some attached to spectacles. Two of Lane's masks also survive in the Lane family records. However, the masks were not popular. They were inflexible, obviously artificial, and the paint chipped and flaked. There are unsubstantiated rumours that a riot of 'Tin Face' patients took place at Aldershot. Whether true or not, reconstruction was certainly preferable.

---

29   For a full description, see W. Muir, *The Happy Hospital* (London: Simpkin, Marshall, Hamilton & Kent, 1918), p.147.

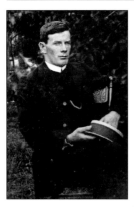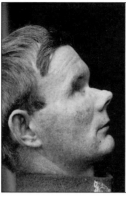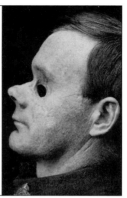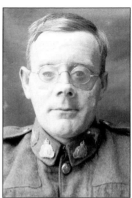

Private Scott, Otago Infantry Regiment. Passing-out photograph; 6 August 1919; 31 January 1920. (RCS)

The Origins of Burns Surgery

The War at Sea

Gillies and his colleagues built on past experience where possible, even if the surgery performed before the war had been inadequately planned and produced poor results. But the reconstruction of a burned face had never been attempted previously, although Thomas Mütter had recorded details of some operations on burns patients in the mid-nineteenth century.[30] Mütter's patients had sustained their injuries up to 23 years before being treated, and were operated upon without anaesthetic. Mütter's use of rotation and advancement flaps was successful cosmetically, at least up to a point, but he reflected that "There are cases in which we must be content with this, while the loss of the function is an evil for which there is no remedy."[31] Gillies' initial work on burns victims was entirely empirical, and he aimed to ensure that functional reconstruction did occur, with successful results.

At the Battle of Jutland on 31 May 1916, the only major fleet encounter of the war, a number of ships were sunk or damaged and the casualties of explosions and fires often suffered severe burns. The injured were transferred to the hospital ship *Plassey* and evacuated to Edinburgh where naval surgeon Cecil Wakeley treated many of them. Wakeley did not favour interventionist treatment. He believed that the use of picric acid dressings, which effectively subjected the skin to a tanning process which created a hard surface, was both damaging and barbaric, due to the pain caused by changing dried dressings.[32] His experience indicated that scarring was made far worse by such dressings, a lesson which had to be re-learned in the Second World War when tannic acid caused a similar problem.[33]

One of the wounded from Jutland became a key subject in the development of modern burns surgery. Magazine explosions and fires were caused both by design deficiencies in British ships, which had insufficient deck armour to protect against high-trajectory plunging shells,

---

30   Thomas Dent Mütter, *Cases of Deformity from Burns: Successfully Treated by Plastic Operations* (Philadelphia, PA: Merrihew & Thompson, 1843). Mütter was of German descent, via Scotland, but born and brought up in the United States; coincidentally, his mother's maiden name was Gillies.

31   Mütter, *Cases of Deformity*, p.17.

32   C.P.G. Wakeley, 'The treatment of war burns', *Journal of the Royal Naval Medical Service*, (1917), pp.156-162.

33   For a full analysis of Jutland and Wakeley's contribution, see A.F. Wallace, 'The development of plastic surgery for war', *Journal of the Royal Army Medical Corps*, 131:1 (1985), pp.28-37.

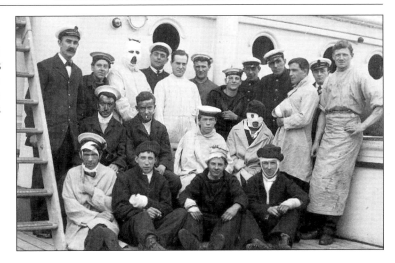

A postcard of casualties aboard the hospital ship *Plassey*. According to crew member Albert Wingrove's diary, 193 men were taken to Edinburgh. Wingrove is standing top left. (Author's collection)

and human error. Gun turrets and magazine hoists were isolated by flash shutters. In the heat of battle the shutters interfered with the smooth supply of ammunition, and they were often left open. In addition, the cordite charges were piled on deck beside the secondary armament turrets. Able Seaman Willie Vicarage from HMS *Malaya* received extensive burns to the face and hands from a shell which ignited one of these cordite piles. Vicarage was transferred to Gillies with severe contracted scars which left him unable either to open his mouth or close his eyes. Gillies embarked on major surgery to graft the affected areas, and discovered that the large skin flaps that he raised tended to roll up. Gillies found that if he sewed the flaps into the rolled shape they naturally assumed, the risk of infection in the large raw areas was reduced. In addition, he discovered that the blood supply along the flaps was significantly enhanced and the tissue death at the end of the flaps diminished markedly. This finding dramatically improved graft survival rates and the speed at which wounds healed. A tube sewn to a new site could be cut from its origin and somersaulted, something which allowed skin flaps to be moved large distances. The technique became known as the tube pedicle procedure, and Vicarage was its first Western subject. He was also the first recipient of a form of eyelid reconstruction which Gillies developed from a procedure first devised by Esser. Gillies named this technique the epithelial outlay procedure, as it reversed Esser's inlay technique, and it has stood the test of time.[34]

Gillies did not take sole credit for the development of the tube pedicle procedure. It was described at the same time by the Russian surgeon Vladimir Filatov in a 1917 article, and Gillies acknowledged his position as a co-inventor of the practice.[35] In terms of its application to large numbers of patients, the procedure was definitely first implemented at Sidcup. However, there was some disagreement in the early 1920s as to who should take the credit for its development in the West. Captain John Law Aymard, the South African ENT surgeon who was attached to both Aldershot and Sidcup at an early stage, claimed in a bitter correspondence with Gillies and *The Lancet* that he was the inventor and that Gillies had stolen the idea. The matter was ultimately decided in Gillies' favour by the General Medical Council, but the episode demonstrates that relations at Sidcup were not as harmonious as its major figures later asserted.[36]

---

34   The procedure is explained further below by reference to a diagram in the notes for another burns victim, Cecil Grayer.

35   V. Filatov, 'Plastic procedure using a round pedicle', *Vestnik Ofalmol*, 34:4 (1917), pp.149-158.

36   After Aymard published his case in *The Lancet*, Gillies wrote (7 August 1920) to confirm that his tube pedicle operation on A.B. Vicarage was performed on 3 October, while Aymard's (on Private B.C. Harris,

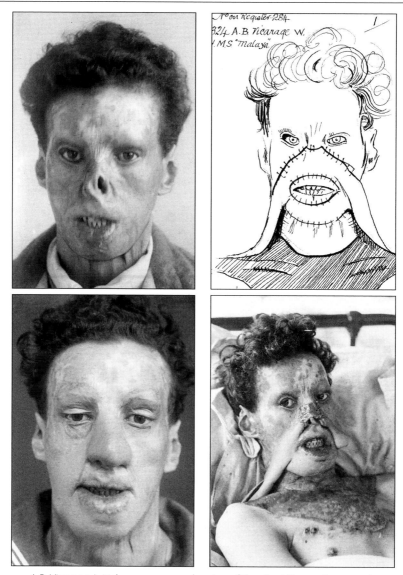

A.B. Vicarage. Initial appearance; a drawing of the chest flap; a photograph
showing the double tube of the flap; final appearance. (RCS)

Like Able Seaman Vicarage, Gunner Yeo of HMS *Warspite* was burnt in a cordite fire and
was initially treated by Wakeley in Edinburgh. A poor copy of a photograph in Wakeley's
account appears in the Queen's Hospital notes. No date for Yeo's injury was recorded at Sidcup,
although it is likely that he received his burns at Jutland. Yeo's contractures dragged down his
lower eyelids, and the eyes appear red and sore in the initial photographs. Yeo's mouth was

7th Middlesex Regiment) was done on the 18th with Captain Seccombe Hett. Gillies tried to defuse the
row by stating: "I am to blame in not informing Captain Aymard at the time he published his rhinoplasty
case in your paper, that he was not the first to evolve the principle of 'tubing' the pedicle." Both sets of case
notes survive and indicate that Aymard's operation failed as a result of infection. Hett subsequently made a
successful reconstruction using the Indian forehead flap technique.

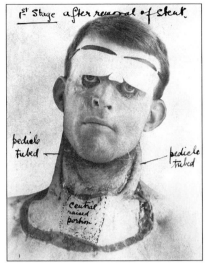

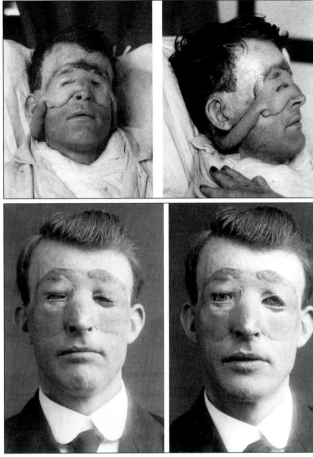

Gunner Yeo. Initial appearance; with tubed chest flap raised; final appearance. (RCS)

also turned down at the corners. Where Vicarage's chest flap covered just the nose and cheeks, Yeo's flap extended across both eyes. Immediately after the operation, Yeo looked as if he was wearing a mask. Some six months after his first operation, he was pictured wearing a broad smile, and photographs demonstrate that he was able to close his eyes by November 1918.

The War in the Air

The North Sea was not the only area of combat in which severe burns were a possibility. The war in the air also provided its share of Sidcup's casualties, including Ralph Lumley (See Colour Section, p.x). As noted earlier, Lumley's accident occurred on his first solo flight. His arrival at Sidcup on 22 October 1917 after the intervention of Sister Agnes Keyser followed a prolonged spell at home, where he had become severely depressed. Perhaps buoyed by the success of his management of Seaman Vicarage and Gunner Yeo, Gillies performed his first operation on Lumley just over a month later. The case was recorded after the war in *Plastic Surgery of the Face*, and began with Gillies' decision to replace the whole skin of the face by a chest flap. Gillies' documented how he created the pedicles on which the huge chest flap was raised, and decided he would need to wait for two months before he created the flap itself. However, Lumley had become habituated to morphine and, "having pinned his faith on the result of the forthcoming operation, he was bitterly disappointed and exceedingly depressed at the thought of having to wait another long period, and it was feared he would not wait so long."[37] As a result, Gillies set aside his maxim of 'never do today what can honourably be put off until tomorrow'.

Disaster followed. The flap failed and became gangrenous and then infected. The chest was covered with a skin flap taken from a volunteer, and it is possible that rejection of this contributed to Lumley's initial deterioration. He died on 11 March 1918. Gillies wrote:

> There is a very pathetic sequel to this most terrible case, in that the patient after having survived the ordeal of the burn, lived and regained a certain amount of strength twenty months after the injury, died as a late result of a plastic operation … In reviewing the case, the attempt to reconstruct the whole face is a procedure which is obviously justifiable, and it would, in a more reposed patient, have succeeded. It is possible that, had the author taken a very firm attitude, and could have persuaded the patient to wait a year, the operation, as planned, would have had more chance of success. The author is convinced that the operation should have been done in piecemeal – perhaps that only one-quarter of the face should have been done at a time. By this means a very presentable result might have been obtained; but it obviously would not have been as good as the single replacement method, and the author feels that his desire to obtain a perfect result somewhat over-rode his surgical judgement of the general condition of the patient.

As always, Gillies did not shy away from the inevitable failures which occurred at Sidcup. Instead, he sought to learn from the mistakes of the past in order to prevent the same situation from arising in the future.

The experience of Norman Eric Wallace was better than that of Lumley's, but still demonstrates the difficulties faced by surgeons presented with extensive burns injuries. Wallace, an RFC artillery observer for the Canadian Field Artillery, was shot down on 19 September 1917. He was transferred to Sidcup from Lakenham Military Hospital, Norwich, on 18 May 1918. As the image of his initial appearance shows, Wallace had been badly burned and his face was a distorted mask. Wallace's file, which contains his operation notes, progress reports, an extensive set of photographs, watercolours and diagrams, is 35 pages in length and documents the 21 operations which Wallace underwent (See Colour Section, p.xi). Free flaps were taken from his buttock, and tube pedicles were raised. Partly concealed by spectacles, the final appearance was reasonable and recorded in the case notes as a considerable improvement. However, as the photograph below illustrates, even after 21 operations Wallace's disfigurement was very severe.

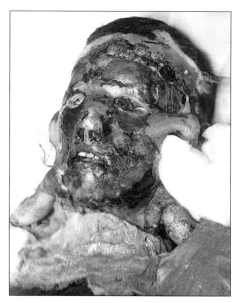

Lieutenant Lumley, RFC. Photograph showing the necrosis of the infected flap. (RCS)

---

37 Gillies, *Plastic Surgery*, p.364. Unless otherwise stated, all quotations in this passage are taken from this source.

Lieutenant Wallace, Canadian Field Artillery (attached to the RFC). Initial appearance. (RCS)

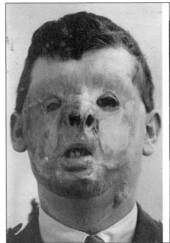
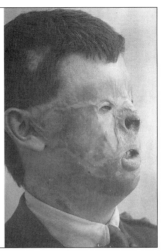

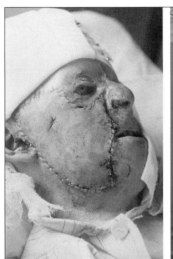
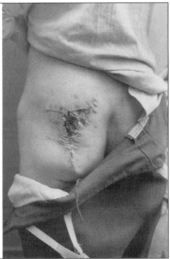
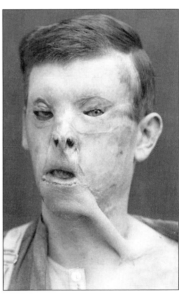

Lieutenant Wallace. Photograph of the donor site; pedicled flap; final appearance. (RCS)

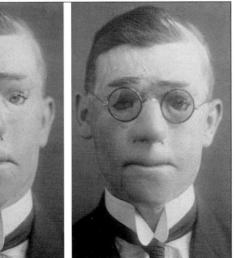

Hope Francis Mulhall underwent just one procedure less than Wallace during his time at Sidcup. His treatment was slightly delayed due to captivity. Mulhall was posted missing on 30 October 1918, and did not arrive at Sidcup until the following January. His notes state that he had been treated by an English doctor in the meantime, but had not undergone surgery. His first operation did not take place until October 1919, a year after he had been captured. After 20 operations, Mulhall's appearance and function was improved significantly. He returned home to Hampshire and lived until 1970. Another patient whose treatment was delayed as a result of enemy capture, Charles Peckham, travelled a far greater distance to get home. Posted missing on 23 June 1918, Peckham had been shot down and taken prisoner. He did not return to England for six months, and was not admitted to Sidcup until January 1919. Peckham underwent treatment for five months, and his records suggested he was a Canadian. In fact, he was an American from Scranton, Pennsylvania. Peckham was evidently unhappy with the treatment he subsequently received in America, as he returned to Sidcup in 1920 to receive more surgery and X-ray treatment on his scars. Gillies performed the surgery.

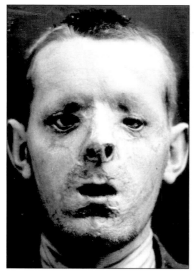
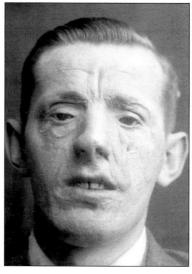

Hope Francis Mulhall. Initial appearance, 14 January 1919; final appearance, 20 March 1922. (RCS)

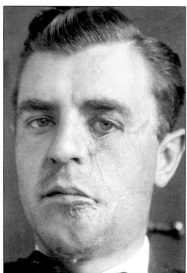
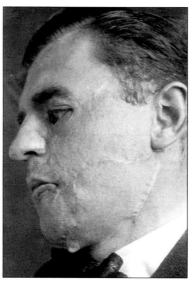

Charles Peckham. Initial appearance, 23 May 1920; final appearance, 22 November 1920. (RCS)

The War on the Ground

Whilst the artillery deployed in colossal numbers across the Western Front was responsible for inflicting many of the facial wounds discussed above, those who served in the artillery branches were also susceptible to burns as a result of explosions. Cecil Grayer was one such patient. Wounded on 22 October 1916, Grayer reached Aldershot in January of the following year and had his first operation in March. His notes are augmented by Tonks' drawings and a pastel. Grayer's burns were confined to the upper part of the face, and involved the forehead and left eyelid. His surgery continued through to his final discharge in March 1918, and consisted of the epithelial inlay technique adapted by Gillies from the procedure first described by Esser (See Colour Section, p.xi). Gillies deduced that the taut, scarred eyelid skin might be stretched by making a mould which was enclosed by an inverted fold of skin. The mould, known as a stent, eventually created a reaction and was extruded, whereupon the newly expanded, inverted loop was everted. Tonks' diagram explained the technique.

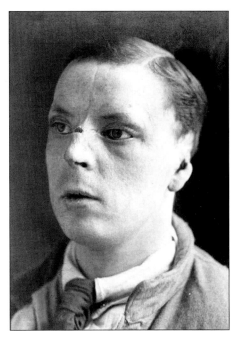

Gunner Cecil Grayer, Royal Field Artillery (RFA). Initial appearance. (RCS)

Secondary Management

Gunner Butt had undergone several operations in Germany whilst a POW there. Gillies wrote that "the left half of his mandible was firmly united to his maxilla; an inadequate forehead flap brought down undersigned and unlined had shrivelled; the forehead defect had been severely pulled together with necrosing sutures; the mouth was scarred and distorted."[38] A handwritten note in Butt's file decried that Butt's was "the sort of plastic surgery one has to fight in one's own clinic as well as in other surgeons." Whilst the final appearance illustrated in the notes was far from perfect, it was at least normal looking and emphasised the value of specialist surgery.

Even the specialists sometimes came to differing conclusions over the outcomes of various patients. The case of Norman Wimbush, 2nd King's Own Royal Lancashire Regiment, offers an example of the negativity of French patient management. Wimbush was wounded at Ypres in 1915, and had been treated by Hippolyte Morestin in Paris and operated upon in London and Neuilly-sur-Seine. Wimbush's treatment had been considered complete and, despite having been declared unfit for service in 1916, he had applied for a renewal of his commission in July 1918. Gillies disagreed that Wimbush's treatment could be considered finished, and four months after his application to return to the war, Wimbush was admitted to Sidcup. His admission photograph demonstrates the significant disfigurement which existed upon his arrival at the Queen's, and 20 operations later Gillies restored the nose and facial contour, as is particularly clear from lateral views.

---

38 Gillies and Millard, *Principles and Art*, p.45.

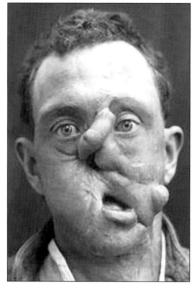
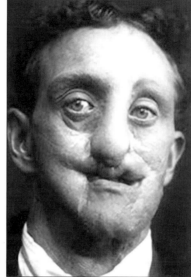

Gunner Butt, RFA, 4 March 1919; 14 April 1924. (RCS)

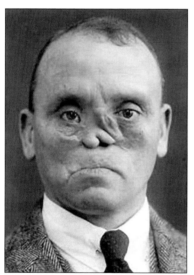
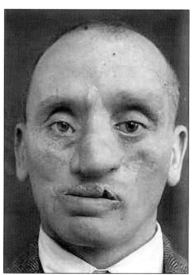

Lieutenant Wimbush. On admission to Sidcup, 23 November 1918; final appearance, 29 August 1920. (RCS)

Tanks

Alongside exposure to a range of facial injuries as a result of collisions with objects within their vehicles, tank crews also risked severe burns. If a tank caught fire, as many did, then so did its occupants. Sidcup treated those who suffered from both wounds and burns as a result of their service with the tanks, including Lieutenant Vanzellor, recipient of the Military Cross as a result of his bravery on 23 March 1918. On that date, Vanzellor had managed to rescue his tank in the face of the German advance. However, on 8 August 1918, when it was the Allies turn to advance, Vanzellor's tank was hit whilst in support of the Canadians. He sustained fractures of the maxilla and nose, with a wound to the right eye and cheek. The contracture of the scar left him with an updrawn lip. No early photographs survive; the first in Vanzellor's file was taken after he had already undergone three operations on his nose. The monocle was used to disguise an artificial eye. Later images show that surgery corrected the sneer.

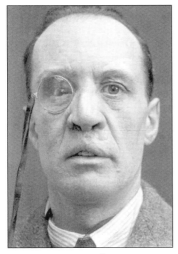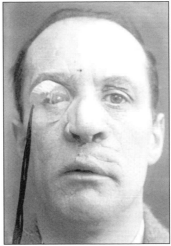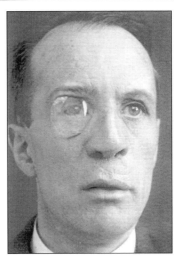

Lieutenant Vanzellor. Prior to corrective surgery, 12 February 1920; two weeks after lip surgery, 29 February 1920; after lip surgery, 17 August 1920. (RCS)

Lieutenant Stanley Cohen also suffered both wounds and burns. Originally from Winchester, Cohen had been in the London University Officer Training Corps prior to the war, and joined the 3/23rd London Regiment as a 20-year-old the week after the declaration of war. First wounded at Loos in 1915, Cohen had transferred to the tanks and was wounded again at Flesquières in November 1917. He was then severely injured at Amiens on 8 August 1918. His tank caught fire, and Cohen sustained burns and a serious injury to his left leg. The leg became infected and had to be amputated.

Over the next three years, Cohen was in and out of various hospitals. He was transferred to Sidcup almost a year after his injury, on 1 August 1919. He later wrote:

> Part of the time there I slept on an open verandah overlooking a fine green lawn and looking towards the old red brick Jacobean house. There was nothing haphazard about Major Gillies' work. He secured photos and made models of the face and had a museum showing his work before and after … He put a graft to cover my nose and four new eyelids. This I believe took four hours and was in the days when ether was used. I think I vomited for a full 24 hours afterwards but all went well and all grafts took and I still have them and scars from whence they came![39]

Cohen learned to use a typewriter during his recovery, but injuries to his hands led to concerns among his attendants that they would have to be amputated. They sought an opinion from Sir Robert Jones, the pioneering orthopaedic surgeon, who said "Something of your own is better than something artificial." As a result, Cohen kept his fingers to go with his new eyelids.

---

39 Stanley Cohen, personal papers.

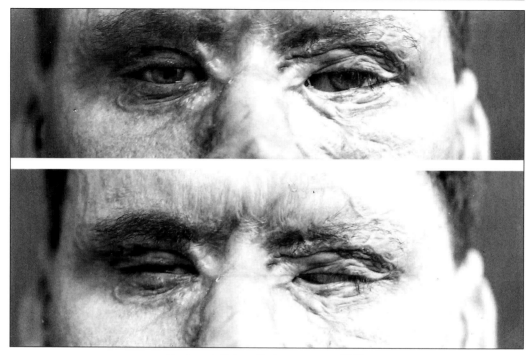

Lieutenant Cohen. Final appearance. (RCS)

Other Uses for the Tube Pedicle

The development of the tube pedicle changed facial surgery immeasurably. It allowed the taking of skin from a distant part, rather than from somewhere near to the site of injury. Thus, skin was taken from the leg, tubed, and attached to the abdomen. Once a blood supply had been established in it, the leg origin was cut and the tube somersaulted upwards to, for example, the arm. After the same sequence, the abdominal attachment was cut, and the tube was applied to the facial defect. The enormous advantage this method possessed over a free graft was the retention of a blood supply into the flap at all times. In addition, it contained both skin and subcutaneous tissue. Gillies also found a new use for the tube in a patient with a deformity not related to injury. Dupuytren's contracture affects the hand. The tissues in the palm become thickened and contract, drawing the fingers into a flexed position. Private Smith, who had been admitted to Sidcup with a facial wound, also possessed a deformity in his hand. Gillies performed a pedicled graft to the palm which was successful. However, Gillies never described this particular case in print, and it was not until the 1940s that the idea was rediscovered.

Failure

Not all those who arrived at Sidcup were so fortunate, as we saw in the case of Ralph Lumley. Men died from pre-existing disease, such as tuberculosis, from the Spanish Flu, from accidental or deliberate overdose of (forbidden) alcohol, from sepsis and occasionally from operative complications. Arthur Albert Mears, a Tasmanian from the 12th Infantry Battalion who was awarded the Military Medal, resided at Sidcup for over a year. His operations generated a wealth of notes, and provide one of the best examples of what George Dorrance so admired about the Queen's

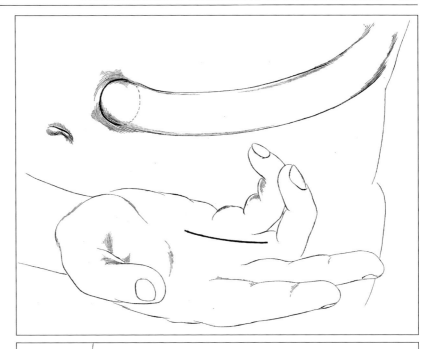

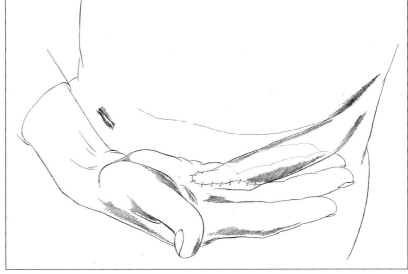

Private W.J. Smith, 13th Royal Fusiliers. Diagrams showing the tubed graft from the abdomen to the left hand. Smith had a cheek wound with a salivary fistula and had lost his right leg. The Dupuytren's contracture was an incidental finding. (RCS)

Hospital: its systematic recording of the progress of surgery (See Colour Section, p.xii). Mears had been wounded near the Menin Road on 20 September 1917. He spent two days in hospital in Boulogne, and arrived at Sidcup on 12 October. He had lost a large part of his mandible. As a result, his tongue overhung the large soft tissue and had become adherent to the extent that he had a permanent dribble of saliva. His case was a surgical triumph. His initial notes are hand-written and contain partly-coloured diagrams by Daryl Lindsay interspersed in the text, a series of photographs, a set of six blueprint diagrams, and a watercolour. Tragically, after his final operation, in which a long piece of rib cartilage, notched so it could be curved into a jaw-like shape, had been inserted, Mears suddenly and unexpectedly died. He had been at Sidcup for over a year.

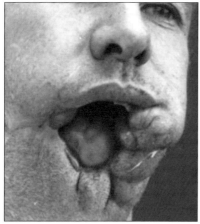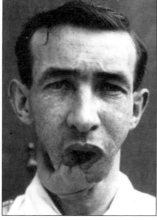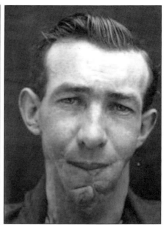

Photographs of Arthur Mears. (RCS)

Mears' funeral was held at Brookwood cemetery. It was a moving occasion, recorded in an official notice for his family:

> The deceased soldier was accorded a full Military funeral, Firing Party, Bugler and Pallbearers being in attendance. The coffin was draped with the Australian flag and surmounted by several beautiful wreaths, sent from:-
> Women of Dulwich Association,
> Mrs F.M. Grayson, Queen's Hospital, Sidcup, Kent,
> L/Cpl and Mrs C. Nelson, and one globe wreath from the comrades of deceased, in Queen's Hospital, Sidcup.
> The Last Post was sounded at the graveside, and the burial service conducted by Chap, Rev. F.S. Suggett, C.F. of the A.I.F. headquarters, London.

A number of Mears' fellow patients attended, listed as Corporals Carne, Duell, Howe and McPherson, and Privates Korose, Axford, Earles, Storrier, Graham and Plumridge. Lance-Corporal Nelson, who provided one of the wreaths, was also a Sidcup patient.

Mears' possessions make a poignant footnote. Apart from a walking stick, the sparse inventory comprised:

> 1 pr Field Glasses, 1 Diary, 1 Pen Holder, 2 prs Gloves, 1 Pencil, 1 Map, 4 Pipes, 2 Cycle Valves, 1 Buckle, Matchbox Holder, Hairclippers & 4 Combs, 1 Fountain Pen & clip, 1 Cigarette Case, 1 Wallet, 4 stamps, 1 Mirror, 2 Private Compasses, 1 Note Case, 2 Paybooks (A.B. 64), 1 Housewife, 1 Penknife (broken), 1 Brooch in Box, 1 Wrist Strap, 4 Razors, Letters, 1 Silk Muffler, 2 Wristlet Watches (damaged), Photos, 1 Wallet, 1 French Map, Post cards, Christmas cards, 1 Hospital bag, 3 Reading Books.
> 1 paybook No.12237 handed to Estates Branch, A.I.F. Hqrs, London. £2.0.6 has been passed to Chief Paymaster, A.I.F. Hqrs, London to be combined with monies due and credited to Pte Mears Ledger Account.[40]

These items were returned to his mother.

---

40 National Archives of Australia, B2455: First Australian Imperial Force Personnel Dossiers, 1914-1920.

Other Clinical Developments: Anaesthesia and X-ray

The surgery performed at Sidcup could never have been performed without anaesthetic. Prior to the invention of anaesthesia in the mid-nineteenth century, surgeons had to work quickly because the operating field wriggled and shrieked. Sedation was confined to almost toxic doses of alcohol. There were no cures for haemorrhage or postoperative wound sepsis. As a result, death was common, and life expectancy after surgery was often short. With the development of nitrous oxide, ether, and chloroform, it was possible to perform surgery under reasonably controlled and unhurried conditions. All the same, anaesthesia in the era of the First World War was still risky. The likelihood of post-operative bronchitis was particularly significant as, thanks in part to their excessive consumption of cigarettes, many of the troops at the front suffered from catarrhal conditions of the respiratory tract. This situation was somewhat belied by a contemporary postcard (See Colour Section, p.xiii) which contained a smoking Tommy with the caption: "The Great Germ Destroyer."

As William Kelsey Fry had found, alongside the risks attached to its use, it was incredibly difficult to administer anaesthetic in the field. Respiratory obstruction was common, either because the tongue and throat were swollen, the muscles which opened the larynx had been lost (which meant the tongue would fall back into the throat), or a combination of the two. Local anaesthesia was used where possible, but the administration of a general anaesthetic to a patient lying flat on their back in the traditional position often required a tracheotomy to get the surgeon out of trouble. Furthermore, the standard method of delivery was by face mask, which was hopeless in cases where the face was the operative field.[41] The surgeons at Aldershot and Sidcup were forced, therefore, to become pioneers in anaesthetics as well as in plastic surgery.

Rubens Wade, the anaesthetist seconded to Gillies, pointed out that plastic operations were lengthy, and often took place on patients who were undernourished as a result of major mouth injuries which impaired their ability to take food. He also outlined the key problem in plastic surgery; that the anaesthetist and surgeon got in each other's way. A mask was not suitable for the delivery of anaesthesia when the operation site lay beneath it:

> The airway is strangely distorted in some part of its course; and, in addition the surgeon must perforce trespass upon the territory usually regarded by the anaesthetist as his own.
>
> Evidently, therefore, there is scope for any and every device that will diminish effort for the patient and anaesthetist, and bring the prolonged strain within the limits of endurance.
>
> An arrangement must also be come to by which the surgeon is spared the disability of disputing the possession of the parts ... For large operations upon the mouth region, intra-tracheal administration in some form has been adopted as a routine ... Ether is the intra-tracheal anaesthetic of choice. It is given under positive pressure, being carried either by a stream of oxygen from a large cylinder or by a stream of air propelled by a small electrically driven motor.[42]

---

41 For head wounds prior to the First World War, anaesthetic was delivered by a tube passed through an oral mouth prop. The first man to use this technique was William MacEwan in 1880.

42 R. Wade. Quoted in Gillies, *Plastic Surgery*, p.23. Unless otherwise stated, all quotations in this passage are taken from this source.

Wade commented "to begin with, the majority of plastic operations are unavoidably long," and the surgeon often had to abandon the operation to help the anaesthetist. Gillies wrote:

> One early bone graft is recalled in which the patient went blue, and I had to help the anaesthetist get the patient's tongue forward and clear the airway. I washed up and continued to chisel the donor bone graft, when the patient went bad again, and the anaesthetist once more had to be helped to keep the patient alive. This happened a third time before the finish, and needless to say the graft did not survive.[43]

In acknowledgement of the advice of Colonel Silk, a senior army anaesthetist who had been sent to Sidcup to advise on the problem of respiratory obstruction for patients in the supine position, Wade pioneered the delivery of anaesthesia to patients who were in a seated position.

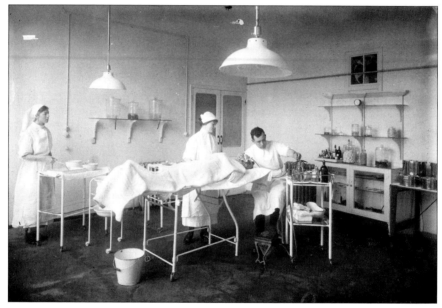

Rubens Wade inducing anaesthesia at Sidcup. The half-plate image allows enlargement – showing that the inducing agent is chloroform. (Author's collection)

There were a number of complications to be overcome. With the patient seated, their blood pressure dropped, or the anaesthetic became too light and difficult to control. Whilst the sitting position reduced the risk of airway obstruction, this was offset by the danger that the patient could wake up. Furthermore, the surgeon, working directly in front of the airway, received a face full of ether every time the patient exhaled. Ivan Magill recalled the situation:

> These reconstructive procedures … went on for hour after hour, and with the surgeon working on the face under aseptic conditions, the anaesthetist had to be entirely out of the field. Without access to the eyes for guidance as to the stage of anaesthesia, and in fact as some were blind, the patients had to be followed by ear. Trying to maintain an adequate airway by remote control and without the aid of suction was a nightmare

---

43 Gillies and Millard, *Principles and Art*, p.25.

… Positive pressure was necessary to prevent blood from entering the trachea, but the surgeon got the blast of the patient's ether-laden expirations and was often enveloped in a spray of blood. On more than one occasion [Gillies], half asleep from my ether, would snap at me, 'Maggie, you seem to get this ether in here jolly well, why can't you take it out again?'[44]

Magill, perhaps the most important figure in the twentieth-century history of anaesthesia, began his anaesthetic career at Sidcup. A short-sighted Ulsterman, he had served in the RAMC during the war and was in medical charge of troops awaiting demobilisation at the time of the Armistice. His wife was a staff doctor on the London County Council and, despite the fact that he had no previous experience of anaesthetics, Magill applied for the anaesthetic post at Sidcup in 1919 simply because it was close to London.

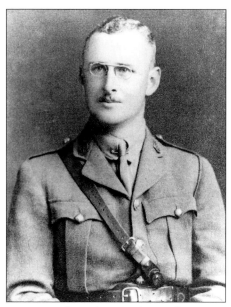
Ivan Magill at Sidcup. (Author's collection)

Magill and Stanley Rowbotham, who arrived at Sidcup at about the same time, devised a simple solution to the surgeon's ether problem. A pharyngeal tube, with an additional angle piece, was passed along with the endotracheal tube so that the expired gases were directed away from the surgeon's face. However, the problem of expiration remained in cases where the pharynx was severely deformed. In those procedures, the pharyngeal expiration tube often proved impossible to position. A solution was found, as Magill described later:

Attempts to find a free channel by means of rubber tubes passed into the pharynx were unsuccessful, until one of these tubes accidentally entered the trachea along with the catheter. The relief which followed left no doubt as to the value of 'two tubes'. Free expiration was ensured without blowing anaesthetic and blood at the surgeon, and the patient's head could be moved into any position without danger of obstructing the airway. Pharyngeal packing about the two tubes effectively walled off the larynx from blood and mucus, which alleviated the necessity of high-pressure anaesthesia. Deliberate occlusion of the expiratory tube was possible when positive pressure was required. A mixture of nitrous oxide and oxygen with a minimal amount of ether was now practical and our postoperative recoveries better.[45]

Magill and Rowbotham also discovered that passage of a single nasal endotracheal tube could often be performed blind, which was an enormous advantage for men with jaw fractures, or in cases where the mouth could not be opened in order to insert a laryngoscope. A soldier boy named Trask, in Magill's words, had always experienced a "miserable recovery" after surgery which used ether. He exemplified the success of Magill and Rowbotham's work. Trask promised that if he

---

44 I. Magill. Quoted in Gillies and Millard, *Principles and Art*, p.60.
45 Ibid.

were only given gas (nitrous oxide) and oxygen, he would smoke a cigarette as he was taken out of the theatre. For his subsequent operations only gas and oxygen were used and Trask kept his promise. Magill recalled him "puffing a cigarette for all he was worth as he was being wheeled back to the ward."[46] Ether often caused patients to suffer from extreme nausea. A New Zealander, Oliver Doidge, recorded his progress in 1920 after his return to Dunedin. His diary reveals that he was very sick from the ether, and the effects lasted over 24 hours.[47] Any reflux of acidic stomach contents into the mouth and nose of patients was both exceptionally painful and highly dangerous.

Magill and Rowbotham reported their experiences at Sidcup to the Royal Society of Medicine in February 1921. They observed that patients were often more fearful of the anaesthetic than the surgery, a point which was later echoed by Second World War plastic surgery teams. Repeated operations, which were the rule rather than the exception at Sidcup, increased the problem. Magill and Rowbotham stressed that nitrous oxide, used in conjunction with local infiltration of novocaine, maintained sufficient analgesia for most lesser operations without the risks or side-effects associated with ether or chloroform. The patient regulated his own gas intake, in much the same way as obstetric delivery is controlled today.

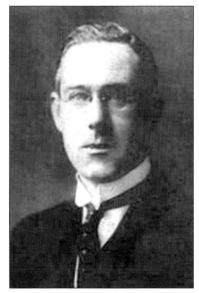

Stanley Rowbotham, from the 1921 hospital Christmas card. (Author's collection)

Whilst Gillies and Magill are the names most remembered as the seminal figures in the development of plastic surgery and anaesthesia, both were essentially figureheads for the teams which produced the results. Pickerill summarised the work at Sidcup in the introduction to his MS thesis. "In many cases," he wrote, "I feel sure that it was a case of necessity being the mother of invention" at the Queen's. He commented further on the healthy rivalry between the sections which stimulated advance, and concluded that "there are very few if indeed any cases now, which, however extensive, would be regarded as beyond restoration by purely surgical measures and from the patients [sic] own tissues."[48] The same desire to advance the practice of anaesthesia drove Magill's team. Magill did not invent endotracheal anaesthesia, but he perfected it, ably assisted by Rowbotham and others. Archie Lane, for instance, made several pieces of anaes-

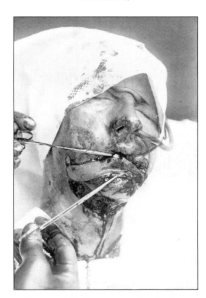

Corporal McCrea: anaesthesia via a nasal tube. (RCS)

thetic equipment to a design created by Rowbotham. The pioneering work of the anaesthetists at Sidcup during the First World War had profound long-term consequences for surgery.

---

46   Ibid., p.61.
47   Diary of Oliver Doidge, courtesy of Malcolm Doidge.
48   Pickerill, 'Facial Surgery', p.2.

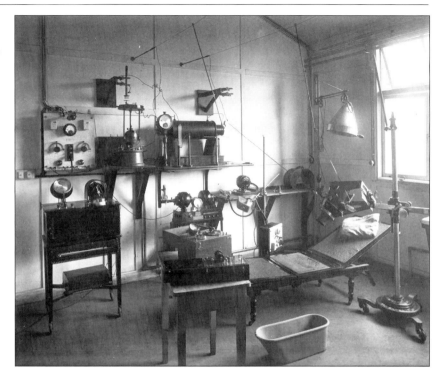

The dental X-ray department at Sidcup. (Author's collection)

Although not a new technique, radiology was also used extensively at Sidcup. Alongside its use for the identification of fractures, which had been common in the early years of the twentieth century, the surgeons at Sidcup also used X-rays to assess the extent of bone loss and to determine the amount and location of foreign material in the wound. Radiographs of the time could be difficult to interpret; the fashion in the period was to make a positive print from the X-ray negative, a step which has been long abandoned in modern practice. In addition, the Sidcup artists made line drawings of the radiographs which proved helpful to the surgical teams.

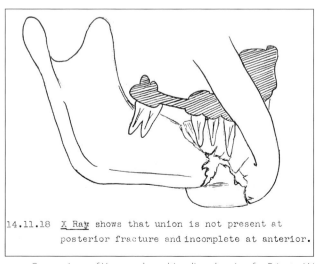

14.11.18 X Ray shows that union is not present at
          posterior fracture and incomplete at anterior.

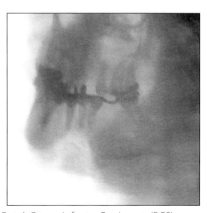

Comparison of X-ray and resulting line drawing for Private J.N. Butel, Otago Infantry Regiment. (RCS)

Overseas: Allies and Enemies

In order to assess the development of facial surgery at Sidcup, it is important to compare what took place in Britain with the developments of the other major nations in the First World War. Comparison with events which took place in France, Germany, and those which involved American surgeons, illustrate clearly the significance of Sidcup as a pioneering institution for the treatment of facial injuries.

France

Despite the impetus given to Gillies as a result of his observations of Hippolyte Morestin at work, the results of surgical intervention on French facial casualties were not of a high standard during the First World War. The problems facing the French surgeons were identical, and were identified almost exactly as within the British military medical services (infection, haemorrhage and scar contracture). Steps were taken to minimise delays in patient transport, but nevertheless these delays remained significant and averaged around 40 days. The second-line service employed by the French was, in addition, little more than a transit stop. Patients on average stayed at the intermediate hospitals for an average of six days, during which time nothing definitive could be achieved. There were also too few medical staff available. At Amiens, for example, Pierre Blot had just eight doctors to assist him. A contemporary American surgeon also commented that the techniques the French surgeons used were crude.

Morestin typified the approach of the French surgeons. He was intensely protective of his work, and he flatly refused to collaborate with his dental technicians. Morestin died shortly after the war, a victim of the Spanish Flu epidemic which swept across Europe in the aftermath of the conflict. He left behind an enormous collection of illustrations of his work in the form of casts, moulages and photographs, all of which have been preserved in the *Musée du Service de Santé des Armées* in Paris. The surviving records confirm the lack of two of Sidcup's hallmarks within Morestin's work: the systematic approach to record keeping; and the ability and desire to analyse poor results in order to develop the practice of facial reconstruction.

The isolation of French surgeons from each other was replicated in a post-war separation of French surgical texts from those of other nations. A number of doctoral theses which describe facial surgery techniques were written in France, both during and after the war. However, without exception they were unillustrated and, as a result, their descriptions of operative techniques are almost impossible to follow.[49] The 1996 television broadcast '*1914-1918: The Great War and the Shaping of the 20th Century*', a joint production between KCET Los Angeles and the BBC, quoted only from French sources.[50] The work of Sophie Delaporte has done much to raise awareness of the contribution of French surgeons to the development of facial surgery across the Channel.[51] The paucity of English-language sources within her work merely reinforces the geographical isolation in which the French surgeons operated.

The best direct insight into the French approach to surgery, and one which lends some credence to the existence of a "stitch the raw edges whatever the tissue loss" attitude of the

---

49 A list of these theses can be found at the following webpage: A. Bamji, 'A Bibliography of Great War Medicine', *The Gillies Archive from Queen Mary's Hospital, Sidcup*, 2015, <http://www.gilliesarchives.org.uk/Qmbiblio1.htm#pt11> (accessed 10 May 2016).

50 A book of the series was released to coincide with the broadcast. See J. Winter and B. Baggett, *1914-1918: The Great War and the Shaping of the 20th Century* (London: Penguin, 1996).

51 Delaporte, *Gueules Cassées*.

Colour Plate Contents

Troops helping to get an ambulance belonging to the 16th (Irish) Division through the mud in Mametz Wood, July 1916. Original photograph by John Warwick Brooke, IWM Q4015; tinted photo-postcard: *Daily Mail* Battle Collection, series 1, no.5. (Author's collection) ... iii

A large fragment of shell casing found on the Somme battlefield in 2001. (Author's collection) ... iii

No.31 of a series of 50 W.D. and H.O. Wills cigarette cards depicting winners of the Victoria Cross. Captain Harry Sherwood Ranken, RAMC was severely wounded in September 1914. He continued to treat men on the front line, but when he finally allowed himself to be evacuated, his condition was desperate. He died on 25 September 1914. (Author's collection) Note: Another card series from Gallaher's illustrated Noel Chavasse and Arthur Martin-Leake, who were two of three double VC winners. ... iv

Pastel portraits of Reginald Evans, DCM and Albert Palmer. (RCS) ... v

'The Plastic Theatre at the Queen's Hospital' by John Hodgson Lobley. (IWM ART 3659) ... v

Shell fragments and a piece of flint recovered from the Somme battlefield; note the razor-sharp point to the flint. (Author's collection) ... vi

Pastels of Walter Ashworth by Henry Tonks before and after surgery. (RCS) ... vi

Private Gardiner, 7th Canterbury Infantry Regiment. Photograph of Tonks' pastel annotated by Gillies to show the soft tissue repair. (RCS) ... vii

Private Williams, 3rd Nigerian Regiment. Pastel by Tonks; photograph from Lane's album, with the dental appliance in place. (RCS and the Antony Wallace Archive, and the BAPRAS Archive) ... vii

Plaster cast of Private F. Hamlett: full face and oblique view. (Author's photograph from a copy of the cast, which was kindly provided by the Royal Australasian College of Surgeons) ... vii

Private Len Tringham. Watercolour by Herbert Cole. (RCS) ... viii

Private Stone. Pastel by Tonks. (RCS) ... viii

Private William Thomas, 1st Cheshire Regiment. Watercolour by Daryl Lindsay. (RACS Archive, Melbourne) ... viii

Opposite: Private Green. The figures show the stages of constructing a new upper lip using a flap taken within the hair line to create a moustache. (RCS and Hocken Library, Dunedin) ... viii

'Newly Blinded' by Francis Leopold Mond. A blind man, with hand outstretched and head raised, is led by a nurse. The painting was reportedly given as a raffle prize in aid of St Dunstan's, and hung for many years in a public house in South London. (Author's collection) Note: Information from David Cohen, from whom the author acquired the painting. The subject bears a strong resemblance to Sergeant Walter Bowen, who was a Sidcup patient. ... x

An eye mask incorporating a glass eye made by Archie Lane at Sidcup. (Author's collection) ... x

Lieutenant Lumley, RFC. Tonks' pastel shows his appearance upon admission. (RCS) ... x

Lieutenant Wallace. Series of four watercolours showing the necrosis of the initial cheek flap taken from the buttock. (RCS) — xi

Gunner Cecil Grayer, Royal Field Artillery (RFA). Diagram demonstrating the epithelial outlay technique adapted by Gillies from Esser's inlay. (RCS) — xi

Notes of Arthur Mears. (RCS) — xii

Hand-coloured photographs of a French soldier with and without his mask. The face beneath the mask is, from a surgical point of view, completed. (Author's collection) — xiii

A diagram of the operation performed on Albert Mears to free his tongue from scar tissue and to reconstruct the jaw. (RCS) — xiv

This wax model – created by Tom Kelsey for Pickerill – was used to demonstrate several surgical techniques. (RCS) — xv

Plaster casts of Storrier, before and after a forehead flap rhinoplasty. (RACS Archive, Melbourne) — xv

A comparison of diagrammatic representation (1). Diagram by Henry Tonks showing first stage of surgery on Spicer. (RCS) — xvi

A comparison of diagrammatic representation (2). Diagram by Herbert Cole of W.G. Brigg. (Hocken Library, Dunedin) — xvi

A drawing and pastel of Grinlington by Tonks; watercolour by Lindsay of Sergeant Lee, Machine Gun Corps; watercolour by Herbert Cole of Gunner Sprout; detailed watercolour by Cole for the frontispiece of Pickerill's book, *Facial Surgery*. (RCS and Hocken Library, University of Otago, Dunedin) — xvii

A postcard of Parkwood Convalescent Hospital. (Author's collection) — xviii

Three paintings by John Hodgson Lobley, which depict the toy workshop, the woodwork department and the business school. (IWM 3756, 3728 and 3767) — xix

David Howard, East Surrey Regiment. Watercolour of original appearance. (RCS) — xx

Albert Parlett as an old man, c.1990. (Courtesy of the Parlett family) — xx

Private Webster. Watercolour by Daryl Lindsay, 10 February 1918. (RACS Archive, Melbourne) — xx

A Devin camera print produced for Gillies by Percy Hennell at Rooksdown Hospital, with the matching photograph dated May 1941. (Author's collection) — xxi

Francis Grayer on admission, 4 June 1917. (RCS) — xxi

The Frognal lawn in 1918, and the same view in 2009. (Author's collection) — xxii

Bruce Fowler. Watercolour by Herbert Cole; Fowler with his daughter, c.1980. (Courtesy of the RCS and the Fowler family) — xxiii

Bob Davidson, RAMC. Tonks' pastel of original appearance. (RCS) — xxiv

Sidney Beldam in the 1960s. (Courtesy of the Beldam family) — xxiv

William Spreckley c.1945. (Courtesy of the Spreckley family) — xxiv

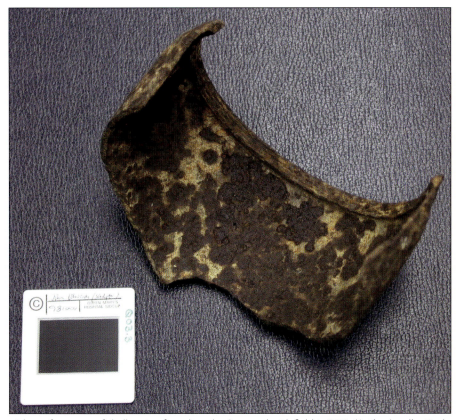

A large fragment of shell casing found on the Somme battlefield in 2001. (Author's collection)

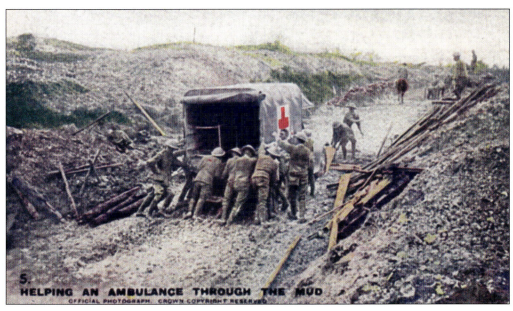

Troops helping to get an ambulance belonging to the 16th (Irish) Division through the mud in Mametz Wood, July 1916. Original photograph by John Warwick Brooke, IWM Q4015; tinted photo-postcard: *Daily Mail* Battle Collection, series 1, no.5. (Author's collection)

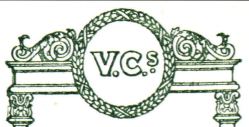

V.C.s

SERIES OF 50

No. 31.

CAPT. H. S. RANKEN, V.C.

Born in Glasgow in 1883. Went to the front in 1914 with the first part of the British Expeditionary Force. After his leg and thigh had been shattered, he continued to tend the wounded under rifle and shrapnel fire, sacrificing all chances of salvation to their needs. When he finally permitted himself to be carried back he died within a short time.

W.D & H.O. WILLS.
BRISTOL & LONDON.

No.31 of a series of 50 W.D. and H.O. Wills cigarette cards depicting winners of the Victoria Cross. Captain Harry Sherwood Ranken, RAMC was severely wounded in September 1914. He continued to treat men on the front line, but when he finally allowed himself to be evacuated, his condition was desperate. He died on 25 September 1914. (Author's collection)
Note: Another card series from Gallaher's illustrated Noel Chavasse and Arthur Martin-Leake, who were two of three double VC winners.

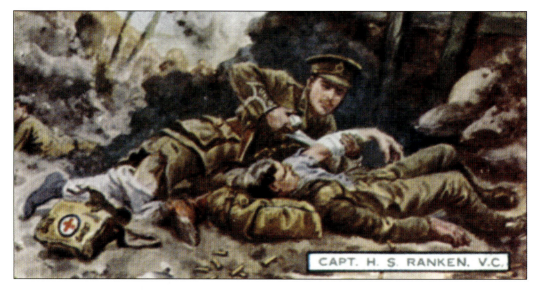

CAPT. H. S. RANKEN, V.C.

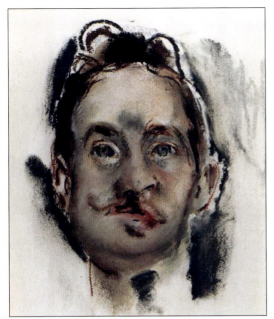
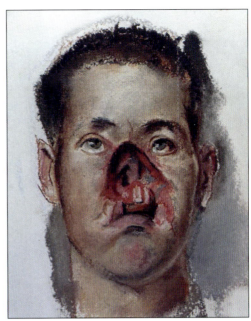

Pastel portraits of Reginald Evans, DCM and Albert Palmer. (RCS)

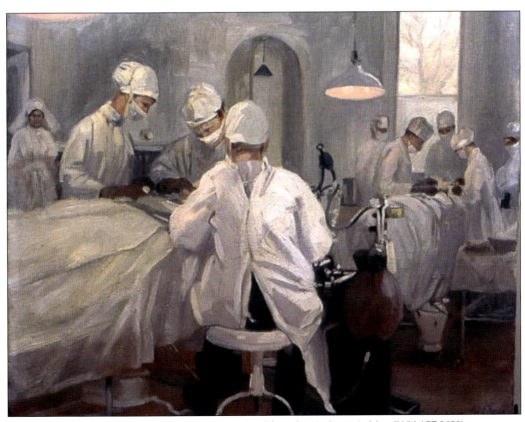

'The Plastic Theatre at the Queen's Hospital' by John Hodgson Lobley. (IWM ART 3659)

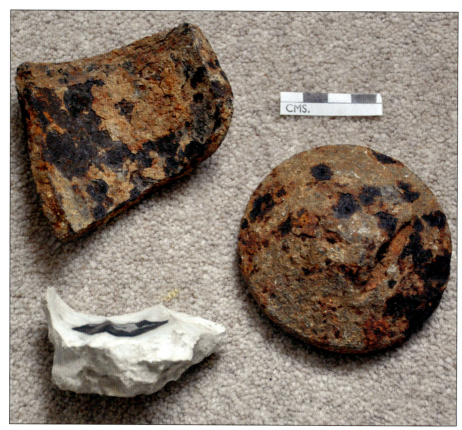

Shell fragments and a piece of flint recovered from the Somme battlefield; note the razor-sharp point to the flint. (Author's collection)

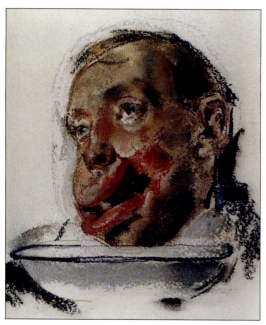

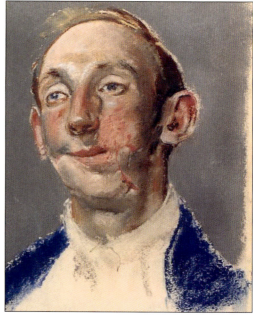

Pastels of Walter Ashworth by Henry Tonks before and after surgery. (RCS)

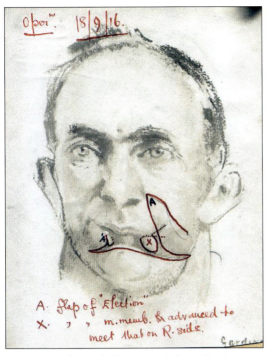

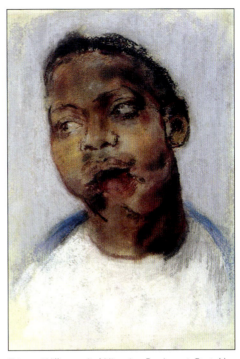

Private Gardiner, 7th Canterbury Infantry Regiment. Photograph of Tonks' pastel annotated by Gillies to show the soft tissue repair. (RCS)

Private Williams, 3rd Nigerian Regiment. Pastel by Tonks; photograph from Lane's album, with the dental appliance in place. (RCS and the Antony Wallace Archive, and the BAPRAS Archive)

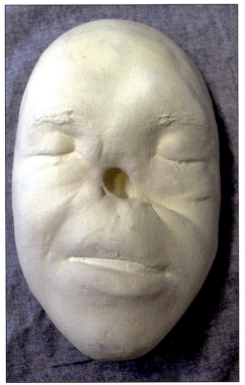

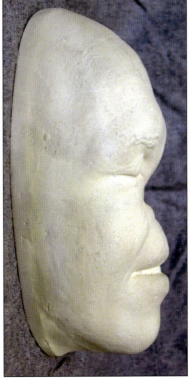

Plaster cast of Private F. Hamlett: full face and oblique view. (Author's photograph from a copy of the cast, which was kindly provided by the Royal Australasian College of Surgeons)

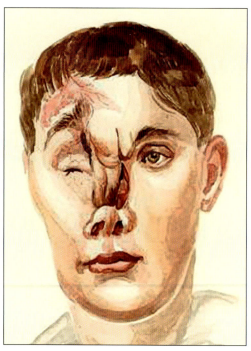

Private Len Tringham. Watercolour by Herbert Cole. (RCS)

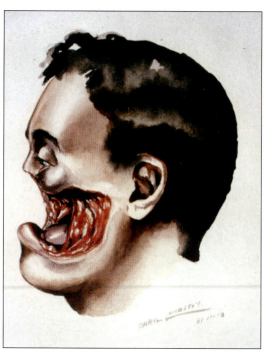

Private William Thomas, 1st Cheshire Regiment. Watercolour by Daryl Lindsay. (RACS Archive, Melbourne)

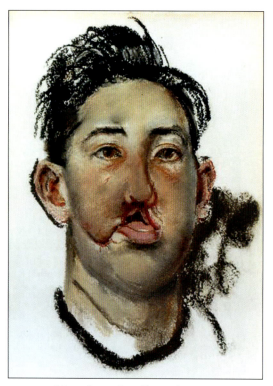

Private Stone. Pastel by Tonks. (RCS)

Opposite:
Private Green. The figures show the stages of constructing a new upper lip using a flap taken within the hair line to create a moustache. (RCS and Hocken Library, Dunedin)

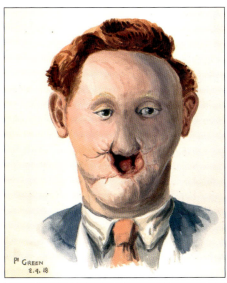

Pt Green
2.4.18

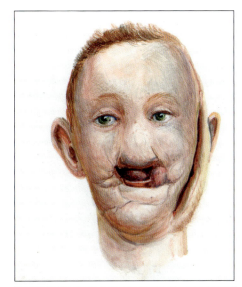

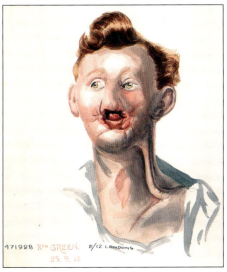

471928 Rfn GREEN. 2/12 LONDONS
23.9.18

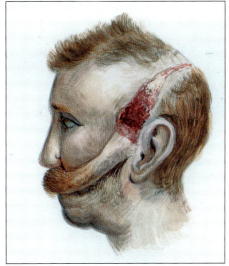

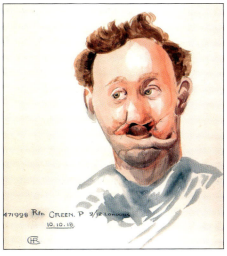

471928 Rfn GREEN. P 2/12 LONDONS
10.10.18.

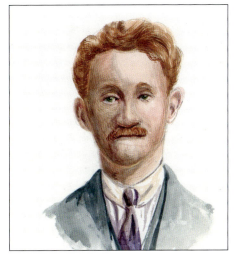

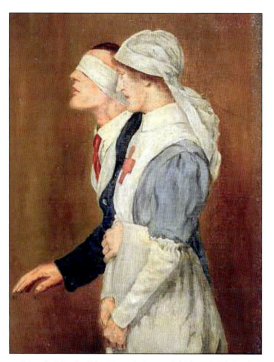

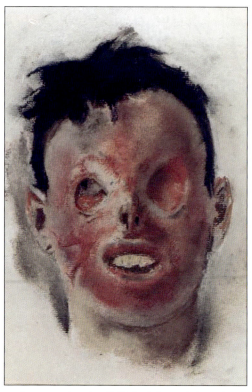

'Newly Blinded' by Francis Leopold Mond. A blind man, with hand outstretched and head raised, is led by a nurse. The painting was reportedly given as a raffle prize in aid of St Dunstan's, and hung for many years in a public house in South London. (Author's collection) Note: Information from David Cohen, from whom the author acquired the painting. The subject bears a strong resemblance to Sergeant Walter Bowen, who was a Sidcup patient.

Lieutenant Lumley, RFC. Tonks' pastel shows his appearance upon admission. (RCS)

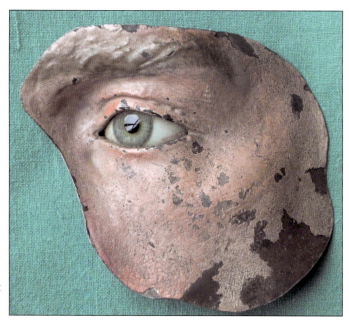

An eye mask incorporating a glass eye made by Archie Lane at Sidcup. (Author's collection)

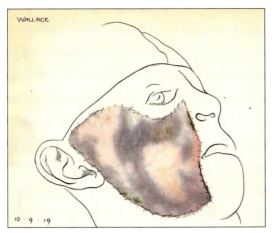
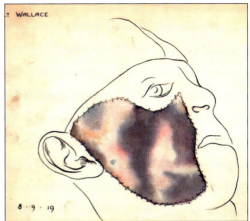
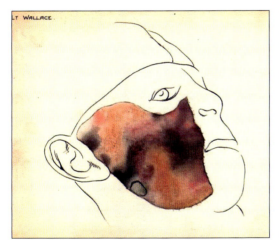
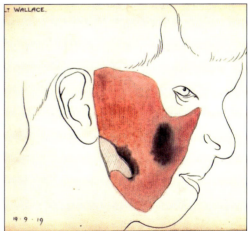

Lieutenant Wallace. Series of four watercolours showing the necrosis of the initial cheek flap taken from the buttock. (RCS)

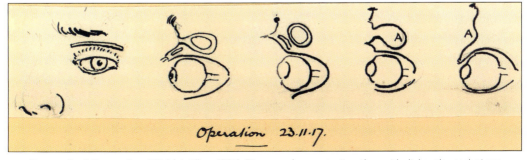

Gunner Cecil Grayer, Royal Field Artillery (RFA). Diagram demonstrating the epithelial outlay technique adapted by Gillies from Esser's inlay. (RCS)

No on Register 588

466 Pte Mears A.A   12 A.I.F.   Age 30   442

Wounded 20.9.17 (3 weeks Boloque Hospital) Admitted 12.10.17

GSW. Large extensive wound causing loss of whole of chin
lower lip + lower jaw from molar region to molar region
Upper jaw fractured.

19.10.17 Operation (Lieut. Bint.) freeing tongue, sequestrotomy
& Extractions

9.11.17 Further operation freeing tongue

26.2.18 Operation (Lieut. Col. Newland) preparatory to
reconstruction of soft parts of chin & lip.
Musculocutaneous flap attached above + below
was made from right Sternomastoid muscle
and its overlying skin. The skin edges were
sutured behind the flap which was then
skin grafted on its deep surface from the arm.
Small Tube drain from the neck.
                              18.4.18 Result quite successful.

18.4.18 Operation (Lt. Col. Newland) 2nd Stage to restore lower
                              lip + chin.

Curved incision made 1½in below the junction of
tongue with skin of the neck. The cutaneous flap
thus marked out was raised in order to form
lining for new lip. The mucous membrane of the
cheek was divided on Each side and the ends
of the curved flap were sutured to the lower
margin of the incision in the mucous membrane
The central portion of the cutaneous flap was

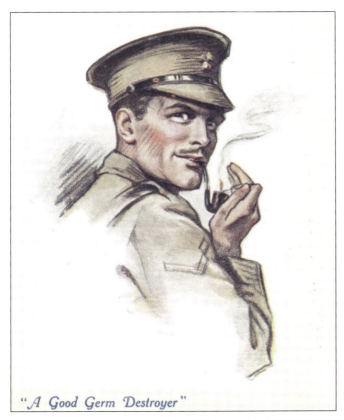

"A Good Germ Destroyer"

A postcard illustrating 'The Great Germ Destroyer'. Smoking was endemic, and many of the common respiratory problems later attributed to gas were smoking-related. (Author's collection)

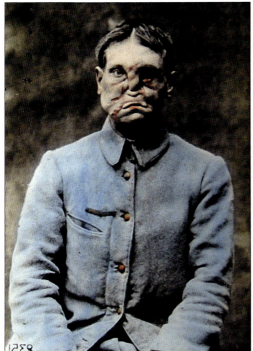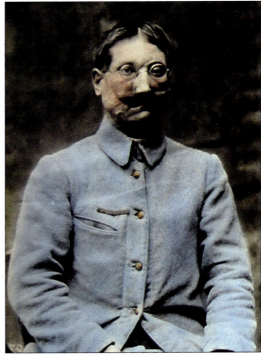

Hand-coloured photographs of a French soldier with and without his mask. The face beneath the mask is, from a surgical point of view, completed. (Author's collection)

pushed backwards and the upper edges sutured.

The incisions were now carried from the angle of the mouth on each side backwards to the ear and downwards just in front of the ascending ramus of mandible. These flaps were raised and slid inwards.

The red margin of the lip was formed from mucous membrane of the cheek which was sutured to the upper borders of the aforesaid flaps.

A large gap still remained. This was closed in the following way: A large semicircular incision was made at the lower end of the right sternomastoid which had been epithelialized at first operation.

This flap and the lower end of the sternomastoid were detached and raised to fill the gap in the lip and chin.   Wounds sutured and 3 drainage tubes inserted.

Note. The cheek flap on right side threatened to slough as the original wound had divided the facial artery.

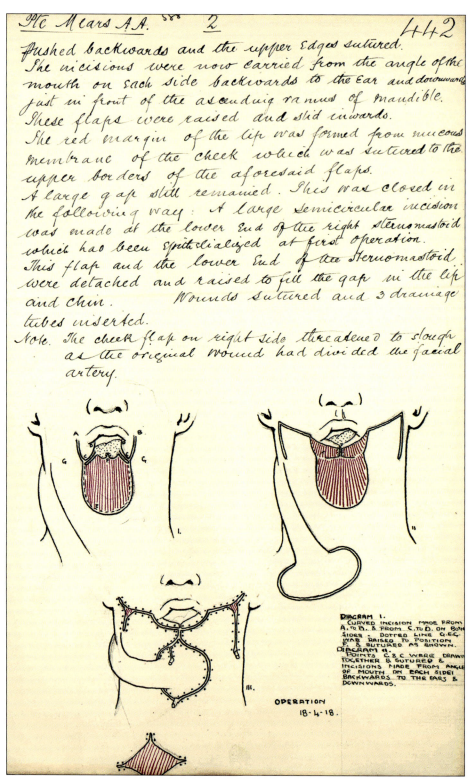

DIAGRAM I.
CURVED INCISION MADE FROM A. TO B. & FROM C. TO D. ON BOTH SIDES - DOTTED LINE G.E.G. WAS RAISED TO POSITION F. & SUTURED AS SHOWN.
DIAGRAM II.
POINTS C. & C. WERE DRAWN TOGETHER & SUTURED & INCISIONS MADE FROM ANGLE OF MOUTH ON EACH SIDE BACKWARDS TO THE EARS & DOWNWARDS.

OPERATION
18·4·18.

A diagram of the operation performed on Albert Mears to free his tongue from scar tissue and to reconstruct the jaw. (RCS)

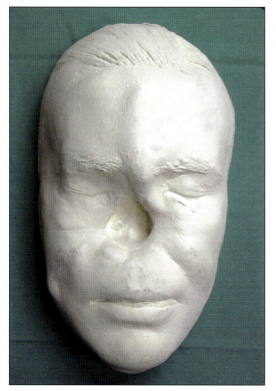
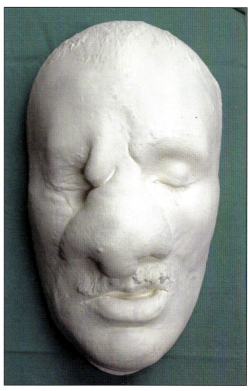

Plaster casts of Storrier, before and after a forehead flap rhinoplasty. (RACS Archive, Melbourne)

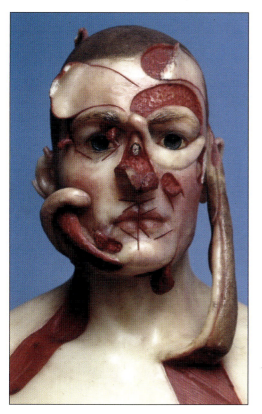

This wax model – created by Tom Kelsey for Pickerill – was used to demonstrate several surgical techniques. (RCS)

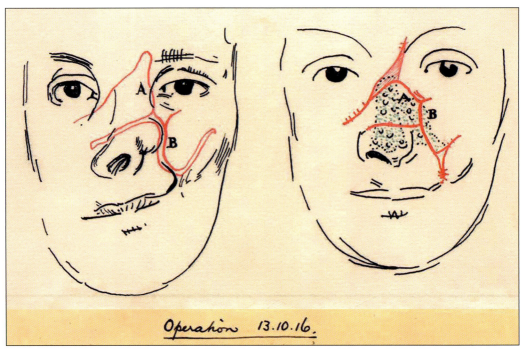

A comparison of diagrammatic representation (1). Diagram by Henry Tonks showing first stage of surgery on Spicer. (RCS)

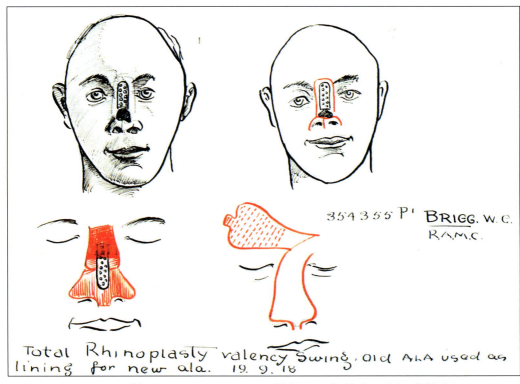

A comparison of diagrammatic representation (2). Diagram by Herbert Cole of W.G. Brigg. (Hocken Library, Dunedin)

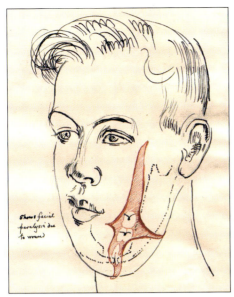

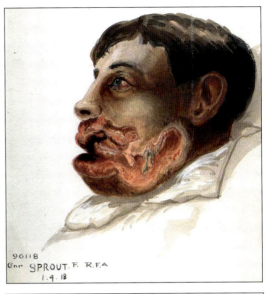

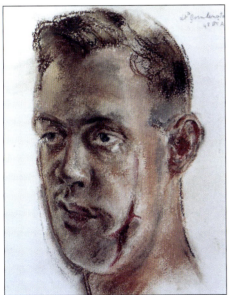

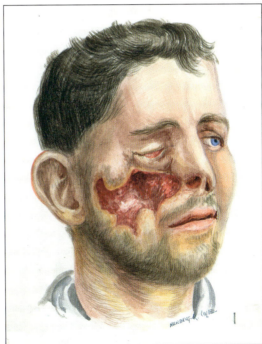

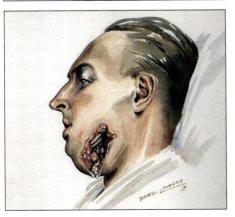

A drawing and pastel of Grinlington by Tonks; watercolour by Lindsay of Sergeant Lee, Machine Gun Corps; watercolour by Herbert Cole of Gunner Sprout; detailed watercolour by Cole for the frontispiece of Pickerill's book, *Facial Surgery*. (RCS and Hocken Library, University of Otago, Dunedin)

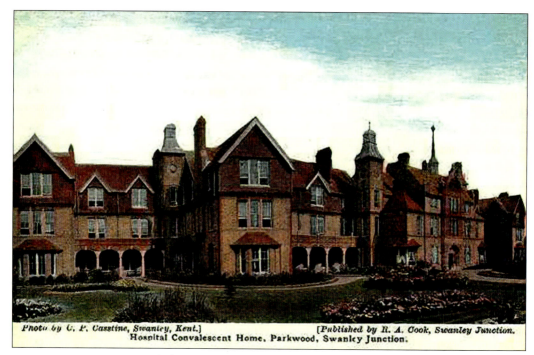

A postcard of Parkwood Convalescent Hospital. (Author's collection)

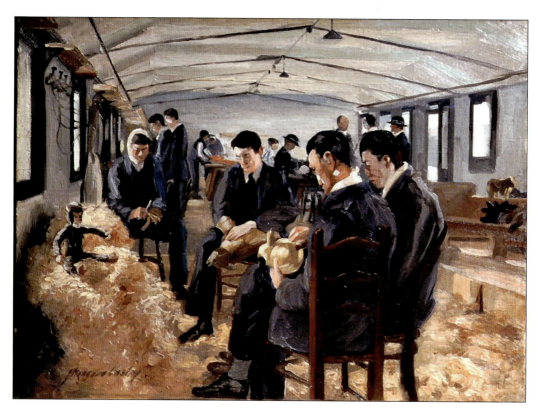

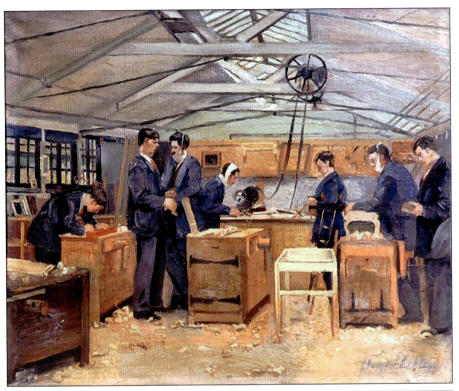

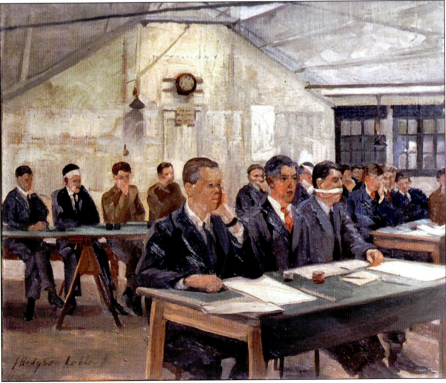

Three paintings by John Hodgson Lobley, which depict the toy workshop, the woodwork department and the business school. (IWM 3756, 3728 and 3767)

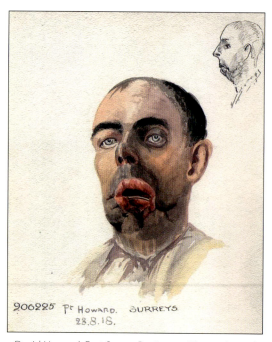

David Howard, East Surrey Regiment. Watercolour of original appearance. (RCS)

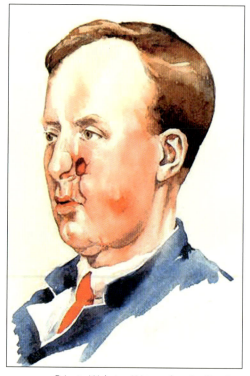

Private Webster. Watercolour by Daryl Lindsay, 10 February 1918. (RACS Archive, Melbourne)

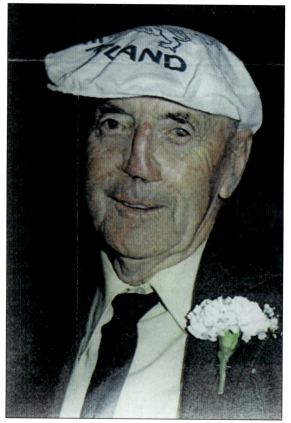

Albert Parlett as an old man, c.1990. (Courtesy of the Parlett family)

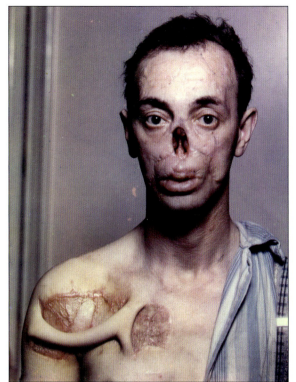
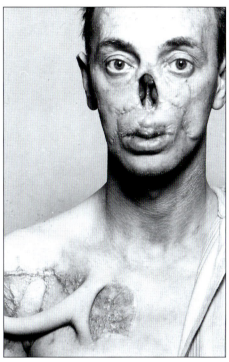

A Devin camera print produced for Gillies by Percy Hennell at Rooksdown Hospital, with the matching photograph dated May 1941. (Author's collection)

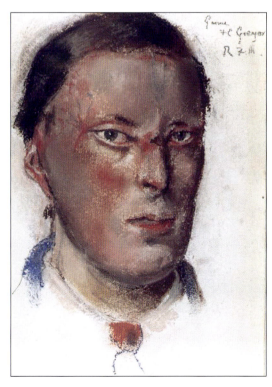

Francis Grayer on admission,
4 June 1917. (RCS)

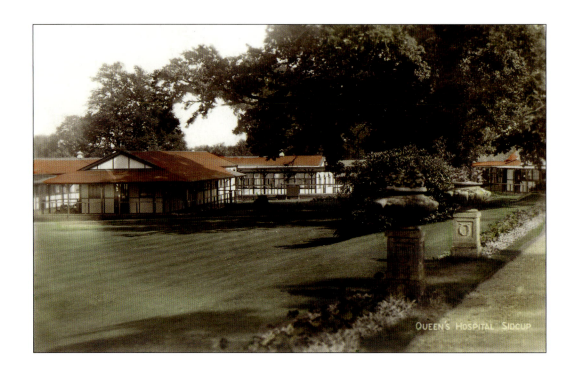

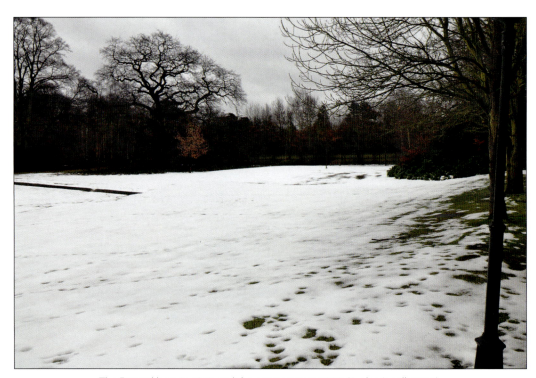

The Frognal lawn in 1918, and the same view in 2009. (Author's collection)

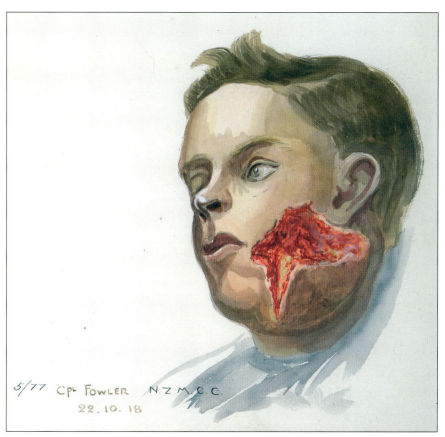

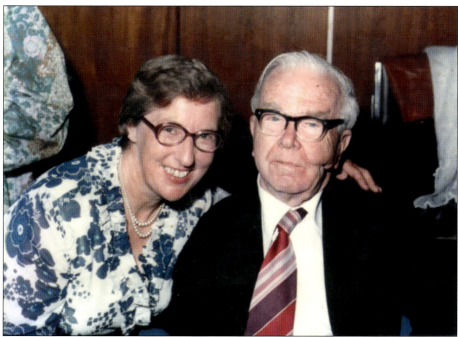

Bruce Fowler. Watercolour by Herbert Cole; Fowler with his daughter, c.1980.
(Courtesy of the RCS and the Fowler family)

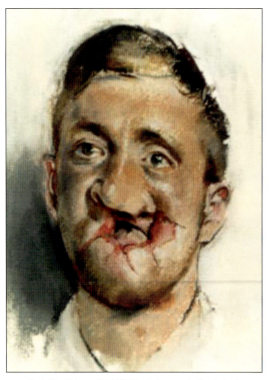

Bob Davidson, RAMC. Tonks' pastel of original appearance. (RCS)

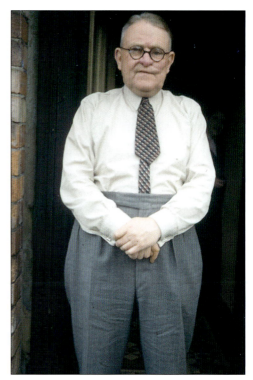

William Spreckley c.1945. (Courtesy of the Spreckley family)

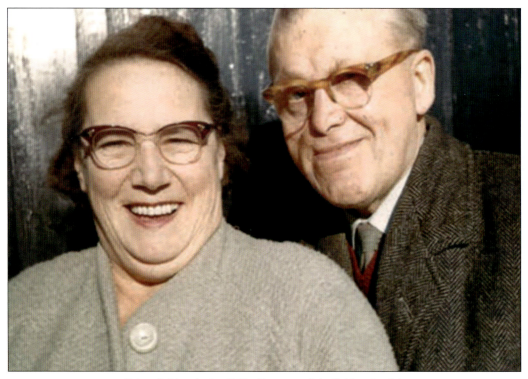

Sidney Beldam in the 1960s. (Courtesy of the Beldam family)

surgeons, appears in Henriette Rémi's account *Hommes sans Visage*.[52] First published in Switzerland in 1942, by which time another horrific conflict was well under way, Rémi's book covers the author's time as a hospital visitor to an institution which specialised in facial injuries. The vignettes within the text also indicate the scope of the horror of those forced to confront facial deformities. Each of Rémi's passages depicts an individual narrative of the difficulties with which the wounded approached their return to public life. The underlying message in Marc Dugain's fictionalised account of his grandfather's experience is the same.[53] Accounts show that the whole service was pervaded by what one might term learned hopelessness. The surgeons had no experience of the massive injuries they encountered and conveyed their despair at the task facing them to their patients, who in their turn became uneasy about having surgery. Furthermore, there was an expectation that disfigurement was to remain profound, and that the reaction to such disfigurement would be a frightening mixture of pity and horror in equal measure. Indeed, the portrayal of this likelihood was almost histrionic. Thus, it became almost an expectation that men would, for their own peace of mind, have to hide from the world. These ideas were exacerbated by the relative isolation of the different units. An Interallied Congress took place in Paris in 1916, from which a review journal was established to disseminate information on individual cases. However, if anything this simply deepened the gloom.[54] The Congress had participants from dental organisations in France, England, Canada, Italy and Portugal, as well as representation from the American Face and Jaw Hospital in Paris. Although the British medical services were represented by the senior physician and surgeon, Sir Wilmot Herringham and Sir Anthony Bowlby respectively, none of the surgeons who later worked at Sidcup were present, and neither was Morestin. Varastad Kazanjian contributed two papers to the journal, and Charles Valadier also submitted a paper, but the only British contribution came from a Manchester dentist by the name of Houghton. Without the opportunity to share direct experience in the operating theatre, and without any apparent drive to make systematic notes, any advances in technique were simply lost in the mass of severe wounds for which a fatalistic attitude prevailed.

Some patients were recorded in photographs, occasionally in sequential sets, but this never became a regular feature of note-taking in France (See Colour Section, p.xiii). Delaporte notes that such records were made at the discretion of the *Médecin du chef*.[55] The sets were added to record books which contained the surgeons' observations, but in the main they were all destroyed after the war. There is no evidence of any concerted effort to regularise note-keeping.

Another factor that inhibited developments in France was the maintenance of strict demarcation between patients. While at Sidcup, there was an officer's block with better facilities and food, in France there was both separation of officers and men and a segregation of junior and senior officers. Officers were managed in single rooms, and thus the opportunities for them to learn from each other's experience of surgery were significantly curtailed.

French treatment was inferior. Surgical services were widely dispersed and patients did not meet each other. The surgeons, once they considered they had finished, left the men to their own devices, unsupported either clinically or with thoughtful rehabilitation. The delicate balance of structure and function which was so important at Sidcup was set to one side, either unconsidered or ignored. Disfigurements were often masked rather than reconstructed; the

---

52 Rémi, *Hommes sans Visage*.
53 M. Dugain, *La Chambre des Officiers* (Paris: Éditions Jean-Claude Lattès, 1998).
54 The *Congrès Dentaire Interalliés* produced a 1,500-page report published in 1917. *La Restauration Maxillo-Faciale* was edited in Paris and ran to 33 monthly issues between April 1917 and December 1919.
55 Delaporte, *Gueules Cassées*, p.77.

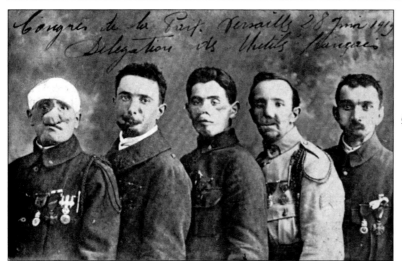

A photograph of the five *gueules cassées* brought by Clemenceau to the signing of the Treaty of Versailles, 1919. Albert Jugon, who was one of the founders of the *gueules cassées* (and who was later to found the French lottery), is fourth from the left. (*Union des Blessés de la Face et de la Tête*)

American sculptress Anna Coleman Ladd was the subject of a short film clip which showed her making masks in Paris for patients from the Val-de-Grâce Hospital.

A group of facially-injured patients was paraded at the signing of the Treaty of Versailles, as if to shame the vanquished nations by exhibiting the consequences of "their" war. Given such offhand and disengaged management, it is not surprising that the French *mutilés* formed their own society, *L'Union des Blessés de la Face et de la Tête*. Established in 1921 as a self-help and support organisation which gave advice and assistance to *les gueules cassées*, the union also offered retreats in society-owned properties to those whose treatment had resulted in life-changing injuries. The surgeons did not help them so they had to help themselves.

No similar organisation evolved in Britain after the war, as a consequence of the different approach to patient management. In England, the vast majority of patients came through the Queen's Hospital. As their treatment involved extended stays in Sidcup for weeks, months or years, the men got to know each other, a point reinforced by the plethora of group photographs. Patients in the later stages of reconstruction acted as models for later arrivals, who could themselves gain comfort from seeing the results of successful surgery. Sensitive follow-up by the surgeons, who were always happy to review patients if they had a problem, supplemented the feeling of solidarity among the British wounded. In addition, the patients were often given a set of their own medical photographs which reinforced their understanding of how much worse the outcome could have been. As well as the camaraderie of the wards, the provision of rehabilitation facilities on site gave men further opportunities to meet fellow patients and make friends. All these factors removed the need for a separate self-help group. It already existed.

The USA

The early American experience of surgery in the First World War is largely fragmentary, and comprises the accounts of surgeons working on behalf of the French in hospitals such as Neuilly. A formal maxillofacial presence came only at the very end of the conflict, and there is only one account which discusses facial surgery in a field hospital.[56] Some of the Americans

---

56 R.P. McGee, 'The maxillofacial surgeon in a mobile hospital', *Journal of the American Medical Association*, 73:15 (1919), pp.1,114-1,118.

had previous experience of facial work, and brought with them new and much needed surgical techniques.

The poet John Masefield recorded a visit to Neuilly in his letters, and noted the staff's "special pride" in:

> face-making … You go out to the front and have both your jaws and your nose blown away and everybody else says 'O Lord, Billy, you are settled as a lady's man'; but not a bit of it, you go to the Neuilly people, and they cut out one of your ribs and make you a new pair of jaws, with excellent teeth and palate … They shewed me some 50 casts of Before and After treatment and really they make human heads out of things that have no single feature left, not even a swelling.

In the dental clinic, Masefield saw:

> A man whose face had been divided diagonally, *comme ça:*- and at the same time shred round to one side. All the lower half of the face was 3 inches lower than it should have been and 2 inches too far to the left. They were engaged in hoisting the lower part back into position and propping it back to the right, with some most ingenious pads and props which were made next door. Then there was a man who had come in with neither nose nor jaw of any kind, and now was quite perfect but for a chin, which was going to be added immediately. They get hold of the man, and clean up the infection of the wound first, and then lay the sort of foundation of his future face by moulding new jaws for him; the jaws they make out of his spare ribs or out of bits of his leg, and when they have got the framework laid the surgeons set to work to put on a new covering of flesh, which they cut from the patients [sic] cheeks or elsewhere, and in some cases they make quite good new lips and noses … The dentists, who are jaw specialists and jaw artists make the frame and the surgeons cover it over. The man who was perfect but for a chin has been under treatment for a year and is now likely to have a few months more of treatment, and may then, for all I know, be recalled to the war.[57]

The official American effort was supposed to have been concentrated in at least three US army centres but, according to the surgeon John Staige Davis, author of a major reference work on plastic surgery, they "did little or no definitive work."[58] Instead, they simply prepared men for evacuation to the United States where the task of reconstruction took place. Davis' view is confirmed by Robert Ivy, who was sent to work at the American unit in Vichy in October 1918. Ivy wrote that "the primary object of treatment of maxillofacial cases was to get the severe ones into as good condition as possible for transfer back to the United States where definitive treatment could be carried out under more satisfactory surroundings."[59] Between September 1918 and January 1919, when the last patient was despatched to America, Ivy and his colleagues dealt with 305 patients. However, they had only performed 137 operations, of which just 30 were plastic procedures.

While Ivy acknowledged the help and advice of Fernand Lemaître, Varastad Kazanjian essentially worked alone. Kazanjian ran the Second Harvard Surgical Unit in Etaples. A dentist

---

57 P. Vansittart, (ed.), *John Masefield's Letters from the Front, 1915-1917* (London: Constable & Co, 1984), pp.120 onwards (diary entries for 3-4 September 1916).

58 J. Staige Davis, 'Plastic surgery in World War I and in World War II', *Annals of Surgery*, 123:4 (1946), pp.610-621.

59 Robert Ivy, *A Link with the Past* (Baltimore, MD: Waverly Press, 1962), p.45.

by training, his initial management was sound.[60] After the war, he wrote a chapter on facial injury for Barling and Morrison's *Manual of War Surgery*. His archive in Boston reveals that, although Kazanjian visited the Queen's Hospital, his isolation in France restricted his ability to disseminate the lessons on offer at Sidcup.[61] Other American surgeons also ventured to Sidcup to observe and learn, including Vilray Blair, George Dorrance, and Ferris Smith. Blair had a distinguished record as a war surgeon and Arbuthnot Lane was an admirer of his work. In fact, much as he had done with Henry Newland, Arbuthnot Lane asked Blair to report back on Gillies in order to be certain that Gillies was the right person to be left in charge of such a large and important unit. Blair told Lane that he had never seen anything like the quality and quantity of work that passed through the Sidcup operating theatres. He was also highly impressed with Gillies, and noted that his relative youth and lack of formal training were far outweighed both by the immense practical experience that Sidcup provided and by the team approach that Gillies had pioneered and fostered.[62]

Germany

A small number of surgeons worked in facial reconstruction in Germany. Jacques Joseph, like Gillies, was an ENT surgeon by training and had considerable experience of rhinoplasty.[63] He worked in Berlin, and was offered a professorial appointment by Kaiser Wilhelm in 1915. However, the appointment came with the stipulation that Joseph would convert from Judaism to Christianity, a condition Joseph was unwilling to accept. Joseph did attain professorial status after the war when the religious condition was dropped, but his suggestion during the conflict that cosmetic repair might influence the mood and character of the patient was anathema to the ideals of Prussian militarism.

The Dutch surgeon, Johannes Esser, worked in Brünn (now Brno) from May to December 1915, having previously been turned down for service by both the French and British. Esser gradually developed his facial surgery skills despite resistance from field surgeons, who took a great deal of persuading that facial patients should be referred to him. His rising reputation led to his appointment at the Imperial and Reserve Hospital No. 8 in January 1916, but his relationship with Anton von Eiselsberg, the director of the surgical university clinic, was a frosty one. Eiselsberg was passionately opposed to the development of plastic surgery as a specialty, and Esser complained that "In every possible way [he] was obstructed in his efforts to create a separate speciality of plastic surgery."[64] Esser felt that his time at the hospital had been wasted, and at the end of the year he accepted an invitation to move to Budapest where the working environment was far more congenial. In 1917, he was invited to move to Berlin, where several

---

60   See J.M. Converse, 'Plastic surgery, the twentieth century, the period of growth (1914-1939)', *Surgical Clinics of North America*, 47:2 (1967), pp.261-278. Converse records: "Gillies has told me of the remarkable condition of those patients received by him at Sidcup who had been treated by Kazanjian at Etaples before their evacuation to England."

61   Kazanjian's signature appears in the Queen's Hospital Visitors' Book, now held in the Wellcome Collection, yet Gillies makes no mention of Kazanjian's visit. On Kazanjian, see H.M. Deranian, *Miracle Man of the Western Front: Dr Varaztad H. Kazanjian, Pioneer Plastic Surgeon* (Worcester, MA: Chandler House, 2007). My thanks to Dr Martin Deranian for providing me with documentary evidence of Kazanjian's contact with Gillies.

62   F. McDowell, *The Source Book of Plastic Surgery* (Baltimore, MD: Williams & Wilkins, 1977), p.407.

63   P. Natvig, *Jacques Joseph: Surgical Sculptor* (Philadelphia, PA: W.B. Saunders, 1982).

64   B. Haeseker, *Dr. J.F.S. Esser and his influence on the development of plastic and reconstructive surgery* (Rotterdam: Erasmus Universiteit, 1983), p.47.

surgeons referred work to him. In Berlin, he pioneered arterial flaps and invented the epithelial inlay technique that was later adapted by Gillies for eyelid reconstruction.

Hans Pichler, from Vienna, managed a reconstructive unit. He would later become famous for treating Sigmund Freud, but his experience up to 1936 was mainly confined to the treatment of injuries to the lower jaw. Pichler's descriptions of his wartime work encapsulate the German experience:

> Those who had escaped death by a 'hair's breadth' arrived in the hinterland with terrible lacerations of the face and enormous wounds in the mouth, full of tooth and bone splinters, dripping with ichorous pus and saliva, unable to speak or to eat and already at this point less concerned about their life than about their human face and their human speech. Thus they were delivered at the beginning of the war, sometimes a dozen at a time, to the clinic of Professor Eiselsberg because this man – in advance of most others – had recognised that in such cases a dental surgeon or surgical dentist would be able to help.
>
> I moved with my dental technician, my two female assistants and two dental chairs into a modest room in the clinic, and now had to clean up, to rinse, to feed and to bandage all day, to make impressions and plaster casts of the shattered jaw fragments, to put them together in the right position and after that to construct prostheses for the jaw and teeth which were to keep them in their correct position. A new firm basis was thus created on which the torn soft parts could be stitched together. This fundamental principle was to prevail and prove successful. When I was allocated a medical man whom I was able to train in cleaning mouths and taking impressions that was already a great step forward. Thus we worked at Christmas 1914 one day after the other till 11pm, and to this day I cannot understand how my staff were able to endure these exertions. I believe it was only the matchless patience and courage of the wounded which kept them going.
>
> This was the beginning of what eventually became the jaw ward of the Surgical Clinic I, which in the course of the war laboriously patched up many hundreds of facially injured. Sometimes for one case alone dozens of prostheses and splints had to be made and twenty or more operations done in order to add to a face what a bullet had left of it.
>
> The war ended, the jaw ward has remained; even today [1935] it still has to deal at times with the consequences of the war, but in the main it still works with the same methods as before.[65]

Reconstruction was primarily done by dentists and dental surgeons like Hugo Ganzer, whose operative experience was extensive, but whose failure to take a medical degree stymied his later career. Pichler's comments are mirrored in other German texts of the period, which contain little mention of *Plastik* surgery and are largely concerned with dental and mandibular realignment and splinting.[66] Like the French, German surgeons worked in isolation and so did not benefit from the lively debate and exchange of experience that was customary at Sidcup. Often, as Esser found in Vienna, the surgical hierarchy stifled collaboration and continued to believe

---

65 H. Pichler. Quoted in *Ärtzte und ihre Helfer im Weltkriege 1914-1918*, ed. by B. Breitner (Vienna: Verlag Amon Franz Goeth, 1936). I am grateful to the late Anne Meyer for the translation.

66 See, for example, C. Bruhn, *Die Gegenwärtigen Behandlungswege der Kieferschussverletzungen. Ergebnisse aus dem Düsseldorfer Lazaret für Kieferverletzte (Kgl Reservelazarett)* (Wiesbaden: Verlag von J.F. Bergmann, 1915-1917).

that facial work could be performed by any general surgeon.

As in France, reconstruction was crude and many men were left with a substantial disfigurement. Ernst Friedrich's polemic *Nie Wieder Krieg* underlines these outcomes through illustrations of disfigured men and ironic captions which indicated that, despite substantial residual disfigurement, their treatment was considered to be complete. Disfigured beggars on the streets were an unattractive sight, and men were treated with contempt. But unlike in France, no self-help group developed in Germany. Men were, at least initially, better supported by the State, which mitigated the financial consequences for those who could no longer follow their pre-war occupation because of their disfigurement.

Conclusion

This chapter has demonstrated the breadth of injuries encountered by the surgeons of the Queen's Hospital. As a result of Gillies' decision to bring all the casualties and surgeons to one place, it became possible to refine previously crude techniques and to invent entirely new ones. By contrast, indi-

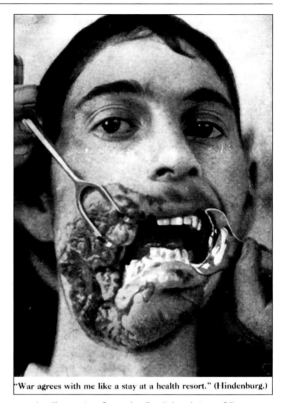

"War agrees with me like a stay at a health resort." (Hindenburg.)

An illustration from the English edition of Ernst Friedrich's book *Nie Wieder Krieg*. The ironic caption underlines the failure to achieve a successful reconstruction. (Author's collection)

vidual surgeons working in France and Germany did not have a large throughput of cases and did not discuss their results or collaborate. In addition, they failed to teach others and, in some cases, were even actively discouraged from specialising in facial work. In terms of surgical technique, Gillies and his team left them behind.

Gillies was acutely aware of and upset by the poor results obtained elsewhere. Several patients had returned to England from POW camps where surgery had been botched, and Gillies had to spend a great deal of time undoing what had been done before he could restart the surgical process. He wrote of one such patient that he was "an example of plastic surgery gone wrong."

These cases were fundamental to Gillies' development of the principle that normal tissue should be restored to normal position, and only then should tissue be brought from elsewhere to fill the gaps. Yet Gillies was far from complacent, and acknowledged his own failings alongside those of other surgeons. He wrote that:

> there were many [instances] in which our results fell far short of the ideal. We notice that if we made a poor repair for a wretched fellow the man's character was inclined to change for the worse. He would be morose, break rules and give trouble generally. Conversely, if we made a good repair, the patient usually became a happy convalescent and soon regained his old character and habits. This seems but to emphasise again the powerful influence that our physical appearance wields over our character. For instance, if my bald head suddenly flourished with a crop of curly red locks and my

receding chin became thick and square, imagine how pleasant my personality would become. This might be offered here as an excuse to all those nice people to whom I have been so rude.[67]

Despite its levity, this quotation contains a disturbing profundity. The resurgence of bellicosity in Germany in the late 1920s and early 1930s was fuelled by an undercurrent of discontentment within the ranks of disabled ex-servicemen, whose sudden loss of State benefits during the collapse of the German economy exacerbated the suffering they had endured, and continued to endure, as a result of injuries which had been imperfectly treated.[68] The images of Dix, Beckmann and Grosz, and the photographs of Friedrich, were thrust upon the public as symbols of unjust loss in a manner that, thanks to the work of the Queen's Hospital, did not take place in Britain.

---

67 Gillies and Millard, *Principles and Art*, p.45.
68 D. Cohen, *The War Come Home. Disabled Veterans in Britain and Germany, 1914-1939* (Berkeley, CA: University of California Press, 2001).

4

A Revolution in Record-Keeping

Harold Gillies' approach to record-keeping was a fundamental component of the surgical advances at the Queen's Hospital. This chapter details the nature, purpose and importance of patient case files, with a particular focus on their inclusion of visual records. In 1920 and 1957, Gillies published two major books on plastic surgery, using the records themselves as an *aide-memoire*. The latter work set out his principles of plastic surgery, which might be considered to have reformed patient management far beyond plastic surgery. Gillies' principles were largely based on his First World War experience, and this chapter deconstructs the evolution of his thinking by relating each principle to specific cases from the surviving records. The patient records from Sidcup have also had an impact beyond the medical world. The visual records created by men such as Henry Tonks and Daryl Lindsay have also played a poignant, visceral role in the remembrance and commemoration of the First World War. Their work provides a unique insight into the experience of war, especially the consequences for those who were affected by the particular circumstances of the Western Front.

The creation of detailed patient records owed a huge debt to Gillies' meticulous standards. Plastic surgery was, in his own words, "a new art" and one which required definition. The work at Sidcup built upon the expertise garnered by the growing team of surgeons, dentists and other staff. Gradually, they learned how to ensure that surgical mistakes were minimised. The level of detail recorded in the surgical notes enabled Gillies and his team to look back at previous cases and modify their techniques accordingly. However, most of the British surgeons abandoned facial surgery at the end of the war; the cosmetic remodelling of faces for aesthetic purposes was looked down upon by doctors, surgeons and the public. Gillies realised that fewer opportunities to experiment with plastic surgery techniques would be available in civilian life. Even in the more dangerous sectors of the British economy, such as the coal and steel industries, there was nothing that produced serious facial injuries in as great a number as industrial warfare. Gillies was eager, to the point of obsession, to ensure the preservation of the Sidcup records for future reference as a teaching resource. The variety of injuries produced by the war, involving every part of the face, provided sufficient base material for almost any conceivable casualty in civilian life. The retention of the surgical records from the Queen's was essential to the establishment of plastic surgery as a specialism.

Visual Records: Artists, Sculptors and Photographers

The records began simply. Early patients at Aldershot were detailed in fairly brief handwritten notes, sometimes accompanied by diagrams drawn by Henry Tonks and a single photograph of the patients' original appearance. As time passed, Gillies and his colleagues realised that facial surgery was unlike the majority of contemporary surgical procedures. Reconstruction was not an in-and-out, one-stop business. Their experiences, coupled with the arrival of men

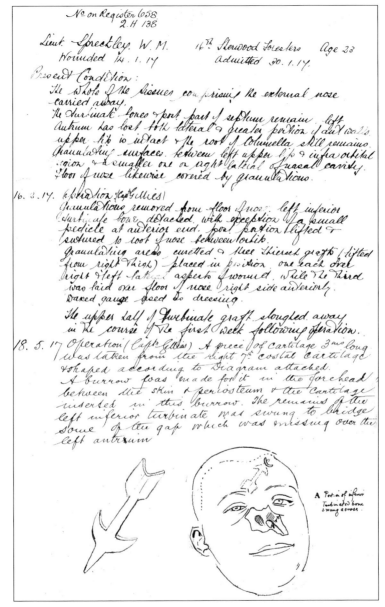

The first page of the case notes of Lieutenant William Spreckley. The notes are handwritten, and the diagram and annotation are by Henry Tonks. (RCS)

who had already received treatment elsewhere, led to the development of staged surgery. As a result, it was necessary to be able to refer back to the details of previous operations, and essential to record these details more precisely. Consequently, the operation notes at Sidcup became longer and more informative. The name of the surgeon was always recorded, and the type of anaesthesia employed was noted.

Gillies' obsession with accurate and comprehensive records was complemented by Tonks' work at Sidcup. The synergy between the ascetic, artistic perfectionist Tonks, and the jocular, polymath surgical perfectionist Gillies was remarkable. Tonks and Sydney Hornswick standardised the methods for recording flap operations. They took notes in the operating theatre and drew up the diagrams later. Drawings by Tonks appear in the notes of Sidcup patients until November 1917, perhaps because by that point Hornswick had demonstrated his competence. Tonks had also been influenced by the offer to become an official war artist, and another competent artist replaced him. Daryl Lindsay, the son of a doctor, belonged to a large family of Australian artists of whom his brother Norman was the most famous. The New Zealand section also recruited an artist, Herbert Cole, from within its own staff. Cole, originally from England, was part of the New Zealand Army Medical Corps and had been transferred to Sidcup in April 1918. After the war, he found modest fame as a landscape artist under the pseudonym Rix Carlton.

In an article entitled 'Five Men', Daryl Lindsay described his recruitment process and initial experiences of life as a medical artist. He wrote:

> My going to Sidcup came about through a casual meeting with Colonel Jock Anderson and Sir Neville Howse at Horseferry Road – they wanted somebody who could draw medical diagrams for [Henry] Newland.[1] Would I go down at once and see Newland? I was due back in France the next day, but they fixed up an extension of leave, and it was not until months later that I discovered I had been 'A.W.L.' for 30 days.[2]

Lindsay reported for duty just as Newland was on his way to the operating theatre, and he watched the surgeon perform the second stage of a nasal reconstruction. He was unsure whether he could "translate what looked like a mess of flesh and blood into a diagram that a student could understand." Newland, however, had every confidence in Lindsay, and persuaded him to stay on.

The latter recalled his first meeting with Tonks as having become:

> aware of being overlooked by a tall, hatchet-faced man, who looked like a cross between a Roman emperor and a wedge-tailed eagle. He asked me what I was doing, and I said 'Trying to draw'. He said 'I'm glad you said 'trying', which is the best that can be said of it; but I think I may be able to help you'.

Tonks offered help in the form of granting Lindsay a day's release each week to study at the Slade School of Art in London. Tonks terrified many of his students: "There were stories of girl students jumping out of second-story windows or wanting to drown themselves at a critical word from the master," wrote Lindsay. However, Tonks admired people who stood up to him. Lindsay, a brash Aussie not afraid to speak his mind, revealed a contretemps with Tonks in class:

> My third lesson from Tonks led me into saying 'I'm sorry, but I don't know what you are talking about. I know the meaning of the words, but not their application to art.' This so staggered Tonks that he stalked from the room and an hour later sent for me. The other students looked at me with sorrow as one condemned to the gallows. It was an interesting conversation – or argument – and ended in my being asked to supper with him the next Sunday night.

---

1   Howse was Director of the Australian Imperial Force's medical services. A British-trained doctor, he was the first Australian to have won the Victoria Cross, which was awarded for his rescue of a casualty in the Boer War at Vredefort in 1900.

2   Daryl Lindsay, 'Five Men', *Medical Journal of Australia*, 18 January 1958, p.62. Unless otherwise stated, all quotations in the following passage are taken from this source.

Tonks' suppers were small and select affairs, and Lindsay soon realised that his admission to the circle had been quite an honour. Under Tonks' fearsome exterior was a man with humour and sympathy for youth, and in 'Five Men', Lindsay rated him the finest art teacher in England in the previous 100 years.[3]

Despite the presence of such talented artists, Gillies was not satisfied. The classic textbooks of Charles Nélaton and Louis Ombredanne demonstrated the limitations of operative drawings. These books were full of stylised diagrams, but contained no photographs. Photographs were easier to understand than diagrams, and during the American Civil War, the appearances of cases at the beginning and end of their surgical experience had been recorded. Yet these images had not been accompanied by information to indicate how the, results had been achieved. At Sidcup, photographs, largely those taken by Sidney Walbridge (1883-1954), were the backbone of the medical records.[4] Walbridge had been a photographer before the war. He was called up in 1915 and joined the Machine Gun Corps attached to the Hampshire Regiment. In December 1916, he was transferred to the RAMC, and from family information it appears that he served at the Cambridge Military Hospital where he presumably encountered Gillies.[5] Walbridge used a plate camera which took full, half and quarter-plate glass negatives, and as time passed the recording process became more systematic and ultimately standardised.[6] A number of surviving images show the head-rest against which the patient was positioned, which allowed for exact comparisons of the stages of surgery. Walbridge recorded each stage of surgery, often from three or even five angles; full face, side, and oblique views were the most common. Where it was necessary to show some functional element, such as the effect of a nerve injury which caused a facial palsy, active and passive views were obtained to demonstrate muscle weakness or recovery of function. For example, a sequence of photographs was taken of patients with burns to the eyelids which showed the patients initially unable to, and ultimately able to, close their eyes. Stereo photography was also used substantially at Aldershot, but was abandoned at Sidcup as plaster casts provided a more accurate representation of the three-dimensional appearance.[7] The experiment with stereo photography was more of a curiosity than a surgical aid.

The surgeons were keen to reconstruct their patients' faces to as close an appearance to the original as possible, and many patients' notes included either pre-war or pre-injury portraits or snapshots of the men. The photographs were used to plan surgery as well as to demonstrate the stages of the surgical process. The use of photographs and plaster casts allowed the production of an accurate template for flaps. While the surviving notes are variable in length and detail, the most complex cases, such as that of Albert Mears, contain a remarkably long sequence of details (See Colour Section, p.xiv). This complexity was new. Surgeons had never recorded their work in such a way before and, by the end of the war, the details provided were sufficient for any surgeon to understand what had been done. The notes were not self-congratulatory, and documented both failures and successes. As with the development of photography as an aid to the written notes, diagrammatic representations of the surgery evolved from Tonks' quick sketches to detailed, annotated drawings by Hornswick, Lindsay, and Cole. The drawings were often reproduced on blueprint paper, to serve as an educational resource for Gillies' team. Before

---

3   This is commemorated by Pat Barker's novel *Life Class* (London: Hamish Hamilton, 2007).
4   Gillies' seminal role in standardising photography was recognised by his election to Fellowship of the Royal Photographic Society in 1952.
5   Rosy St Brooke, personal communication.
6   After the war, Walbridge had a photography studio in South London, but nothing is known about him.
7   A large collection of stereo cards survives in the Army Medical Services Museum, but they are unaccompanied by medical notes.

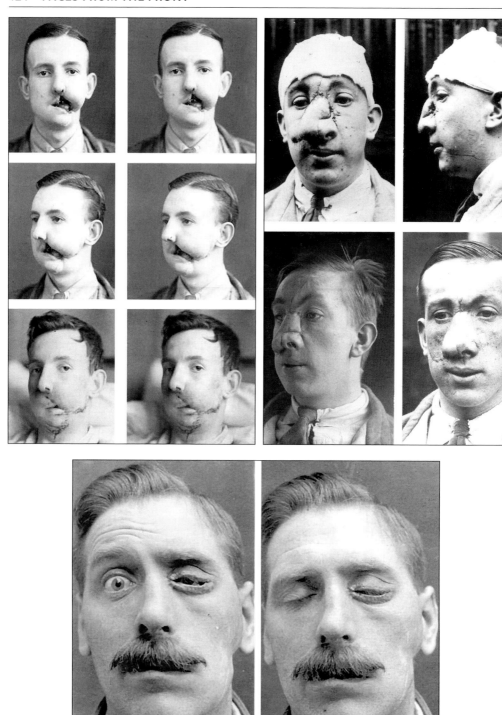

Above and overleaf: The scope of photography at Sidcup. Stereo photographs of Cecil Smith; photograph page of Day showing different face views; photographs of Dawkins showing his facial palsy, with the left view demonstrating loss of function, as he attempts to raise his eyebrows; demonstration page showing the ability to close eyes following the epithelial outlay technique in a burns patient. (RCS and the author's collection)

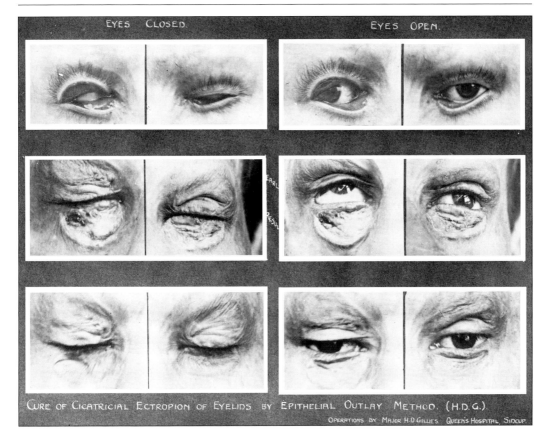

EYES CLOSED.   EYES OPEN.

CURE OF CICATRICIAL ECTROPION OF EYELIDS BY EPITHELIAL OUTLAY METHOD. (H.D.G.)
OPERATIONS BY MAJOR H.D.GILLIES. QUEEN'S HOSPITAL. SIDCUP.

this work began, there was no significant reference work that showed either the real results of plastic surgery or how those results were achieved.

As noted above, the visual recording work at the Queen's Hospital was not restricted to two dimensions. While the artists recorded what they saw, Kathleen Scott, noted sculptress and widow of the polar explorer Robert, was prevailed upon by Tonks to model new faces at Sidcup. Her initial reaction at Sir John Ellerman's hospital in Regent's Park was unfavourable. Her diary for 1918 recorded:

> October 1st. I went to Ellerman's hospital to fix about modelling faces. I saw a man without any mouth, and am to model him ... October 5th. At the hospital I worked on the man with no mouth – rather bad. They asked me, if I could stand it, and I replied confidently that I could, and I did, but I was very unwell when the tension was over ... October 19th. I am to model a chin for a man at the hospital. I feel terribly like God, the creator. The surgeon said with a smile 'Don't make it too long, or we shan't have enough to cover it.' Sad! It's a fantastic world ... November 4th. At the hospital I worked on a man with a wonderful face and no nose. These men with no noses are beautiful, like antique marbles.[8]

---

8   K. Scott, *Self-Portrait of an Artist, from the Diaries and Memoirs of Lady Kennet* (London: John Murray, 1949), pp.167-168.

Nº on Register 588

466 <u>Pte Mears</u> A.A   12 A.I.F.   Age 30   442

Wounded 20.9.17 (3 weeks Boloque Hospital) Admitted 12.10.17

GSW. Large extensive wound causing loss of whole of chin lower lip + lower jaw from molar region to molar region Upper jaw fractured.

19.10.17 Operation (Lieut. Birt) freeing tongue, sequestrotomy + Extractions

9.11.17 Further operation freeing tongue

26.2.18 Operation (Lieut. Col Newland) preparatory to reconstruction of soft parts of chin + lip. Musculocutaneous flap attached above + below was made from right Sterno-mastoid muscle and its overlying skin. The skin Edges were sutured behind the flap which was then skin grafted on its deep surface from the arm. Small Tube drain from the neck.

18.4.18 Result quite Successful.

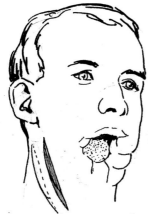

18.4.18 Operation (Lt. Col Newland) 2nd Stage to restore lower lip + chin.

Curved incision made 1½in below the junction of tongue with skin of the neck. The cutaneous flap thus marked out was raised in order to form lining for new lip. The mucous membrane of the check was divided on Each side and the ends of the curved flap were sutured to the lower margin of the incision in the mucous membrane. The central portion of the cutaneous flap was

Above and overleaf: A series of diagrams of the operations performed on Albert Mears to free his tongue from scar tissue and to reconstruct the jaw. (RCS)

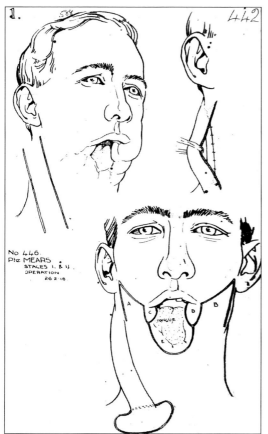

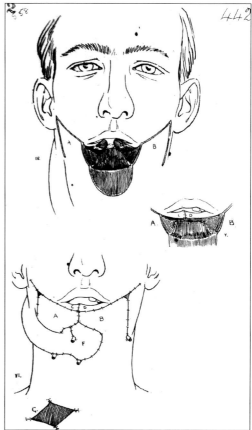

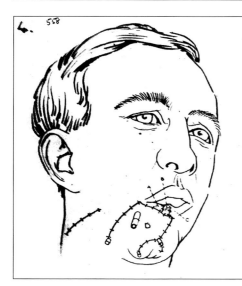

No 446.
Pte MEARS   STAGE III.

OPERATION FOR LOSS OF LOWER LIP & CHIN

DIAG I.
    A & C . Flaps of mucous membrane
    B. Flap of skin turned up to form lining to lip
    D. Sterno-mastoid flap detached at upper end

DIAG II.
    Showing flaps A. B & C turned up.

DIAG III.
    Same as DIAGS I & II with flap D turned down.

DIAG IV.
    Flaps sutured in place. Drain tubes. Wound
    left by division of upper pedicle sutured.

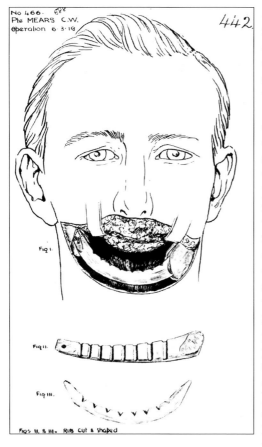

No 466.
Pte MEARS C.W.
Operation 6. 3.19.

442

Fig I.

Fig II.

Fig III.

Figs II. & III. Rib cut & shaped

Scott appears to have modelled a few men as a form of portraiture, but she did not remain at Sidcup for long.[9] Nonetheless, as a consequence of her work, along with that of Derwent Wood at Wandsworth, Gillies realised that working in three dimensions had substantial advantages.

While photographs and paintings might capture the essence of a problem, it was much easier to visualise what needed to be done on an accurate model (See Colour Section, p.xv). Gillies drew on photographs, and even upon photographs of Tonks' pastels, but by first mapping out the incisions on a plaster cast the surgeons were able to recreate them in the flesh with a far higher degree of accuracy. By chance, a patient who had lost half of his face overheard a discussion between Gillies and a colleague about Gillies' wish for someone with anatomical knowledge who could make models and implants to hang his grafts on. The patient, who was unable to speak, gestured for paper and pencil and wrote down the name of an old friend of his, John Edwards. Stationed on the east coast, Edwards was alarmed when he received a summons to report to the War Office, where he found Gillies waiting to take him to Sidcup. Edwards recorded his work there in an album. The collection of images was found one day by Edwards' young son, who read it secretly under the stairs. He was discovered and admonished as the contents were deemed unsuitable for young eyes. None of the family has seen it since.[10] The casts he made were used for more than hanging grafts on. The artists, having made quick life sketches during surgery, used Edwards' casts to complete their paintings. Daryl Lindsay was photographed in his studio doing precisely that. Some of the casts were even painted in a lifelike fashion, perhaps because the mannequins were intended for display in the hospital's museum.

Masks were also made up from the casts. Ward Muir described his process, in which the cast was filled with Plasticine to recreate a normal contour, from which another cast was taken. A thin metal plate was then beaten out over the second cast. The mask making process was a highly skilled task undertaken by some of the dental technicians who possessed a broad range of talents. Archie Lane, who after the war qualified as a dentist and practised in Orpington, made many of the dental splints and appliances.[11] He also constructed a number of the so-called 'Tin Faces', two of which survive. Lane compiled albums of his work, like Albert Norman at Stamford Street, which document the various facets of plastic work and detail interesting cases.

9   Scott's son, Wayland Young (Lord Kennet), recalled seeing some of the faces as a child, but did not know what had happened to them. Lord Kennet, personal communication.
10   John Edwards' daughter Thirza, personal communication.
11   His albums are held in the BAPRAS Archive.

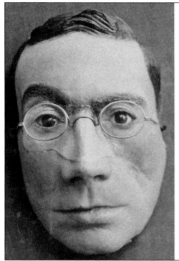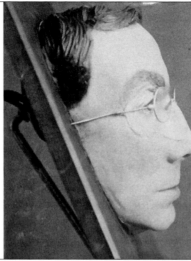

A photograph from the album of Archie Lane showing a painted plaster cast with applied mask. (BAPRAS Archive)

The albums included admission photographs, intermediate stage pictures, and several cast and mask series. They also contain a large selection of dental prostheses and splints, some of which were clearly derived from the splints devised before the war in the United States and Germany, and some of which were new designs. Lane's albums represent the most complete record of the technical work performed at Sidcup, and some of his illustrations appeared in the chapter on facial injuries in the Official History of the Medical Services.[12]

Teaching models were also created to demonstrate the various surgical procedures undertaken at Sidcup. Tom Kelsey, a modeller attached to the New Zealand section, was responsible for making two wax models used to teach surgeons about flaps, pedicles and bone grafts (See Colour Section, p.xv). He also made a small number of moulages which are now in the possession of the Oral Surgery Department in Dunedin. Two of his post-war wax models, which detail dissected structures in the neck, have also survived and are in the possession of the Anatomy Museum in Otago University. Close inspection of the models reveals that one portrayed Lenin and the other Stalin. It is unclear whether this was a joke, or an expression of Kelsey's political beliefs.

Record-keeping went beyond individual case notes, and Gillies oversaw the establishment of a museum while the Queen's Hospital was still functioning, which was described in a report of 1930:

> One special feature of the Queen's Hospital was the Facial museum. This was designed to contain as complete a collection as possible of examples of the work done in these branches of surgery. Here were kept wax models, plaster casts, diagrams and coloured sketches of every sort of facial injury taken at different times in the history of the individual cases, and showing therefore the amelioration achieved through restorative treatment. This museum formed a work of permanent historical value to all students of facial injuries.[13]

---

12 H.D. Gillies and B. Mendleson, 'Injuries to the Face and Jaw', in *Official History of the Great War: Medical Services; Surgery of the War*, ed. by W.G. Macpherson, A.A. Bowlby, C. Wallace and C. English, volume 2 (London: His/Her Majesty's Stationery Office, 1922), pp.40-102.

13 BAPRAS Archive: Anon. Report on the work of the Queen's Hospital, 1917-1929. Privately printed, c.1930.

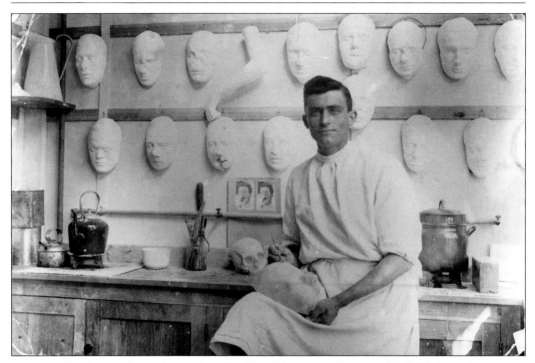

Tom Kelsey in his studio at Sidcup. (Auckland War Memorial Museum, PH-CNEG-C28348)

The museum's collection was highly valued, and the hospital's Secretary, Sir Charles Kenderdine, suggested it should be preserved by the RCS. He negotiated its relocation in 1923 with Sir Arthur Keith, anatomist to the College, where it became part of the collection of the Hunterian Museum. It comprised about half of the completed cases dealt with at Aldershot and Sidcup. Sadly, on 11 May 1941, during an air raid on London, the College was struck by a high-explosive bomb. About half of the Hunterian collection, including all the Sidcup museum items and all of Charles Valadier's records from Boulogne, was destroyed. Fortunately, Tonks' pastels had been removed from the College, together with other works of art, and so survived the catastrophe.

A significant proportion of the case files escaped damage from the explosion because they were not there. Gillies had retained them for two reasons: to write his seminal textbook *Plastic Surgery of the Face*, with sections devoted to the different anatomical areas; and because there were still men undergoing treatment at Sidcup in 1923. Gillies may also have retained the files because he had developed a personal attachment to – and a professional use – for them. The files enabled Gillies to refresh his memory of operative details and progress, at a time when copies were not available. The text of *Plastic Surgery* drew heavily on his personal recollections of the cases which go beyond what is recorded in the notes. However, some of the later, and more intricate, cases could not be included in the book. Gillies began to devise what he saw as the essential principles of plastic surgery from further consideration of many of these cases.

The Principles of Plastic Surgery

Gillies thought long and hard about the principles which underpinned his teaching. They were finally set down in 1957 in *The Principles and Art of Plastic Surgery*. He and his collaborator on the book, Ralph Millard, chose their title with great care.[14] Where *Plastic Surgery* simply described cases, illustrated with the trademark diagrams and photographs, *Principles and Art* was discursive and anecdotal. The later book comprised a record of Gillies' surgical journey, and included discussion of specific cases, all underpinned by the principles illustrated by particular patients. The text demonstrated Gillies' mind at work. In that respect, it was entirely different from a traditional dry surgical manual which simply gives instructions for a procedure. *Principles and Art* provided notes on what the surgeon could do, and also discussed what they should not.[15] A lecture Gillies gave in the 1930s provides a perfect example of the humanity which pervaded Gillies' work. He stated that, "in the beginning when this deformity was first tackled I was completely nonplussed, for a very devout senior surgeon abjured me not to operate. In his opinion these patients had earned their deformity and it was not for man to cure them. But I ask you, how could we leave them like this?"[16]

Gillies did not seek to conceal mistakes in either of his published books. The case files contain reminders of the mistakes made at Sidcup, sometimes alongside suggestions of what should have happened, and Gillies drew heavily on these examples to make his points in the text. While some revision of the basics happened as a result of his extensive experience of casualties during the Second World War, and his recording techniques were enhanced by the technological advances of colour photography, the replacement of the glass plate camera by sophisticated 35mm film cameras, and cine photography, many of the principles within Gillies' work can be traced back to individual cases from the First World War.

Although many of those principles seem obvious today, they were revolutionary at the time. "Plastic surgery," wrote Gillies, "is a constant battle between blood supply and beauty." He commented that he considered the principles to be applicable as a philosophy for life as well as for surgery.[17] He began by setting out the starting point: "Observation is the basis of surgical diagnosis." Certainly, every case from Aldershot and Sidcup was thoroughly observed. As if to underline his multidisciplinary approach, Gillies also suggested that there was "no better training for a surgeon than to be taught observation by a physician." The second principle, "diagnose before you treat," seems obvious, but experience at Sidcup had revealed to Gillies that what might be visible on the surface often gave no clue as to what lay beneath. The third principle required the surgeon to "make a plan and a pattern for this plan. Use paper, bandage or jaconet shaped to the defect and carry out a pretence operation in reverse. Do not rush in with a piece of skin hoping it will fit."[18] Lieutenant Frederick Stacey of the Royal Naval Division provides a good example of this principle. Stacey's notes contain a photograph carefully annotated by Gillies, with the outline of a forehead flap drawn in. A further page contains photo-

---

14 The two corresponded at some length over the title. The correspondence is not in the BAPRAS Archive.

15 The style of *Principles and Art*, although it encapsulated Gillies' personality perfectly, did not appeal to Mark Bonham Carter of Collins, who wrote: "In our view the fairly long insertions about his personal life and particularly those which deal with his jokes, letter, etc., interrupt the course of the narrative and should be drastically cut. Further, we feel that the book is written in a style which is so elaborate and facetious that it gets between the reader and what the author is saying. Sir Harold does not appear to recognise the difference between a story which is told by him to an appreciative audience of friends, and a story written and addressed to a series of unknown people." See letter from Mark Bonham Carter to George Greenfield, Gillies' literary agent, 9 July 1957, Gillies' correspondence. (Courtesy of Susie Winter) Collins turned down the opportunity to publish the English edition.

16 Lecture given to the *Berliner Medizinishe Gesellschaft* in 1938, reproduced in H.D. Gillies and R. Millard, *The Principles and Art of Plastic Surgery* (London: Butterworth & Co., 1957), pp.103 *et seq.*

17 Gillies and Millard, *Principles and Art*, p.49. Unless otherwise stated, all quotations in the following passages are taken from this source, pp.49-54. Emphasis in original.

18 Jaconet: a lightweight cotton cloth with a smooth and slightly stiff finish.

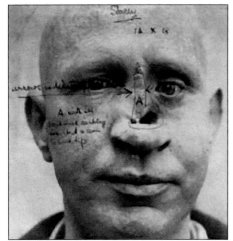
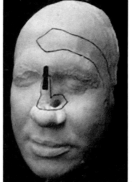
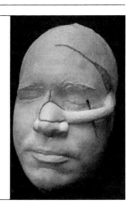
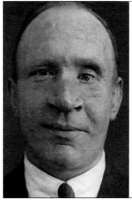
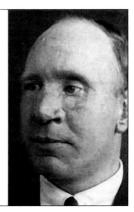

Lieutenant Stacey, Royal Naval Division,
Anson Battalion. Photograph showing
Gillies' annotations; the three-
dimensional appearance of the forehead
flaps; the final result. (RCS)

graphs of plaster casts onto which the flap was drawn, and from which the paper pattern was traced and cut. The pattern was always slightly larger than necessary. Like a fired pot, the flap or graft could shrink once the bruising and swelling settled, and it was better to have to reduce an over-large graft than be required to start again because it was initially too small and had distorted.

Gillies' fourth principle was to: "Make a record. Start with a diagram in the notes … while you operate have special methods recorded by artists or Leica … Follow up the case with the camera, for that is where most of us slip up."[19] The careful use of standardised photographs and the evolution of diagrams have been discussed above, but it is worth reflecting on distinctions between early and later technical drawing. Tonks' swift freehand sketches evolved into the draughtsman-like drawings of Hornswick and Lindsay, to which Lindsay provided detailed annotations (See Colour Section, p.xvi).

Gillies was happy to try new technology as soon as he could. His notes from Rooksdown Hospital, where he worked during the Second World War, were supplemented by boxes of several thousands of negative strips. He was also a pioneer of cine photography in the operating theatre, and used a three-lens Devin camera to produce non-fading colour images. However, he was only too aware of the risks of failure, and so entreated his readers to observe his fifth principle:

---

19   The Leica was a 35mm camera which first appeared in the 1930s.

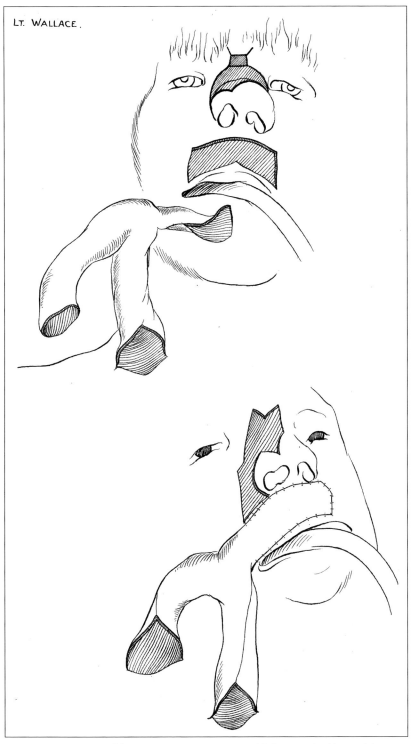

LT. WALLACE.

A comparison of diagrammatic representation (1). Diagram by Hornswick demonstrating the raising of tube pedicles for Lieutenant Eric Wallace, Canadian Field Artillery. (RCS)

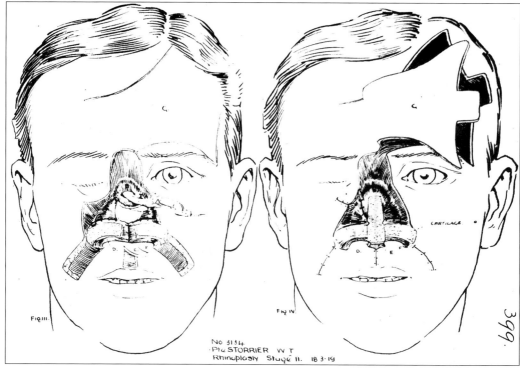

A comparison of diagrammatic representation (2). Diagram by Daryl Lindsay of Storrier. (RCS)

The lifeboat. It is impossible at times to be sure that a flap will fit or look well or even survive … It is as well to have a reserve plan in the form of another flap or skin graft … Having made all the plans conceivable for a case, it often happens that at operation the actual plan adopted is a different one. This is humiliating until one reflects that it is on the steps of these discards that the final variation is made possible.

Undoubtedly, this principle derived from the fact that Gillies and his colleagues had started facial reconstruction effectively from scratch. As has been discussed, existing texts were inadequate to deal with the types of injury seen at Sidcup, and thus in the early days a great deal of experimentation was necessary. Having an alternative option mitigated the risk of failure and reduced the likelihood of revision surgery.

Facial surgery was a delicate task and demanded a level of skill which went beyond the stitching of, for example, a large cut on the leg, which might be adequately done by a new trainee or even a student. "A good style will get you through," wrote Gillies. "Surgical style is the expression of personality and training exhibited by the movements of the fingers; its hallmark – dexterity and gentleness."

Gillies' seventh principle was born of some of the patients who arrived at Sidcup having been operated upon elsewhere:

Replace what is normal in a normal position and retain it there. If some of the bones of the face have got out of place … it is incumbent on you to put them back in place and hold them there … If the soft tissue defect is too large for primary closure without distortion, it is better to retain what is left in normal position and so define the defect to be filled.

Gillies specifically mentioned Private Bell, a man referred to him by Valadier, as an example of this principle. Bell's injuries, which involved significant tissue loss, had been dealt with by primary closure. He arrived with no upper lip and a distorted nose. Gillies recorded how his first move had been to cut the healed scars to allow the edges to flop back to where they should have been, and to work on from there by replacing missing tissue from elsewhere. In the case of Rifleman Moss, where the damage was too extensive to be repaired, Gillies inserted an adjustable splint to push the soft tissues out to the right position.

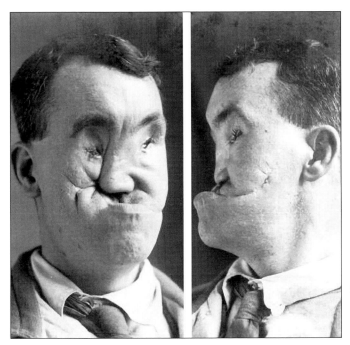

Rifleman Moss. Drawing by Tonks of the adjustable splint inserted by Gillies to push out the collapsed face, between two photographs from the notes of the before and after appearances. (RCS)

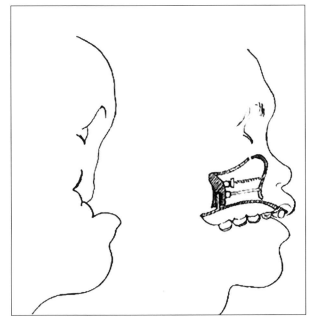

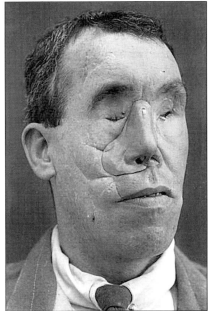

Complex defects had to be dealt with in the correct order. As Gillies stated, "Treat the primary defect first. Do not let concern for the secondary defect endanger the final result. *Borrow from Peter to pay Paul only when Peter can afford it*. When Mahomet is a long way from the mountain, try to move the mountain to Mahomet." Gillies transposed pedicle flaps long distances; areas where soft skin suitable for a face could be found included the inner part of the arm, the chest, abdominal wall and buttock. The tubes could be transplanted into an intermediate site if it was too far to move it in one go, but closure of the wound created by raising the flap was of secondary importance. The ninth principle was also important to remember in this regard: "Losses must be replaced in kind … thus the eyebrow is grafted from the hairy scalp, thin skin for an eyelid and thick for the palm." The cases of Len Tringham and Percy Green, also outlined in Chapter 3, are classic examples. Tringham's first, and failed, nasal reconstruction had been performed in Birmingham with a forehead flap whose tip was within the hairline. Apart from the fact that the flap was unsupported and unlined, and thus collapsed, the nose had a hairy tip. Likewise, use of the hairy skin for transfer to the inside of the mouth created an unpleasant problem. Conversely, Henry Pickerill's upper lip reconstruction deliberately used skin from within the hairline in order to create a moustache and to conceal the underlying scars. The reconstruction of Private Button's upper lip was performed on 22 January 1919 "as in the case of Pte P. Green."

By the end of the war, patients arrived at Sidcup within days or even hours of having received their injury. As a consequence, some of the wounds were almost as they had been generated: raw, irregular and very difficult to comprehend. The surgeon had to start somewhere, and Gillies recommended they "Do something positive. When a lacerated lip is a jig-saw puzzle, look for landmarks and if you can find two bits that definitely fit, put them together – at least you will have made a vital *first move*".

Principle eleven was to "never throw anything away. In plastic surgery never throw anything away until you are sure you do not want it." The principle today is exemplified by the severed finger, which can only be re-attached if it has been saved. Gillies applied this principle between operations, as well as during them. The notes record rib cartilage removed for nasal bridge reconstruction for one patient as being too large. It was cut down, and the residual piece was

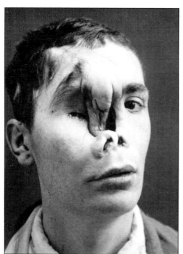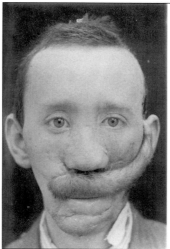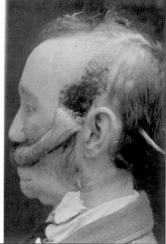

Photograph of Private Len Tringham showing a poorly planned forehead flap; a photograph of Private E. Button, RAMC showing Pickerill's reconstruction of the upper lip using a flap taken from within the hairline to create a moustache. (RCS)

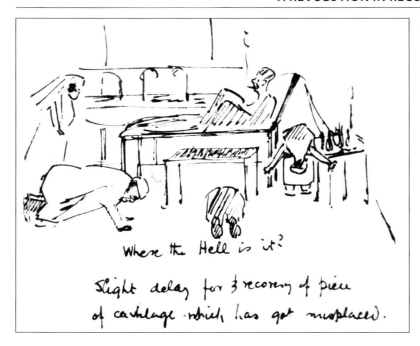

A sketch by Gillies after the loss of a cartilage graft in theatre. (Author's collection)

used in another patient. Cartilage was quite slippery, and occasionally escaped as it was being trimmed. Gillies drew an amusing cartoon of the surgical team rummaging on the theatre floor to find a piece that had flicked off the table. The piece was, after a careful wash, used in the surgery, and happily the patient did not get an infection.

Perhaps as a result of his initial difficulties when trying to follow the techniques in the old books, Gillies became insistent that surgery could not be done by rote, using exactly the same approach regardless of the patient. There were too many variables: infection, the amount of bone loss, the state of remaining teeth and many more. Outward appearances could be deceptive, so although two injuries could look very similar, damage to the underlying structures might be very different. What dictated the approach to be taken depended on principles one and two. Therefore, he wrote: "Never let routine methods become your master. Routine methods must be mastered, but never let them master you. The answer to the question, 'How do you make this or do that?' should be, as in all surgery, 'Show me the case!'"

Gillies' surgical approach involved consultation and discussion within the surgical team. Even Henry Tonks, whose surgical skills must have been rusty, took part in planning discussions with Gillies and William Kelsey Fry. The drawbacks of isolation were very clear to Gillies, leading him to recommend that the surgeon "consult other specialists … The reaction of one man's mind to another's is increased by the stimulus of sharing mutual problems. In planning, two heads are better than one – in execution, gain the co-operation of the appropriate regional expert." This attitude underpinned Gillies' collaboration with, even reliance on, the dental surgeons, dentists and technicians at Sidcup, whose experience in dealing with the hard tissues outweighed his own. Likewise, while he was keen to teach techniques to surgeons from elsewhere, he was equally keen to pick up tips from them, as evidenced by his adoption of some of the bone grafting ideas that Fred Albee had tested at Neuilly in France. This principle was one of the first recorded examples of collaborative work in surgery, commonplace today but unknown in the autocratic teaching hospitals of the early twentieth century where the surgeon was the supreme ruler. Furthermore, Gillies' principle of consultation extended to the patient, who was considered part of the team as a specialist in and of himself.

Meticulous as he was, Gillies had a reputation for being very slow. If a trainee's sutures did not please him, he ordered that they were taken out and redone. "Speed in surgery consists of not doing the same thing twice," he said. "It's the old story of the hare racing back and forth at terrific speed while the tortoise, without retracing one step, slowly crosses the finish line."

Gillies' penultimate principle related both to the surgery itself, and to the necessary splinting, physiotherapy and mobilisation of, for example, a jaw that had become fixed. It also epitomised the post-operative support offered at Sidcup to the patients as they recuperated. "The after care is as important as the planning or the surgery itself – Or, for that matter, the surgery itself! … How futile it is to lose flap or graft for the lack of a little postoperative care." Gillies might have added that pre-care was equally important. It was futile to operate on an infected wound, and great care was taken to cleanse wounds and clear all signs of infection before surgery began. It is also apparent that there was a growing awareness that anaesthesia needed to be managed very carefully. If a patient had a chest infection, the surgeons elected to wait for its clearance.

The last of the principles echoed the fourteenth: "Never do today what can be honourably be put off till tomorrow … *When in doubt, don't!* … If there is the slightest danger, that manoeuvre had better be left for another and safer day … It is well to remember that *Time*, although the plastic surgeon's most trenchant critic, is also his greatest ally." The case of Ralph Lumley, described in Chapter 3, who was severely burned after his aeroplane caught fire after a crash landing, epitomised failure as a result of haste, and was the source of this last principle. Lieutenant Spreckley, who had lost his nose, had a large cartilage-supported graft turned from his forehead. Gillies wrote, "the new bloated columella stuck ahead like an anteater's snout and all my colleagues roared with laughter … but hasty judgement leads often to the discard of a principle the soundness of which may later be proved." Sure enough, Gillies' policy was vindicated. The swelling subsided, excess fibrous tissue was removed, and the end result was very respectable.

The Lasting Importance of the Sidcup Portraits

Photographs could be taken in seconds, but the construction of colour paintings, whether in pastel by Henry Tonks or in watercolour by another artist, took time. Painting required thought and care, and the use of colour added an entirely new dimension to record-keeping at Sidcup. The surviving records from Sidcup contain a number of different drafts of Tonks' diagrams; he pasted the original sketches onto a page and re-drew the detail later on a separate sheet. The work was made easier by the use of photographs and plaster casts to guide the finished portraits, which meant that the artists did not have to watch their disfigured subjects move, hear them talk, or suffer the smell of infection. A photograph of Lindsay at work shows the artist's use of a cast as an *aide-memoire*.

Tonks was employed by Gillies not primarily as a painter, but to create diagrams which demonstrated how operations were performed. His surgical training made him ideal for the task. His pastels were often worked up from operative drawings, as in his portrait of Lieutenant Grinlington (See Colour Section, p.xvii).[20] Daryl Lindsay's watercolours were meticulous, drawn with a firm hand. They appear more photographic and less vivid than Tonks' pastels. However, Lindsay's social interaction with Tonks would not have occurred had Tonks had been dissatisfied with the paintings. Herbert Cole did not show the same fluidity of line in the portraits filed in the notes, yet the smaller paintings he produced to illustrate Pickerill's

---

20   Grinlington returned to serve at the front and was killed at Passchendaele. He is buried at Nine Elms
       cemetery, just west of Poperinge.

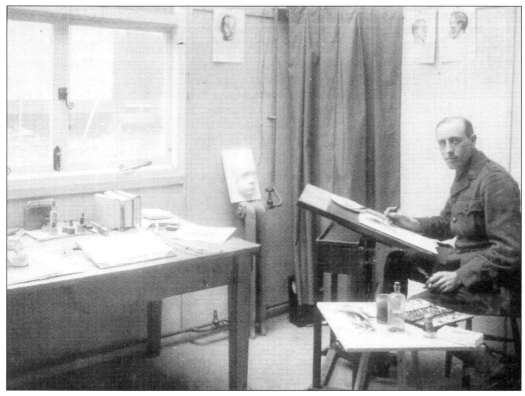

Lindsay at work on a watercolour in his studio. (RACS Archive, Melbourne)

textbook were excellent, executed almost as miniatures in fine detail (See Colour Section, p.xvii). The remainder were little more than journeyman works for reference only.

The purpose of the pastels and watercolours has been debated extensively by historians, partly as a result of their dramatic impact on the viewer. I believe that Tonks' works are simply painting exercises of captive subjects. Seeing all of Tonks' work in one room at once, mirroring Tonks' own studio at Sidcup, is a moving, even stupefying experience. The portraits are haunting, expression-filled images which seem to capture the personality of their subjects. The portraits were not commissioned, nor did the men give permission to have them done. The paintings were a working part of the surgical record. As Simon Schama has written, "it was Art not for Art's sake … but for life's sake."[21]

Many at the time thought that images of deformity should be concealed, just as many believed that the facial casualties themselves should have been. Tonks did not want his pastels to go to the IWM, which had first call on the work of official war artists. He was adamant that they should not be available for the vicarious gratification of a bloodthirsty public. The Sidcup museum was, he considered, somewhere that visitors came, gawped and shuddered, so the pastels went to the RCS with the hospital's museum collection. Seventy-three pastel portraits and drawings by Tonks are held today in the RCS, and a further three are in the collection of the

---

21 S. Schama, *The Face of Britain: The Nation through its Portraits* (London: Penguin/Viking, 2015), p.530.

Slade School of Art, part of University College London.[22] The New Zealand records acquired by the Queen Mary's archive contained 103 watercolours, the majority by Herbert Cole, with three by Daryl Lindsay. There are also 68 Lindsay watercolours in the RACS, Melbourne, and 39 others by Cole in the Hocken Library, Dunedin, although the majority of the latter are copies.

Despite Tonks' concerns over public display, a few public representations of facial injury were painted. Perhaps the most famous of these were the angry caricatures of Otto Dix. In *The Skat Players*, Dix captured the emotions of revulsion and contempt of those who had made no sacrifice. Other artists, such as George Grosz, also portrayed facial injury, with many of the pictures depicting the anti-war ethos that gained traction following the conclusion of hostilities. Most depictions of facial injury intended for public consumption, whether official or otherwise, did not appear until after the war. Friedrich's book *Nie Wieder Krieg*, published in 1924 and translated into French, Dutch and English, is perhaps the most graphic. The relative paucity of facial injury units ensured that public exposure to the subjects themselves had been limited. A few illustrated accounts appeared in the public domain, but even the Official History of the war skipped over the worst of the deformities and concentrated on dental work. Only 17 of the 58 illustrations within its pages are photographs of faces, while there are 20 examples of splints and dental prostheses.

Nowadays, these works are valued as evidence of the physical effects of war, and have been placed on public display frequently in recent years. The visual records from Sidcup are a crucial component of understanding the consequences of the war experience. Tonks' work has appeared on public display, notably in a 1994 exhibition at the Barbican Gallery entitled 'A Bitter Truth', and at the Venice Biennale in 1995. An exhibition at the National Army Museum in London in 2007, 'Faces of Battle', showed a number of Herbert Cole's paintings and photographs from Sidcup and was well-received. A number of newspapers refused to publish any of the more graphic images, but a BBC '*Timewatch*' programme, centred on the last day of the war on the Western Front, showed viewers one of the most destructive injuries seen at Sidcup. Some of the Sidcup watercolours were displayed at Tate Britain as part of the exhibition entitled 'Watercolour' in 2011. Pat Barker featured on the '*South Bank Show*' with some of Tonks' pastels in 2012 following the publication of the second of her novels which focused on Tonks, and the National Portrait Gallery's 'Portraits of War' exhibition in 2014 included a panel of four pastels.[23] In 2014, the RCS displayed all of Tonks' pastels together, juxtaposed with the work of Julia Midgley, a modern artist who illustrates injury. Some pastels also featured in a recent television series on the history of British art. Exhibiting these brutal images of the consequences of war encourages better understanding of the effects of artillery and small arms fire.

Conclusion

The records of Harold Gillies and his colleagues evolved from brief and simple notes at Aldershot to thorough and detailed logs of the surgical procedures undertaken by the team at Sidcup. Written and typed notes were underpinned by diagrams, photographs and colour work. Records with these characteristics are now the norm, but a hundred years ago, they were revolutionary. The Sidcup records contain tens of thousands of pictures, and the photographs added a new dimension to surgical notes as they represented the most modern form of

---

22 John Bennett, 'Henry Tonks and plastic surgery', *British Journal of Plastic Surgery*, 39:1 (1986), pp.1-34. Bennett lists 72 pastels. However, during a major conservation exercise on the Royal College of Surgeons' portraits in 2010-2011, a second pastel was discovered on the reverse of another.

23 Pat Barker, *Toby's Room* (London: Penguin, 2012).

portraiture. Had colour photography been available, Gillies would undoubtedly have made use of it as well. Instead, the colour work had to be attained by old-fashioned painting, an echo of the illustrations of Goya or of Sir Charles Bell's depictions of the Napoleonic Wars. The creation of coloured representations afforded the surgeons the advantage of viewing natural colour, so the full character of the wounds could be properly understood. Gillies' sixteen principles depended for their development on the thoughtfulness of a careful and committed surgeon, based on immaculate, comprehensive, multimedia records. The notes from the Queen's Hospital stand as a template for modern surgery.

5

Rehabilitation, the Patients' Experience and Public Perceptions

Facial surgery at Sidcup encompassed reconstruction rather than repair. As a result, treatment often involved a series of operations and took place over long periods. This chapter assesses the implications of these prolonged stays at the Queen's Hospital, including the careful management of surgical beds by relocating patients to convalescent beds in the locality while they recovered, and the development of a comprehensive system of rehabilitation to prepare soldiers for their future lives. Patients wrote home during their long stays, and often sent family members a postcard which depicted the hospital. These communications, coupled with the recollections of staff, provide vivid testimonies of the daily routine of hospital life, and shed light on the psychology of disfigurement and the emotional impact of war. New patients gained important reassurance of the benefits of treatment from their encounters with those who had already undergone procedures. The length of treatment also meant that the costs of care were high. The chapter explores how the press was used extensively to attract publicity and funds. The manner in which the press reported the development of Sidcup influenced public perceptions and encouraged Londoners rich and poor to give money to support the hospital.

The establishment of the Queen's Hospital transformed the management of patients with facial injury. In addition, the staff of the hospital brought to their work a clear recognition of the psychological trauma of disfigurement, and an appreciation of how it might be ameliorated by reconstruction. As well as receiving medical treatment, patients participated in social and sporting activities which formed an important part of the process of rehabilitation. The attitudes and experiences of the patients are outlined in personal accounts written by them or told to their relatives, some of which challenge the presumption that facial disfigurement by injury caused depression and despair.

Public Responses to Facial Injury

The Queen's Hospital was located on what had been a country estate, although it was not far from the village of Sidcup. By train, the hospital was just three-quarters of an hour from the centre of London. Patients with severe facial injuries, often sprouting flaps and tubes of skin, were encouraged to go into the village or even up to London. Some patients were sent further afield for convalescence. Horace Sewell was sent to a convalescent home in Burnham-on-Crouch. As previously noted, the town's residents petitioned for the men to be excluded from the town.[1] At Aldershot,

---

1   Horace Sewell, letter to Reginald Pound, 17 March 1963. Quoted in R. Pound, *Gillies: Surgeon Extraordinary* (London: Michael Joseph, 1964), p.52.

military regulations stipulated that convalescents took exercise by marching through the town. Gillies recorded that the Sergeant-Major would pray for rain so that he did not have to conduct his charges through the streets. The chorus of 'It's a Long Way to Tipperary' was a signal for anxious mothers to call their children in from play.[2]

Despite the entreaties of the press to take pity on the mutilated (and the newspapers pulled no punches when describing the appearance of men who were almost expected to provoke revulsion), there was local resistance to the appearance of these disfigured men. The standard hospital uniform of blue suit and red tie offered some warning, and some benches on the way into Sidcup were painted blue to alert the public that they might get a shock if they looked at those seated upon them. The patients of the Queen's Hospital were forbidden from drinking alcohol, which meant that visits to the local hostelry were not allowed. A Rest Room was established in Sidcup High Street in an empty shop; it served non-alcoholic drinks, and was open

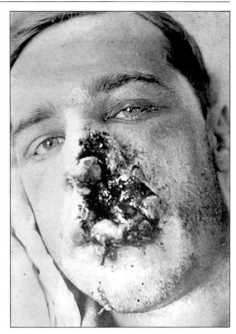

Horace Sewell. Initial appearance. (RCS)

to the patients of other military hospitals in the vicinity. Whilst some of the men, as one might expect, found ingenious ways to circumvent the alcohol ban, it meant that there was no possibility that they might upset local residents on a night out. Conversely, it also meant that the ordinary populace did not have the opportunity to become familiar with, and inured to, the sight of disfigured men. However, alongside the fear and loathing there was compassion. As a girl, Miss Dorothy Martin of Eltham stood outside New Cross station with her sister and collected cigarettes in tins for the "poor wounded soldiers." They then hopped on the tram and headed "down a leafy lane" to deliver them to the front entrance of the hospital.[3]

Members of the hospital staff were susceptible to the same responses to the wounded as the public, and many found it hard to look at patients with damaged faces. Ward Muir at Wandsworth struggled to conceal his dismay when he discovered that he "must fraternise with his fellow-men at whom he cannot look without the grievous risk of betraying, by his expression, how awful is their appearance."

"Hideous is the only word for these smashed faces," he continued:

> the socket with some twisted, moist slit, with a lash or two adhering feebly, which is all that is traceable of the forfeited eye; the skewed mouth which sometimes – in spite of brilliant dentistry contrivances – results from the loss of a segment of jaw; and worse, far the worst, the incredibly brutalising effects which are the consequence of wounds in the nose, and which reach a climax of mournful grotesquerie when the nose is missing altogether.

He described such men as "broken gargoyles."[4]

2   Pound, *Gillies*, p.36.
3   Dorothy Martin, personal communication.
4   W. Muir, *The Happy Hospital* (London: Simpkin, Marshall, Hamilton & Kent, 1917), p.143.

Emily Bayne also recalled the trauma of post-operative care. A nurse trained prior to the war at the Woolwich Union Infirmary and who had been to France with the Scottish Women's Hospital, Bayne had transferred to Sidcup to care for the Canadian patients. Her job often involved sitting for days with men who had developed infections, applying hot towels to sweat the fever through. Many soldiers would recite favourite poems, or passages from the Bible, to take their minds off the pain.[5]

Many of the war's poets wrote about faces and torment, but there was a lighter side. The irrepressible humour of even the stickiest situation was recorded by the likes of Bruce Bairnsfather, himself wounded and returned to Blighty, and by the cartoonists of the hospital and ambulance journals. While these responses are often interpreted as putting a gloss on things there is clear evidence of black humour among the casualties. Gillies recalled one of his patients who used to go up to London in his mask, and upon his return happily held up several fingers to indicate how many passers-by he had frightened in the capital when he removed it. There was a spectrum of patient behaviour and adjustment, between those who could cope and those who could not, rather than a shared experience of facial injury.

The horror induced by the mere thought of facial injury ensured that the world's first ever hospital dedicated to the treatment of facial wounds attracted enormous media coverage. Both national and regional newspapers sent reporters to see the hospital for themselves, and they were clearly disturbed and moved by what they saw. Harold Begbie, a reporter for the London *Daily Chronicle*, was allowed into the operating theatre in December 1917. The experience was too much for him. "I begin to feel – How hot it is!" he wrote. "My mouth is dry. Yes, it is wonderful, most wonderful, this science of surgery. A miracle; but I can't stand it. Let me get out. What a disturbance I should make dropping down in my surplice. Have I the strength to walk across the room? Yes, if I go now. Now, now; as quietly as I can." Begbie wrote his report based on photographs shown to him later.[6]

Reports in the press encouraged contributions to the Sidcup fund through the publication of stories which focused on the physical and psychological difficulties associated with facial injuries. A cutting from the *Sunday Chronicle* provides a typical example through its description of a visit to Sergeant Bates by his wife. Bates had made light of his injury, and his wife was clearly unprepared for his disfigurement. The Matron warned her, "with an infinite pity in her face … what Sergeant Bates in his agony of mind could not write." Supported by one of the nursing sisters, Bates tried to turn his damaged side away from his wife. However, "deliberately choosing the other, she went right up to the bed, and with a hand on each shoulder, kissed him – ever so lightly – on the worst scar of all."[7] The daughter of another patient at Sidcup, in correspondence with the author, commented that her father always positioned himself for the camera by turning his injured side away, emphasising the long-term effects of facial injury.

The audience for such moving stories was huge. Some 15 million people read a daily or Sunday paper. These articles, reproduced with variations throughout the country and often accompanied by sympathetic illustrations, kept the contributions rolling in. The Queen's Hospital, despite its development for war casualties of the nation's army, was funded almost entirely from voluntary contributions. It was not alone in this regard. The voluntary arrangement was mirrored by other institutions which sprang up to assist in the treatment of war casualties

5   Emily Bayne's daughter, personal communication.
6   Recorded in Pound, *Gillies*, pp.51-52. Begbie's article was reproduced in the *Adelaide Register*, 26 April 1919.
7   LMA: H02/QM/Y/01/005 Hospital Press Cuttings book. There was a real Sergeant Benjamin Bates treated at Sidcup, but the case file does not match the description in the article.

unlikely to return to the front, such as the facilities provided for the blind at St Dunstan's and the Star and Garter Home in Richmond.[8] A small hospital for officers, located in Regent's Park and affiliated to Sidcup, was funded by the shipping magnate Sir John Ellerman. Captain Budd spent several months there with his two black eyes and damaged nose. On his arrival in London by train from Southampton, he wrote: "it was rather touching to find that there was an enormous crowd of sympathisers gathered at the station gates to meet the Hospital trains as they arrived, and numbers of people ran forward and threw in packets of cigarettes, etc, as we drove quickly away."[9] Budd required prolonged treatment, and he recorded one of the most detailed patient accounts of surgical treatment during the First World War. He had a plaster cast taken, "a strange and uncomfortable process, especially when the hardened plaster was pulled away giving one a most extraordinary feeling of being sucked all over one's face until the air got under at one corner when the whole thing lifted off easily." The cast was remodelled with wax and covered with a thin metal foil sheet, so that the exact shape of the skin flap to be taken could be determined. A piece of rib cartilage was removed at Budd's next surgery, but he developed a chest infection and a persistent cough.

The treatment for this was unorthodox:

> one evening after a particularly tough bout of coughing the sister in charge got windy and fetched the M.O. to see me. The result of his visit made the cough almost worth while [sic] as he immediately said, 'I think this calls for Champagne and Oysters', and sure enough I had a half bottle of champagne and a dozen oysters for my supper, and believe me that did me a world of good. I can recommend that medicine to anyone who is in a similar predicament, at any time![10]

Unsurprisingly, such a regimen was restricted to officers only.

The Lancet joined the press in their enthusiasm for the Queen's. It published several illustrated articles by members of the Sidcup staff, and commented favourably on the results in November 1917:

> Among our wounded sailors and soldiers none, perhaps, deserve our sympathy and compassion more than those who have suffered grievous facial injuries, in many cases of such a nature as to render them at first unrecognisable. Surgical skill properly applied avails to relieve immediate suffering, but cases of this character require continuous and special care during a long period of convalescence. Surgery today can effect cures to a large proportion of cases which two or three years ago would have been considered hopeless instances of facial mutilation … The clinical outcome is already wonderful.[11]

A month later, the same journal underlined one of the key principles developed by Gillies and his team; that both structure and function mattered. "Every reader will agree that the ingenuity

---

8   The British approach was in marked contrast to the State-organised services that developed in Germany. This dichotomy is discussed in D. Cohen, *The War Come Home. Disabled Veterans in Britain and Germany, 1914-1939* (Berkeley, CA: University of California Press, 2001).

9   BLSC: Budd Papers, LIDDLE/WW1/WF/REC/01/B43. This repast was translated to Sidcup by Howard Brenton in his play *Dr Scroggy's War*. Unless otherwise stated, all quotations in this passage are taken from this source.

10 BLSC: Budd Papers, LIDDLE/WW1/WF/REC/01/B43.

11 These references are saved as cuttings in the Queen's Hospital record book in the London Metropolitan Archive, H02/QM/Y/01/005 (first quotation dated 3 November 1917; second dated 5 December 1917).

and skill of the operators are worthy of the highest praise. The results are both wonderful and suggestive, and it is difficult to say which is the more remarkable – the improvement in the cosmetic appearance or the benefit in many cases to the functional utility." Such effusive commendation of Gillies' efforts emphasises the recognised importance of the work which was undertaken at the Queen's both during and after the war, and touches upon both the psychological and physical impacts of facial injury upon the men who suffered them. It was crucial, therefore, that Gillies and his team created an environment in which the wounds, both visible and invisible, of their patients were catered for.

The Daily Routine of Hospital Life

The surviving Sidcup notes describe the medical and surgical progress of more than two-and-a-half-thousand men. However, they are dry surgical summaries and give little indication of what daily life was like for the staff and patients of the Queen's. Some injuries were fairly straightforward, but many were not. Men came in with injuries that required careful attention not just once, but on multiple occasions. The brevity of the notes themselves demonstrates the significant workload of the staff: "a splint is required"; "dentures are to be made"; "a persisting infection needs treating." The complexity of the surgical process meant that men were at Sidcup for weeks or months, and returned over several years.

Some official photographs of the staff and patients survive from the First World War era, but few contemporary accounts of their experiences. The photographs include a number of formal group shots of medical and nursing staff, images of the ward interiors, and less formal pictures of the men. Royal visits were also recorded, and the dental technician Archie Lane compiled two albums which contain a few group photographs. In addition, several orderlies, nurses and patients took their own photographs, some of which survive in family albums. Some photographs, in particular the ward photographs taken at Christmas time in 1917, were reproduced as postcards and some recorded some of the more homely aspects of life at the Queen's Hospital.[12]

There was plenty of time for letter writing as the men waited for surgery. As had become common practice for military hospitals, postcards were printed for staff and patients to send home. Sidcup appears to have produced more than any other hospital, both to offer variety to the men whose stays were prolonged and, more frequently, to be bought as souvenirs. One complete set of 12 was taken home to Wales by Frank Whipp, and is beautifully preserved.[13] Few were actually written upon, and the messages recorded were largely banal. Frank Garrod's message home to Bury St Edmunds is a typical example: "Dear Maud and Will, Eff & Bob, Leslie George & Flo. Beatie and everyone. Trust you are all keeping O.K. as for me I am keeping fine and well as can be. When are you going to write don't forget to drop a line soon. Heaps of love from Frank."[14]

George Brooks of the Australian Machine Gun Corps was transferred to Sidcup from the Australian hospital at Dartford with a cheek wound. In November 1917, he sent a series of postcards from Ward 3 back to his family in Australia, with one unusually detailed message spread across three cards:

---

12   An album compiled by one of the nurses contains several full and half-plate images. (Author's collection)
13   The set is now in the author's collection. More than 70 postcard views of the Queen's Hospital were produced – including a single hand-coloured version of the black and white original. No other hospital produced such a large range.
14   Postcard in the author's collection.

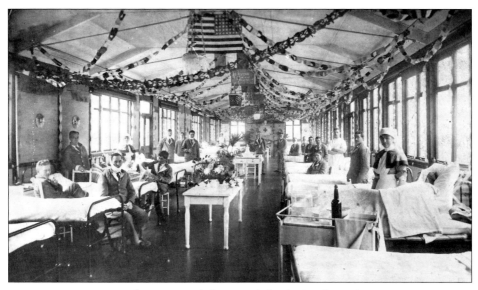

A Christmas ward photograph. (Author's collection)

I came to this hospital yesterday. So I have got this set of cards to let you see what the place is like as you will see it is a very nice place. This is a view of one of the wards the same as the one I am in. They only deal with face wounds here and I can tell you there are some very unpleasant sights to see some of the faces but the work they do here is marvellous. It is supposed to be run by the Queen and she is often here paying visits. I don't know what they are going to do with me but I don't think they will have much to do. This place is nearer London than Dartford. I like this place very well & I think I will soon be fixed up. So it may not be so long before I am on a trip home. I am enclosing a Christmas and New Year Card I think it is very nice & I am sure you will like it. You will see it is especially printed for the hospital. But it will be rather late for Xmas when it arrives.[15]

Brooks was right: at the end of January 1918, he was discharged from Sidcup and transferred to Harefield Hospital to await transport home. His Christmas card was a photographic ward scene which depicted the patients by their beds.[16] It seems to have been a standard format, made up for all the wards, but in George's case there was an additional second group photograph taken outside the ward. Two of the dental surgeons, Captains C.F. Rumsey and E.G. Robertson, were pictured alongside their patients. Another of George's photographs confirms that there was a white Christmas at Sidcup in 1917.

   Although the intense pressure of the war years eased, patients who had initially been treated with little success at other units were referred to the Queen's Hospital after the Armistice. For the next seven years men returned to Sidcup for further surgery, and for dental treatment and appliances. Although Sidcup was near enough to London, many patients came from further afield and stayed for months or longer. There were long delays between operations. In addition,

---

15 George Brooks, personal papers.
16 The author has one original and two other Christmas ward postcards are held by Bexley Local Studies centre.

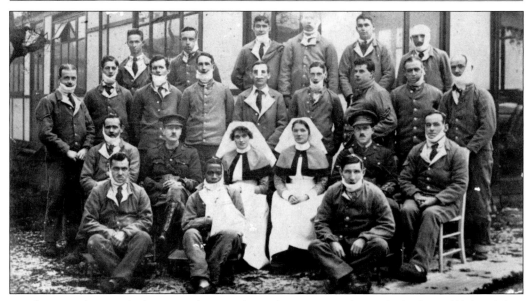

A Christmas photograph of patients taken outside Ward 3. George Brooks is in the back row, fifth from left.
His friend Joseph Hickey stands in the front row, fifth from left. The Nigerian soldier Private Williams is seated
on the ground, towards the left. Surgeons Rumsey and Robertson are seated either side of the ward sisters.
(Courtesy of the Brooks family collection)

now and again a procedure went wrong and required revision. Men who shunted back and forth between the Queen's Hospital and the various outlying convalescent units had time on their hands (See Colour Section, p.xviii). The rotation gave them a change of scenery, but there were long periods in which nothing much happened.

Aside from the postcards, the very few remaining accounts of the patients and staff at Sidcup also display little emotion. Captain Budd's observations of hospital life offer some insight into the tedium of waiting for the next procedure, and are dominated by thoughts of food. He wrote:

> I can still look back on the breakfasts we had, and wonder how we got through them! There were always two huge dishes placed on the side board, one piled high with fried eggs and the other with bacon, and all comers just had as much as they felt like. No bally rationing, since the Hospital ran its own chicken farm, and probably, for all I know its own piggery as well![17]

Champagne and oysters may not have been on the menu as they had been during his time at Regent's Park, but the standard of the food served at the Queen's was evidently to Budd's satisfaction, although the officers' food was a cut above that for other ranks.

Despite the frequent operations, the nauseating effects of the anaesthetics, the pain from injury and infection and, not infrequently, the wiring together of the jaws to allow bone grafts to set in the right position, the patient experience at Sidcup was a convivial one. John Glubb was wounded three days after the Queen's Hospital officially opened, and had been tagged with a Gillies label. In his case it was not enough to ensure his direct evacuation to Gillies' team. "At Rouen," he said, "I had been marked with a label, 'Cambridge Hospital, Aldershot', which was

17   BLSC: Budd Papers, LIDDLE/WW1/WF/REC/01/B43.

the chief place for face wounds. But on the boat they said there was no room there, so I was sent up to London. When we got to Waterloo, a man came in and gave us all tickets for hospitals. Mine was the 3rd London General."

Glubb was there for three months, in which he received no medical attention and his wound became infected. However:

> At last, in November 1917, three months after I had been hit, I was transferred to a new hospital for face injuries at Frognal, Sidcup, in Kent … Here things were very different. My broken and septic teeth were extracted and my wound cleaned. The problem then was how to reunite the broken fragments of my lower jaw bone, which were still hanging loosely in my mouth. The solution adopted was to set the broken bones of the lower jaw and then cement it to the upper jaw, which thereby acted as a splint … As most of my lower jaw had gone, I was shown an album of photographs of handsome young men and asked to choose the chin I would like to have![18]

As Begbie wrote: "the cheerfulness of every one is the unconquerable soul of man. Wherever I go in this beautiful garden I find men with bandaged faces, or men whose faces have been mended. They are perfectly happy. They are laughing and jesting."[19] Nellie Cryer, a nurse who had begun her career in Manchester before moving to Sidcup when the Queen's Hospital opened, concurred. She believed that "there could not have been a more appropriate place for those kind [sic] of patients."[20]

George Brooks also wrote fondly of his time at Sidcup in his memoirs. He recalled "a wonderful place with men with facial wounds from all countries," including an Irishman named Hickey who had lost his nose but not his mischievous sense of humour. Efforts to create a new nose had not initially been successful, so a suitably coloured aluminium replacement had been made. Hickey:

> seldom wore it in hospital, but one day he had to leave to visit London. The sister saw to it that he was well dressed, nose and all. However, on his return, he was minus his nose. Sister exclaimed: 'What have you done with your nose, Hickey?' 'Sure and it fell off and a dog run away wid it' said he. Of course, it was in his pocket. We had some bad cases there but humour played its part to cheer them up.[21]

Even though drink was forbidden, leisure and fun were encouraged by the staff. Photographs survive of fancy-dress parties and picnics at the Queen's, and at Christmas in 1919 the patients were treated to a play written and performed by their comrades. *The Patients Dream*, or *A Visit to the Theatre*, was written by Norman Wimbush and set in "a Facial Hospital in Nightmareland." The small cast included Lieutenant J. Steel as the anaesthetist Captain Odours, and Private J.B. Jordan as the patient. The advertisements on the cover further exemplify the black humour of the patients: "Are you satisfied with your face? If not, come to the Beauty Parlour, X-ray now" read one. Just below it was another: "Are your Friends satisfied with your face? Probably not. See above."[22]

---

18   J.B. Glubb, *Into Battle* (London: Cassell, 1978), pp.193-194.
19   Recorded in Pound, *Gillies*, pp.51-52.
20   Nellie Cryer, 'The most rewarding years of my life', personal reminiscences sent to the *Reader's Digest*. (Author's collection)
21   George Brooks, personal papers.
22   Souvenir Programme, Queen's Hospital Thespian Society, Friday 19 December 1919. (Author's collection)

SIDCUP GALVANIC SOAP

Mr. S. W. ANK writes: "I had no life in my ears, but after using your soap, I can now flick flies off my nose with either ear."

BUY IT TO-DAY.

WEAR A PEDICULE

and do away with a ticket-pocket.

MAKES AN EXCELLENT PIPEHOLDER.

Join the League of Rations

and help us to abolish bullybeef and mince

Why Buy Fags?

Smoke O.P. Cigarettes and SAVE MONEY.

Queen's Picture House.

Next week, the great Success

THE

Drunkard's Drink

In 3 reels and 1 stagger.

The great PUSSYFOOT Drama.

HIGHEST PRICES PAID FOR

OLD RIBS

Send your disused Ribs to the Original Firm,

Messrs. ADAM & EVE, GENESIS ROAD, PARADISE, N.

Original Production, for the first time on any Stage, of the great, blood-thirsty, soul-stirring, humorous and Musical Drama by   W. INDUP

"THE PATIENT'S DREAM"

OR

"A VISIT TO THE THEATRE"

In 1 Act and Several Groans.

Time -   -   -   -   -   - THE PRESENT
Scene - A FACIAL HOSPITAL IN NIGHTMARELAND

CHARACTERS.

Major Bullybeef, R.A.M.C., *A Surgeon* ... MAJOR STAPLETON
Captain Odours, R.A.M.C., *An Anaesthetist* LIEUT. J. STEEL
Pte. MacNabb, R.A.M.C., *An Orderly* LIEUT. J. K. WILKIE
Sister Stitchem, *A Dear*   ...   ... PTE. HOWARD
A Patient, *A Poor Devil*   ...   ... PTE. JORDAN

Produced by Mr. N. N. WIMBUSH.

Scenery by RAPHAEL & TITIAN.   Dresses by REQUEST.
Cigarettes by ABDULLA & Co.   Moustaches by ACCIDENT.

NOTE.—The Management of this Theatre are not responsible for the truth of the Advertisements. The public patronise the Firms at their own risk.

N.B.—The Audience is respectfully requested not to throw bricks at the Actors. All Bricks are urgently required for the Housing Scheme.

EDUCATION!   EDUCATION!!   EDUCATION!!!

Billiards Taught.   Dancing Instruction.
Whist.   Trigonometry.   Tea-Making.
Learn to Drive————We Supply the Car.
Tuition in GOLF, PONTOON and EUCLID.
Learn a Foreign Language————French, Bad or Swahili.

JOIN THE SCHOOL OF INSTRUCTION TO-DAY.

WHO SUPPLIED SAMSON

With the famous Jaw - bone which enabled him to slay umpteen Philistines? If YOU wish to be a Bible Hero and

SLAY PHILISTINES

get your next Jaw-bone from us—

Messrs. YALE & PADDLE, Bone Sawyers & Dope Dealers, NINETEENTH AVENUE.

SEE YOURSELF

AS YOU REALLY ARE

Get your Photo taken at the

X RAY DEPT.

The human body contains more than 200 Bones. Our Photos show them all.

ARE YOU A CONVINCING TALKER?

IF NOT, USE OUR SPLINTS.

Send no money. Call personally.

Messrs. Splutter & Stutter

Gas Engineers, WESTMINSTER.

If you have nothing to do any forenoon, why not spend

A HAPPY HALF-HOUR

At the Throat Clinic.

Do not fail to see our Field Officer with the Mirror on his Eye.

ARE YOU SATISFIED WITH YOUR FACE?

If not, come to

The Beauty Parlour,

X-RAY ROW.

N.B.—As an additional attraction customers are allowed to converse with the charming lady proprietors during treatment.

ARE YOUR FRIENDS SATISFIED———— WITH YOUR FACE?

(Probably not. See above.)

You may not be a Beauty, but you might be worse.

The programme for the 1919 Christmas show. (Author's collection)

The autograph books of nurses and patients bear witness to the literacy of wounded men. Poetry was popular: well-known poems were often quoted alongside an inscription or drawing, and original, inventive verses were produced. The 3rd London General Hospital's journal, initially under the editorship of Ward Muir, offered another, more public outlet for many poems. The prose and verse in the journal were relatively mawkish. However, some of the cartoons were superb. J.H. Dowd's 'The Doings of Donovan' were even reprinted in a single volume by *Country Life*.[23] The 3rd London's journal was professionally produced and printed, and sold

---

23 J.H. Dowd, *The Doings of Donovan in and out of Hospital* (London: Country Life, 1918).

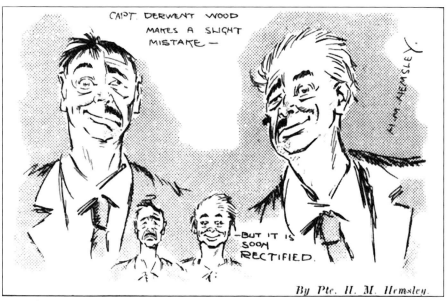

CAPT. DERWENT WOOD
MAKES A SLIGHT
MISTAKE —

—BUT IT IS
SOON
RECTIFIED.

By Pte. H. M. Hemsley.

A cartoon from the 3rd London Hospital journal making fun of Derwent Wood's 'Tin Noses' workshop.
(Author's collection)

at four pence an issue. Other hospital journals were sustained by advertisement revenue from local shops and firms. Most contained a mix of sentimentality and grim humour. Although a number of hospitals produced their own journals during the war, no evidence of a journal produced at the Queen's Hospital has been found.

For the more active patients, football, cricket, and sports days were arranged. The short report on the hospital's work printed in 1929 included a photograph of the hospital football team captioned "patients whose features had been restored." The placid and solemn demeanour of the footballers in their team photograph is belied by Albert Collins' tale of violence and bodily harm on the field. He recalled the team winning matches and the fights afterwards; the team's success was unsurprising given that several of the players had been professional footballers before the war.

Private Joe Kassler of the 1st Auckland Infantry Regiment was awarded a silver goblet for victory in the 100-yard sprint at one of the hospital's sports days.[24] In addition, there was the card school, of which Frank Whipp was an enthusiastic member, whilst both patients and staff members ran books for the races. These amenities helped the men to endure their long sojourns with great patience and, in some cases, substantially lighter wallets.

Nevertheless, some men tired of the long, tedious days of waiting, of repeated anaesthetics that made them sick, and of the postoperative pain, relieved by morphine or cocaine which also produced nausea. These men gave up on surgery, and case notes bear witness to arguments between surgeon and patient. Men defaulted from follow-ups, behaved badly, and insisted on being discharged.

One set of notes records a battle of wills which lasted several months between the surgeons and a patient who had had his mandible largely removed by a bullet, as well as a fractured

---

24 The goblet now resides in the BAPRAS Archive. It was found by a police diver at the bottom of the
    Waikato River in New Zealand in the 1970s, and was kindly returned to Britain by Tim Fuller.

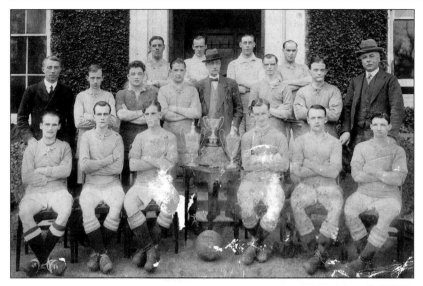

A photograph of the 1921 football team. (AWA and the BAPRAS Archive)

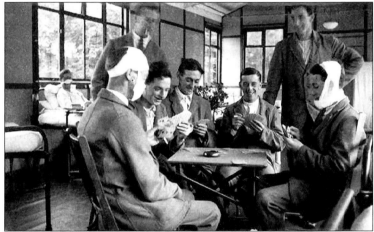

Patients in a Queen's Hospital ward, as photographed by Frank Whipp. (RCS)

humerus which would not unite. Wounded in 1917, he also had the misfortune to develop diphtheria. After five years, and seven operations, the patient refused any more:

> 26.9.22 Patient has remained in hospital awaiting treatment, but has refused operations under orthopaedic and plastic surgeons. He is not to be given any further option re operative treatment.
> 11.10.22. Patient was ordered to attend the dental department on 8th Oct to see Sir F. Colyer, but failed to attend.
> 20.10.22. For final discharge as all necessary treatment has been refused … refusal not considered reasonable.

Not all cases reached such an impasse. Gillies was a cheerful man who tried to put men at their ease, and who would follow the patients' wishes in some instances. Budd recalled such an occurrence in the aftermath of his "major op." Following the operation, Budd's "beautiful new nose looked more like a short piece of cucumber slipped on my face," and was surrounded

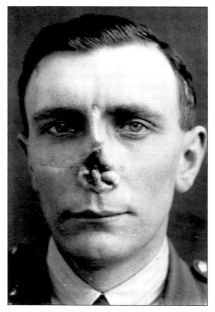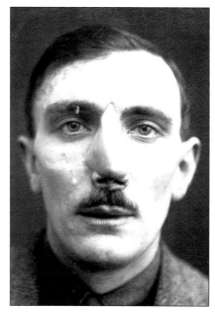

Captain J.G.H. Budd, 5 May 1919; 15 December 1919. (RCS)

by swelling which took a long time to return to normal. After the swelling had settled, Gillies trimmed off the "kink." On this occasion, Budd was sedated with a local rather than general anaesthetic, "for which I was glad, since it avoided the discomfort of the usual preparations and of the unpleasant aftermath of an ordinary do with A.E.C. [air, ether, chloroform] and the like." Unfortunately, shortly after the procedure, the tip of Budd's nose began to "show signs of trouble and it was decided another trim up was required" to aid Budd's breathing and remove a piece of cartilage from the bridge.

To Budd, "this did not seem to be much more of a job than the last," and he asked Gillies to repeat the local anaesthetic:

> After some demur he agreed to try it that way, and I shan't forget that operation in a hurry. I had 1½ hours on the table, never any pain, but always expecting it the next moment and at the end both I and all the people assisting in the operation were really exhausted. I remember my relief when I hear the words 'and now for the hairs of the horse, my boy' and I knew that it was only a matter of stitching up.[25]

Once the stitching up had been completed, at the end of six operations, Budd's treatment at Sidcup was complete.

Mindful of the long gaps between procedures, Gillies and his colleagues realised from the outset that boredom would be one of the worst enemies of their patients. R. Tait Mackenzie expressed a similar concern in a short book written in 1918:

> In England and France, where great numbers of wounded were thrown on the community at once, the country houses, given by the public-spirited owners as auxiliary Red

---

25 BLSC: Budd Papers, LIDDLE/WW1/WF/REC/01/B43.

Cross Hospitals, too often became nurseries of the 'hospital habit'. Men who came to them keen, well-disciplined, and alert, too often lapsed in an atmosphere of indulgence and hero worship into disorderly loafers.[26]

As a consequence, in addition to periods dedicated to leisure and entertainment, thought was given to useful activities which would occupy Sidcup's patients and set them up for civilian life.

Many classes were established at Sidcup to prevent the development of "an atmosphere of indulgence." The 1921 Hospital Report listed all the occupations being taught at that time, ranging from boot repairs to coach building (see Table 5.1). The artist John Hodgson Lobley painted several classes at work (See Colour Section, pp.xviii-xix).[27] Needlework was also practised. Bill Hollins, a member of the notorious hospital football team, made two beautiful pieces as cushion covers. However, as he was so ashamed of his "women's work," Hollins hid them away.[28] To be fit only for "women's work" was a blow indeed. Other handiwork items produced by the soldiers included bead necklaces made from rolled paper, some of which were created from cigarette packets.[29] These items were often presented for sale.

Table 5.1: Occupational Activities to July 1921

Course	Number on course
Toy making	322
Woodwork	253
Commercial	120
Beadwork	67
Boot repairing	23
Poultry farming	22
French	9
Dentistry	5
Hairdressing	4
Cinema operating	4
Bookbinding	3
Motor engineering	2
Draughtsmanship	1
Watch/clock repairing	1
Photography	1
Horticulture	1
Coach building	1
Other foreign languages	Not listed

26 R. Tait Mackenzie, *Reclaiming the Maimed: A Handbook of Physical Therapy* (London: Macmillan, 1918), p.105.
27 These paintings are now in the IWM.
28 Bill Hollins' daughter, personal communication.
29 Private Herne, West Yorkshire Regiment, made two necklaces. These were kindly donated to the author by his daughter, Pauline Curwen, and are now in the BAPRAS Archive.

The produce from Sidcup's most popular class, toy making, was also sold. Sidcup toys were sold at many outlets for the benefit of the hospital, and were widely praised for their quality. Sales were held in London and regularly advertised in the daily newspapers. A contemporary newspaper report said:

> The Queen, Princess Mary and Princess Helena Victoria paid a visit on Sunday to Chelsea House, Cadogan-place, and inspected there an exhibition of children's toys and beadwork and woodwork articles made by the soldier patients of the Queen's Hospital, Frognal, Sidcup. Several articles were selected by the Royal party for purchase.
>
> Princess Helena Victoria was again present yesterday when a very successful sale was held. The toys were all animals of the regulation 'woolly plush' order, with movable limbs and a finish equal to those seen in any toy store. The 'Teddy Bear' no longer ruled, though he was well represented. There were elephants (numbers of them white), dogs, ducks, and even camels. Many varieties of monkeys, chimpanzees, and apes also reproduced in woolly plush. The Queen chose a small grey chimpanzee among other things. Many of the elephants had springs cunningly arranged in their legs, and bounded behind their purchasers in a manner hardly becoming the elephantine dignity.[30]

Alongside the financial rewards for the hospital, the article also acknowledged the psychological importance attached to the classes. In some extreme cases, it explained, where sufferers had become depressed to the point of contemplating or even attempting suicide, the work had brought 'a powerful counteracting interest'.

Some of the occupations taught in classes at Sidcup were designed to keep men from the public eye. We do not know which men chose to learn cinema projection, but the job involved arriving before the audience, from whom they were hidden in the projection booth, and leaving after it. Poultry farming likewise enabled men to live away from major conurbations. Of course, teaching the men this trade had another significant advantage, because it provided the hospital's chicken farm, essential for the production of the eggs that comprised much of the sloppy diet administered by tube to those who could not take food because of their injury, with a renewable source of free labour.

Gillies did his best to humour and encourage his patients, although some of his colleagues were less than impressed with his methods. As noted above, Tommy Rhind, a young surgeon from New Zealand, was uncomfortable with Gillies' jocular approach to his charges. However, for every negative observation of Gillies' methods there were 10 which espoused the benefits of his style. Men responded well to the light-hearted banter and respected Gillies for not talking down to them. The whole ethos of rehabilitation, set out even before the Queen's Hospital opened, was testament to Gillies' nuanced understanding of the challenges which faced disfigured men. His approach counterbalanced the usually horrified reaction of family and friends at first sight of the injured man. The offer of photograph sets to patients, so that they might recall their appearance before, during and after treatment, acted as a form of positive reinforcement. Men might look odd, but far less so than they would have done untreated. The photographs were a constant reminder of their progression. Teaching men to cope with their disfigurement through humour was just one of the approaches taken at Sidcup.

In addition to providing men with photographs of their treatment, the staff at Sidcup also ensured that the men's physical appearance was taken care of. Albert Collins, a local boy who

---

30 LMA: H02/QM/Y/01/005 Newspaper cutting from *The Times*, 19 December 1919.

joined the staff of the Queen's Hospital at the age of 13 in 1919, was part of the grooming process. He was the lather boy, responsible for lathering up the faces of patients in readiness for the cut-throat razor of head barber, Freddie Scott.[31] With deep scars, missing areas of cheek, pedicles, and flaps, shaving the faces of men at Sidcup was not easy, and it was some time before Collins graduated to shaving. Special shaving techniques were used. Patients whose eyebrows were to be reconstructed had their scalps shaved except for a strip across the front, within the hairline, which would later be used as a flap. The solders, with typical humour, referred to their tube pedicles as sausages.

The Psychology of Disfigurement and of War: Causes of and Reactions to Injury

The Sidcup records contain some cases of self-inflicted injury. The commonest form of self-mutilation was an injury to foot, wrist or trigger finger. A few men shot themselves in the face, including George Webster (See Colour Section, p.xx). Born near Shrewsbury in 1887, Webster became a bank clerk and was recorded as a boarder in Bolton in the 1911 census. He signed up in Derby on 21 May 1916, and was posted to the East Kent Regiment in January 1917. Webster's Casualty Form baldly states: "Wounded. 'Self Inflicted'," just two months later, and ends with his transfer to England from the 8th Stationary Hospital in Wimereux on 13 June. The final entry reads: "GSW Face (S.I.) Whilst Insane." Correspondence suggests that Webster was indicted for a disciplinary offence, but that action on this was abandoned as a result of his mental state.[32] Unfortunately, his pension records have not survived and we do not know what motivated his actions. Another case, that of James Nash, Duke of Cornwall's Light Infantry, was so unusual that it was unclear whether the wound was a deliberate attempt to emulate the subject of Wilfred Owen's 'S.I.W.' or an accident. Nash received a vertical gash from chin to forehead, the repair of which was remarkable.

Others did not live to see the end of their treatment. David Howard was wounded in February 1918, and admitted to Sidcup in August of the same year (See Colour Section, p.xx). He had lost his lower lip and part of his jaw. After nine procedures, he was found dead in a local cottage by one of the surgeons on Boxing Day 1920. The cause of death was given as acute alcoholic poisoning. Alcohol was forbidden at the hospital, and from the available records it is unclear whether Howard chose to end his life. In peacetime Howard had been a chimney sweep, a profession which required regular contact with the occupants of the houses he visited. It is impossible to know whether a fear of the reaction he might provoke in his customers influenced his actions immediately before his death.

Post-traumatic stress disorder (PTSD), as it is now known, war neurosis or neurasthenia, was recognised even before the concept of shellshock was invented during the Great War. Shellshock resulted in major psychological disturbance and was thought to be due to the concussive effects of shell bursts, although there was no evidence of physical damage to the brain which supported this position.[33] Many soldiers suffered from shellshock. Contemporary reports indicated that 34 per 1,000 casualties from the front in 1916 suffered from neurosis and some 20 percent of 160,000 claimants in 1918 received their pension for functional nervous and mental disease. By 1921, this figure had doubled. Several texts, including Harvey Cushing's

---

31   Scott was also the hospital's unofficial bookmaker.
32   TNA: WO 363/W644, Army Service Record File for George Eliot Webster.
33   In 2014, evidence from warfare in the Gulf suggested that there was, after all, microscopic brain damage which might be the cause of shellshock/PTSD. See J. Ryu et al, 'The problem of axonal injury in the brains of veterans with histories of blast exposure', *Acta Neuropathologica Communications*, 2:153 (2014), <http://actaneurocomms.biomedcentral.com/articles/10.1186/s40478-014-0153-3> (accessed 26 January 2016).

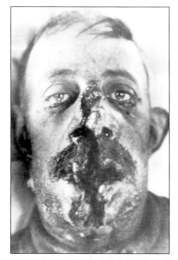 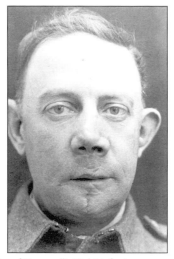 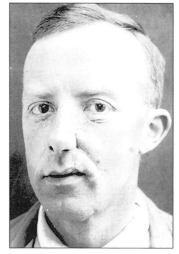

James Nash, 1/5 Battalion, Duke of Cornwall's Light Infantry.
Photographs before and after repair. (RCS)

Private Webster after surgery,
22 July 1918. (RCS)

From a Surgeon's Journal, illustrated the contorted postures adopted by soldiers who could no longer face life in the trenches.

Contemporary reports conveyed a curious class distinction in the depiction of men suffering from mental illness. The common soldier was portrayed, by MacCurdy for instance, as prone to hysterical behaviour. Officers, meanwhile, developed anxiety states. As W.H.R. Rivers noted in his introduction to MacCurdy's book, "Dr MacCurdy explains this fact by differences of education and responsibility which produce a different mental outlook towards the two chief means of escape from the rigours and horrors of warfare."[34] MacCurdy suggested, unsurprisingly given the stress imposed on a front line soldier, that the first symptom of shellshock was an undue sense of fatigue. Those who could not cope began to suffer disturbances in their sleep, with the appearance of severe hallucinatory nightmares. Some sufferers would then hope for injury or death, and would often court this through reckless behaviour. The final breakdown was precipitated by a near-miss shellburst, which either resulted in concussion or the burial of the victim. As a rule, sufferers were not physically harmed.

Outside the medical profession some scorn was expressed towards those who showed no sign of physical disability. Inside the medical profession, the management of patients varied greatly. On the one hand there was the kind, analytic approach of Rivers at Craiglockart as outlined by Siegfried Sassoon and immortalised in Pat Barker's *Regeneration* trilogy.[35] On the other hand was the more direct, 'pull yourself together' treatment practised by Lewis Yealland, a neurologist at the National Hospital for Nervous Diseases in London.

Discussing the case of an "emotional Irishman" who had been shot in the back and suffered from rigid paralysis of the right arm and head drop, Yealland wrote:

> I said 'You have been sent here so that you may have your arm and head cured. You must be very tired of walking about in such an attitude … Five months is a long time

---

34 J.T. MacCurdy, *War Neuroses* (Cambridge: Cambridge University Press, 1918).

35 S. Sassoon, *Sherston's Progress* (London: Faber & Faber, 1936); Pat Barker, *Regeneration* (London: Viking Press, 1991).

for such a disturbance to exist, and it has been five months of misery, I am sure. I would sympathise with you were it not for the fact that you will be cured in an hour'.[36]

In fact, the cure took three hours. Torture with electric shocks and humiliation were the main planks of Yealland's treatment.

Only three Sidcup facial patients were formally recorded as shellshocked. However, the case files indicate that there was some psychological disturbance among those with facial injuries. Rifleman Louis Ripps was a prime example. Photographed by the *Daily Mirror* with the Queen at his bedside in 1917, Ripps suffered from injuries to both his face and head. He returned to Sidcup several times with unexplained neurological symptoms, which included apparent fits. Despite a number of exploratory operations to try and determine an "organic" cause for his symptoms, none was ever found.[37]

Post-war psychological disturbance was not necessarily caused by injury. In Webster's case, the opposite was true, as his psychological disturbance clearly led to his injury. While there is unequivocal evidence that the war experience could be traumatic, those who suffered severe mood swings or were prone to violent behaviour may have been predisposed to post-war mental illness.

Harold Cullimore's granddaughter reflected upon the war's effect on her grandfather in a letter to the author in 2002. She wrote:

> He … went on to marry Beatrice Stone [a nurse at the hospital] and they had 7 daughters and one son. He became a postman and window cleaner and died in his late 80s or early 90s … I didn't go to his funeral. My mum didn't tell me or my 2 sisters that he had died until it was all over. She said that all his children had hated him and were scared of his brutal ways, apparently he used to drink a bit of cider and bash my granny quite regularly and he would hit the kids and shut them in the cupboard under the stairs.[38]

Cullimore's case notes provide evidence that he had been a difficult patient: "8.10.21. Patient is anxious about his health and is hypochondriasis [sic]. I have pointed out that his health is largely dependent on the repair of his mouth and jaw, but he insists his nerves are too bad to undergo a series of operations." A year later, Cullimore refused further treatment because of a dispute with the Ministry of Pensions over a grant to his mother.

Such behaviour may in many cases be attributed to what would now be termed PTSD, but it transpires that 'Gramp Cully' had possessed violent tendencies prior to the war. Cullimore attended the literacy class organised by Lady Gough, the widow of Brigadier General Sir John Edmond Gough VC, and his manuscript survives. "I'm a native of Gloucestershire," he wrote:

> [and] was born in the parish of Iron Acton in the year 1895. My father died when I was about the age of seven. Having a strong boyish will and temper, I often quarrelled with one or other of my brothers. During a fit of temper one morning, when I was about fourteen years of age, I struck an older brother with my clenched hand. The result of this action caused me to leave home and to live with a friend. A few months later my friend removed to another district and, not wishing to return to my home I decided to

---

36   L.R. Yealland, *Hysterical Disorder of Warfare* (London: Macmillan, 1918).

37   Royal College of Surgeons (RCS) Archives: MS0513/1/1/30 1746, Ripps, Louis – Rifle Brigade 7th.

38   T. Browne, personal communication, 21 June 2002.

enlist as a soldier. By this time I had reached the age of fifteen and I was stronger and bigger than many youths three or four years my seniors.[39]

Cullimore's age was discovered at his medical, but he blagged his way through and was enlisted at a recorded age of 18 years and three months. He served in Malta and China before being recalled with his regiment for action on the Western Front. He was shot by a sniper on 17 February 1915. His military records do not survive so, unlike some men whose service was punctuated by misdemeanours, we do not know whether army life had suppressed his violent instincts. Clearly, an aggressive past preceded his war service. At best, one could argue that Cullimore's personality did not aid his adjustment to civilian life.

It is impossible to say with confidence whether it was the war or the injury which caused PTSD. Some men were badly affected by their war experience whilst some appeared not to be. Whether or not they had received any major physical injury does not seem to have been a significant factor. Personality, resilience and the underlying spirit of the age compelled some men to get on with it. To the acclaim of the press at the time, Gillies and his team did all they could to support the physical and psychological recuperation of the men in their care. However, after the war was over, the mental scars of the battlefield remained.

Today, we have a better understanding of the causes of PTSD, but even so there are inexplicable anomalies in the overall picture. Thus, some symptoms attributable to stress or injury may be magnified by a perception that anyone put through the same situation will develop them. In the nineteenth century, there was an epidemic of psychogenic back pain attributed to rail travel, the so-called syndrome of railway spine. In the First World War a cardiac syndrome known as soldier's heart was extensively investigated; the symptoms, first described by Da Costa in the American Civil War, turned out to have no organic basis. More recently, the so-called Gulf War Syndrome produced a constellation of symptoms attributed variously to the stress of battle or exposure to toxic agents. However, it transpired that some of the same symptoms were also apparent in men who had never served in the Gulf theatre.[40] In the field of wartime facial injury it is apparent that the airmen burned in combat and treated at the Royal Victoria Hospital, East Grinstead in the Second World War, had a range of adjustment to their injury. The "Guinea Pigs" displayed responses from withdrawal to devil-may-care extroversion. While these responses may have been modified by psychological or medical interventions, I believe that pre-existing personality traits influenced adjustment.

Once the flow of new casualties from the fighting dried up, the Queen's Hospital began to fade gently into obscurity among the public. The gradual rundown of the plastic surgery work led to an arrangement with the Ministry of Pensions to admit general medical and surgical cases. In 1924, these were supplemented by the admission of patients with neurasthenia. No records of this work remain. In the following year the eight remaining facial patients were transferred to Queen Mary's Hospital, Roehampton. For the patients, the transition from wounded hero to gargoyle was not always easy. Some men never came to terms with their injuries and never left the hospital, opting to stay on as orderlies and porters after the war. Even the mortuary technician was an ex-patient. Jocky Anderson of the Black Watch, who claimed to have had more operations than anyone else, was one of those who remained. He celebrated his fiftieth operation by defying the hospital's alcohol ban. He went out, got roaring drunk and, on his return to the ward, smashed every window.

---

39 BLSC: LIDDLE/WW1/GA/WOU34, My Personal Experiences of the Great War, Essay from Lady Gough's class, January 1922.
40 Simon Wesseley, personal communication.

Conclusion

Men with facial injuries were, through reconstruction and rehabilitation, able to return to their communities without necessarily encountering rejection by family, friends and the public. Through the provision of useful occupational training, tailored to the circumstances of the patients, the process of rehabilitation was often successful. Men were kept busy with work experience and leisure activities. The misery predicted by some press articles did not reach the proportions predicted. The positive attitudes of the surgeons, the camaraderie that developed between the men who encouraged and supported each other, and the benefit to new arrivals of seeing the changes wrought by surgery in those who had come before them, all contributed to the convivial atmosphere at Sidcup. Nonetheless, some men were traumatised by their injury and felt unable to move far from the safe environment of the hospital.

6

The Legacy of the Queen's Hospital for Surgeons and Surgery

Daryl Lindsay described the relief of one of Sidcup's Australian surgeons when the Armistice was declared on 11 November 1918. He wrote:

> It was the day of the armistice, 1918. The Colonel [Henry Newland] had been to the dispensary, and we met on the ramp and passed the time of day. 'Interesting news, Lindsay', he said, and might have been commenting on a minor topic in *The Times*. But as he spoke he was unconsciously snapping some tubes of tablets in his hands, and the tablets were falling on the ramp. It was, I think, a deeply-felt suppressed emotion of a man who had seen the war in all its phases, and now it was over.[1]

Yet for those at Sidcup, the task was not complete. The Queen's Hospital did not close at the end of the war, and surgical work continued to take place there until 1925. But the specialty of plastic surgery, although it had undergone rapid and extraordinary growth in response to the demands of the conflict, almost disappeared in Great Britain once the backlog of cases had been cleared. Harold Gillies and Tommy Kilner kept the surgical pot simmering for another 20 years, until the demands of a second global conflict sparked another upswing in demand for facial reconstruction. This chapter will explore the careers of those who worked at the Queen's Hospital, chart the gradual dispersal of Sidcup's surgeons across the world, and explain why many of them returned to non-plastic surgical work after the war. It will also evaluate the worldwide legacy of facial surgery at Sidcup during the First World War, in terms of technique, education, and psychology.

The Effect of the Armistice on Facial Reconstruction Work

The Armistice did not immediately end the plastic surgery work of the Queen's Hospital. New casualties arrived almost up to the last minute of the war, and the surgical processes which had begun still had to be finished. However, it was not long before the Dominions' contingents began to return home with their patients and records. By the summer of 1919 they were all gone. In May 1920, the War Office handed control of the hospital over to the Ministry of Pensions, and general medical and surgical cases were admitted. Gillies and his British colleagues continued their facial work.

---

1   D. Lindsay, 'Five men', *Medical Journal of Australia*, 18 January 1958.

The reputation of the Queen's Hospital had been firmly established during the war. The American George Dorrance, who had gone to France at the end of his attachment, said "[The] hospital holds an enviable position; the originality of the surgeons, coupled with their excellent technic [sic], established principles in plastic surgery which will last forever."[2] Patients were referred to Sidcup from other hospitals for a second opinion well into the 1920s.

The reputation of Sidcup was so widely recognised that referrals were not always made at the suggestion of a doctor. Gillies himself recalled of a particularly case when:

> At a cocktail party in London … one of my officer patients, on whom I had been working for no less than a year, was approached by the charming hostess. She led him off to one side and confidentially whispered, 'They say this fellow Gillies is quite good. He could set your face right again. Why don't you go to see him?'[3]

In addition, the patients themselves were often keen to be reviewed. Major Northey, 1st Gurkhas, had first been admitted in October 1917. He had been wounded in March and, according to the notes, had "a large depressed scar region of angle of ascending ramus left jaw due to loss of tissues— bony and soft— in this region." In June 1921, he wrote to Gillies:

> I am writing to ask if you will kindly have just a look at my face any time. — I have got a few weeks leave & would much like to come & look you up again. I am very fit and well, thanks to your skilful [sic] treatment, and have no trouble really at all with my jaw.
>
> One or two enthusiasts have volunteered to still further diminish the scars a good deal and 'round off' my cheek by massaging or some such means, but I thought that I would rather not let any one touch it, until I had shown it to you. — As a matter of fact, I am absolutely & perfectly content with the whole thing as it is, and the scars don't worry me at all. Anyhow I would like just to show it to you just once to show you how things are getting on. Every body [sic] always says what a wonderful job you made of it.— Hope you have not forgotten your violin with excess of work, etc.— With kindest regards to Mrs Gillies.[4]

Gillies fixed an appointment, decided against action, but resolved to monitor the situation. Eventually, Northey returned in 1923 and Gillies inserted an abdominal fat graft to pad out the cheek. During the early 1920s, the occasional civilian also began to appear among the admissions at the Queen's. All that is known of the circumstances surrounding Sister McGee's broken nose is that the records state she was hit with a golf club. Albert Parlett, who was only 16 when he was first admitted to Sidcup, lost his nose in a bottle fight. His reconstruction was a success (See Colour Section, p.xx).

Many of those referred to Sidcup after the war were difficult cases in which surgery elsewhere had gone wrong. As a result, the surgery at Sidcup not infrequently failed to produce good results. Bone grafts failed and failed again; cosmetic repairs occasionally looked worse than the original. Some problems simply defied Gillies and his colleagues. Despite their best attempts to repair injuries of the cheek, where the zygomatic arch of the maxilla below the

---

2   G.M. Dorrance, 'Observations on the work at Queen's Hospital in England, *The Dental Summary*, 39 (1919), p.866.

3   H.D. Gillies and R. Millard, *The Principles and Art of Plastic Surgery* (London: Butterworth & Co., 1957), p.43.

4   RCS Archives: Gillies Archives, Letter in Northey's case file.

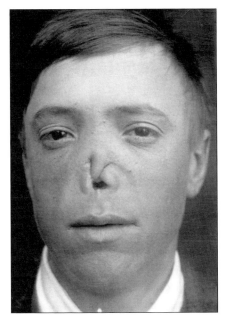 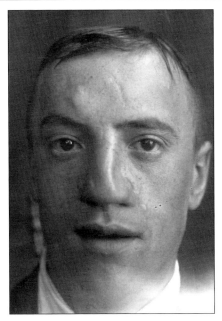

Albert Parlett, aged 16 on admission, August 1923; following completion of surgery after seven operations, 22 July 1924. (RCS)

eye had been lost, the reconstruction of a reasonable eye socket was rare.[5] In addition, reconstructive surgery for nerves was non-existent. Men whose facial nerves had been severed by a shell fragment suffered from persistent facial paralysis, although partially successful experiments to transpose muscles which allowed patients to close their eyes did take place. A great deal of the later work was dental rather than facial. Men came with little superficial injury but major bone loss, particularly of the mandible. Due to their injuries, many had developed stiffness or complete fixation (ankylosis) of the jaw joints and were unable to open their mouths. Function was paramount in such cases and the cosmetic aspects were often ignored.

William Arbuthnot Lane did not achieve the recognition he had sought for his perceived role in the establishment of the hospital:

> What pleased me most during the war was the organisation of Queen Mary's Hospital at Sidcup, for the treatment of the deformities of the face resulting from wounds ... I realised that our hospital would be much improved by competition, so I approached the directors of the Canadian, South African, Australian and New Zealand hospitals. They all responded that the section in each were quite satisfied with their existing staff. I then approached these gentlemen socially and pointed out to them the advantage that would accrue to them and all if they joined us and competed amicably with one another. They all agreed and finally we had huts allocated to each with their own medical staffs. This competition brought out many men who were excellent at plastic

---

5   It is possible that the surviving records at Sidcup overstate this problem. Many of the maxillary fractures were transferred to Sir Frank Colyer at Croydon War Hospital and only the worst cases were retained at the Queen's.

work and also vied with each other in advancing this special form of surgery. The result of their activities was remarkable. Nothing was more painful than the sense of loneliness of those mutilated, since these deformities repelled even their wives and children. I understood that many, faced with the horror of the situation, committed suicide rather than meet those they were engaged to.

When peace had been declared I expected that [Sir Alfred] Keogh would have been given a practical expression of the debt his country owed to him for his invaluable work during the war, but to my amazement such monetary and titular rewards were allotted to such of the fighting generals whose activities were only too frequently less appreciated by the nation than his merited. Men that save life never get the same appreciation and reward as those whose business it is to destroy life.[6]

Arbuthnot Lane's disappointment with the lack of recognition for the work of the army's medical services in Britain was matched by an equally selective acknowledgement of those who had operated in France. The end of the war in November 1918 brought to an end the work of the British-run hospitals on the Western Front, and the flamboyant Charles Auguste Valadier wound down his work at the 83rd General Hospital in Wimereux. His throughput had been far smaller than that at Sidcup, but the British authorities never gave his work the recognition it deserved. Valadier had provided most of his own equipment and worked for nothing, had started Gillies' career as a facial surgeon, and was as generous with his records as he had been with his time and money. Less than three weeks after the Armistice, Colonel Elliott wrote from the 8th British Red Cross Hospital in Boulogne to Sir Arthur Keith at the RCS:

I had a talk this afternoon with Valadier in his department at the hospital. He is showing greater generosity in the matter of our War Office Collection than any officer with whom I have had dealings in France. Everything that he possesses in his collection is being given to you without reserve, and you will have the power to allow anyone to make copies or duplicates from any of his material ... Long ago he promised me that his collection should be given to London, and he has upheld his word with the fullest honesty. He might quite fairly have asked that his collection should be divided between America, Paris and London, so that his work might be made evident in each of these three places. But instead of doing so, he has given all to London, though London has throughout treated him with a persistent contempt that would have prompted most men to the petty revenge of refusing to give their work to London. I do hope that when this collection reaches you, as it will in January, that you will persuade those in authority to prove their gratitude to Valadier in some effective way. He has deserved well of you.[7]

Valadier's records included wax and plaster casts, moulds, photographic negatives and prints, which Elliott noted were "all fully labelled and described." In return, rather grudgingly, he was offered an honorary knighthood. Sadly, Valadier's career nosedived after the war. He gained notoriety as a dilettante, shortened his working day and passed over all but the easiest work to his colleagues. He charged enormous fees to those who could afford to pay them and, with the

---

6   Quoted in T.B. Layton, *Sir William Arbuthnot Lane, Bt.* (Edinburgh: E. & S. Livingstone, 1956), pp.110-111.
7   RCS Archives: Letter from Thomas Renton Elliott to Sir Arthur Keith, 27 November 1918. (Courtesy of Dr Sam Alberti, RCS)

aid of a large inheritance from his mother, he lived the high life. Valadier spent large sums at the gaming tables until his death, sick and penniless, in 1931.[8]

The fate of the Facial Museum at Sidcup was discussed at some length by the staff at the end of the war, and it was decided in 1921 that a selection of material should join Valadier's collection at the RCS. Sir Charles Kenderdine managed to delay the move on the grounds that there were still 250 patients at the hospital and the specimens were of value to the surgeons.[9] However, the number of patients decreased, and in March 1922 the Facial Museum was transferred. Following the departure of the last facial injury cases to Roehampton, a large ultra-violet ray department was installed for the treatment of ulcers, tuberculosis of the skin and old wounds. Treatment in the sun was popular, but by 1929 the Ministry of Pensions had clearly lost interest in Sidcup as 470 of its 550 beds lay vacant. As war pensioners were "necessarily a diminishing class" according to the hospital report, the Ministry moved out the patients and laboratory and closed down the hospital altogether. It was more than just the men and equipment that were removed, as noted in a structural survey completed in 1947. Some government-sponsored asset stripping also occurred, as "the owners removed a quantity of joinery of historic interest including the chestnut panelling in the billiard room, the early 17th Century mantelpiece in the dining room and the mantelpiece in the Long Gallery."[10]

With the patients and equipment gone, arrangements were made to sell the site. The freehold was vested in the charity which had originally administered the hospital, and two of the trustees, Kenderdine and Surgeon Rear-Admiral Hill, laboured for some months to negotiate a sale to the London County Council. After considerable haggling over the price, the two parties agreed on a total of £29,000. The proceeds were transferred to the Star and Garter Home at Richmond, with a provision to draw on the fund for the purpose of providing welfare for ex-Sidcup patients enshrined in the terms.

The final arrangements over investment of the proceeds took until 1931. At their conclusion, there was a palpable sense of sadness at the end of an era, as Hill wrote to Kenderdine:

> My dear Sir Charles,
> I am enclosing the copy of the Minutes of the last meeting of the Queen's Hospital (Sidcup) Committee duly signed as requested. I must repeat my sense of indebtedness to you as Hon Secretary and Treasurer for all the work you have done and enabled the transfers to be carried out so smoothly. It is quite sad to think … *C'est tout fini.*[11]

Kenderdine's reply indicated his relief, tinged with anger that, like Arbuthnot Lane, his own contribution had not been fully recognised. He was particularly upset that the St John's Ambulance had not accorded him any honour, and he treated the Government's response with contempt:

---

8   Xavier Riaud, *Pionniers de la Chirurgie Maxillo-Faciale* (Paris: L'Harmettan, 2008).

9   Correspondence between T.H. Goodwin (War Office), Sir Charles Kenderdine (Queen's Hospital Management Committee) and Sir Arthur Keith (Royal College of Surgeons). (Courtesy of Dr Sam Alberti, RCS)

10 Bexley Local Studies Centre: Papers of Doctor Andrew Bamji, Survey report on the structure of Queen Mary's Hospital, 1947. Sadly, the fine staircase was secretly (and illegally) removed during alterations to the house in the 1980s and replaced by a poor-quality pastiche.

11 Correspondence in the records of Queen Mary's Hospital Roehampton, transferred to LMA (H02/QM). Unless otherwise stated, all quotations in these passages come from this source.

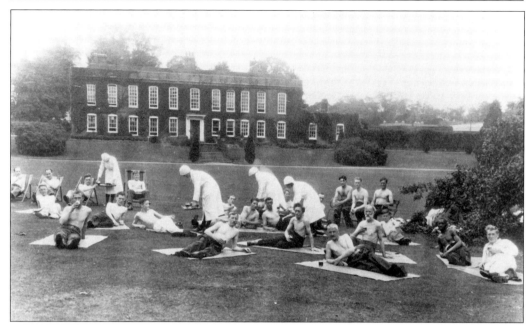

The Frognal lawn, with tuberculosis patients sunbathing. (Author's collection)

Thank you very much for your kind remarks. The winding-up has been a long job, as I knew it would be, although I think the ladies thought it could be accomplished by a stroke of the pen.

It has been a pleasure to me as the founder and organiser of the whole concern from start to finish, and I am rather proud of the remarkable work that has been accomplished there. It has now all faded out and been forgotten. In any case I have got the happiest remembrances of the dear old place where I spent the best years of my life and the sincere thanks of yourself and Lord Clifton for my efforts. I also received a short letter of thanks from the Secretary to the Ministry of Pensions, which I consigned to the W[aste] P[aper] B[asket].

Kenderdine's letter made reference to the remarkable work which had been accomplished at Sidcup. The official statistics provide further evidence to the achievements of the surgeons of the Queen's Hospital. Up until 1921, a total of 11,752 operations had been performed. In later accounts, this figure was incorrectly interpreted as 11,000 patients, and did not take into account the repeat surgery which had been required in many cases. A further four years of work after 1921 saw more patients, both new ones and readmissions, pass through the Queen's.

Sidcup was unique among British hospitals due to its specialisation in facial reconstruction. The 3rd London General Hospital, which housed Derwent Wood's 'Masks for Facial Disfigurement' workshop and undertook some dental work, is an example of one of the small number of hospitals which undertook some facial surgery as part of their general work. The Christmas 1916 edition of the hospital gazette described the 3rd London General's work in great detail, even including the clinic times of the dentists. However, the work appears to have been largely confined to splinting. The facial work was discussed by two surgeons in 1940, but their introduction makes clear that no case notes had been available. Therefore, the content of the book was the result of their own memories and fragmentary photographic material.[12] Sir Frank Colyer, who held an honorary position at Sidcup, ran a unit at Croydon to which some of Sidcup's jaw patients were sent.[13] Some work, again mostly jaw surgery, had also been done in Birmingham, Manchester and Leeds. In Edinburgh, a burns unit had been run by Cecil Wakeley that took in men from Jutland. Wakeley published a series of papers about his work, and some of his patients made their way south to Sidcup.[14] None of Wakeley's clinical notes survive. The paucity of records was exacerbated by the destruction of all British medical notes by the Ministry of Pensions on the basis that, by 1928, all pension computations had been completed and there was no need to retain them. Fragments of medical reports survive in some soldiers' files in the National Archives.

The Diaspora of Surgeons

Sidcup has been rightly acknowledged as the birthplace of modern plastic surgery. Gillies was determined to ensure that lessons would be learned from the war casualties, and immediately set to work on his first textbook, *Plastic Surgery of the Face*. It was published in 1920 and set the standard for facial reconstruction for the next 30 years. The book was almost entirely based on Sidcup's military patients. As a result of its organisation, illustrations, and the detailed nature of its outcome analysis,[15] *Plastic Surgery of the Face* became the reference work of choice, and through it Gillies began to outline what he viewed as the key principles for the work. In contrast, the other major reference work of the period, John Staige Davis' *Plastic Surgery: Its Principles and Practice*, contained no military cases despite the author's expressed hope that it would aid surgeons dealing with wounded soldiers.[16]

Most of the Queen's Hospital's surgeons and dentists returned to their pre-war posts and abandoned facial reconstruction. In three cases in particular this was surprising. Bedford Russell, who assisted Gillies with the editing process for *Plastic Surgery*, continued to work at Sidcup on a sessional basis, but in private practice he reverted to ENT surgery. He wrote to a friend in April 1920 that "I have been let loose on the ears, noses and throats of a long-suffering and unsuspecting public … Luckily I still draw food bar gold from the Queen's Hospital, Sidcup where I've been making noses with Gillies for the last 12 months – very fascinating work it is too."[17] Bertram Mendleson ("Mendelson" in all the Sidcup staff records), who helped write the section on facial injury in the Official History, returned to his dental practice just off Harley Street, and Gilbert Chubb, who was credited by Gillies with the development of wire fixation of bone grafts, returned to his original specialism of oto-rhino-laryngology. However, Chubb also continued to work at Roehampton. Whilst these men did not pursue plastic surgery after the war, their experience of plastic surgery work did inform their work in their post-war careers.

---

12 W. Warwick James and B.W. Fickling, *Injuries of the Jaws and Face* (London: John Bale & Staples, 1940). Curiously, the book makes no reference to the work of the Queen's Hospital.

13 J.F. Colyer, 'A note on the treatment of gunshot injuries of the mandible', *The British Medical Journal*, 2:1 (1917), pp.1-3.

14 C.P.G. Wakeley, 'The treatment of war burns', *Journal of the Royal Naval Medical Service*, (1917), pp.156-162; 'Skin grafting in the treatment of war burns', *The Lancet*, 191:4943 (1918), pp.736-737; 'The treatment of burns in naval warfare', *American Journal of Surgery*, 33:3 (1919), pp.61-63.

15 Many of the outcome analyses within the text were incomplete – a result of the fact that the book was written and published before many of the patients had been discharged.

16 J. Staige Davis, *Plastic Surgery: Its Principles and Practice* (Philadelphia, PA: P. Blackiston's Son & Co., 1919). For a comparison of Davis' and Gillies' works, see M.F. Freshwater, 'A critical comparison of Davis' principles of plastic surgery with Gillies' plastic surgery of the face', *Journal of Plastic, Reconstructive and Aesthetic Surgery*, 64:1 (2011), pp.17-26.

17 Letter from Russell to 'Gus', an obstetrician friend, 16 April 1920. (Author's collection)

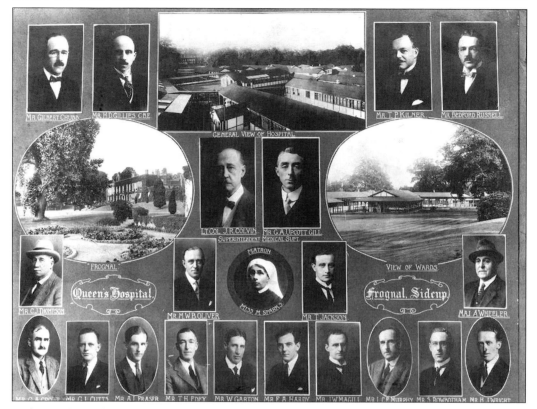

The 1920 hospital Christmas card, with portraits of the surgical staff. Gilbert Chubb is top left, and Bedford Russell is top right. A.L. Fraser – one of Gillies' two original dental colleagues at Aldershot in 1916 – is in the bottom row, third from left. (Author's collection)

By the end of 1919, all of the overseas staff had left Sidcup. Fulton Risdon and Carl Waldron established a plastic surgery presence in Canada, as did Henry Pickerill in New Zealand. In the United States, Vilray Blair, Ferris Smith and George Dorrance all established units. However, the more important drive came both from Davis, who had completed his textbook on plastic surgery without exposure to the mass of military casualties, and surgeons such as Varastad Kazanjian, Robert Ivy, and C.W. 'Bobs' Roberts, who had seen service in France but were aware of the organisational success of Sidcup. Great strides were made in the development of services in the United States, led by surgeons who had acquired experience at Sidcup. It may be argued that the more tolerant attitude of American surgeons and the American public to the development of cosmetic surgery underpinned the successful expansion of plastic surgery there. The Australian service petered out as Henry Newland completed work on the returned Sidcup men. Newland returned to Melbourne, where he continued to manage the Australian patients who required ongoing treatment, but otherwise he gradually reverted to general surgery.

Pickerill continued treatment of the New Zealanders who occasionally re-referred themselves to his surgery at Dunedin. However, his post-war story was one of discontent. Within a short time Pickerill ditched his appointment in the Dental School, abandoned his wife and left for Australia where he married one of his trainees. The move did not work out, and he returned to New Zealand where his domestic changes saw him ostracised by colleagues. Assisted by his new wife, Cecily, Pickerill continued to do facial work but did not train any surgeons. He operated on children with cleft lips and plates, but left much of the aftercare to nurses and only attended his small hospital weekly to operate and see new patients. His post-war textbook, *Facial Surgery*, ungraciously failed to acknowledge any of the other Sidcup surgeons.[18] In contrast, Gillies' book scrupulously gave credit where it was due, and recorded Pickerill as the inventor of a number of procedures. John Law Aymard also returned home embittered. He never forgave Gillies for, as he saw it, stealing credit for the tube pedicle from him. Whilst Aymard's family recall that he had retained many of his detailed case notes, sadly they were stolen and their whereabouts are not known.[19]

In 1921, there were only two recognised plastic surgeons in England: Harold Gillies and Thomas Kilner. There was only a small demand for cosmetic surgery, which was certainly not on widespread offer in the voluntary hospitals. Furthermore, there were only a limited number of people who could afford cosmetic surgery. Such work was inevitably done privately and was still perceived as less than suitable for quality surgeons. The two men entered into partnership, but their relationship soured in 1925 when the Sidcup plastic surgery unit was moved to Roehampton. Kilner agreed with the move, but Gillies did not. The disagreement between the two surgeons was aggravated by what Richard Battle has referred to as Kilner's unwillingness to "play second fiddle for ever."[20]

Gillies had a major hospital appointment at St Bartholomew's Hospital, but did most of his work privately. He consulted in Harley Street and performed many of his operations at St Andrew's, a small hospital in Dollis Hill, north-west London. Business picked up, and Gillies began to struggle with his workload. In 1930, he took on a new associate, one who also happened to be a New Zealander. Rainsford Mowlem joined Gillies almost by accident. He had completed his surgical Fellowship in 1926, and happened to meet Gillies whilst he acted as locum for a sick colleague prior to his return home.[21] Archibald McIndoe, also a New Zealander, reached London the following year by way of the Mayo Clinic in Rochester, Minnesota, where had been spotted by the eminent Leeds abdominal surgeon, Berkeley Moynihan. Clearly impressed with McIndoe's skills, Moynihan had spoken with great enthusiasm about the development of a Postgraduate Medical School at Hammersmith Hospital in London, and suggested that McIndoe was precisely the kind of surgeon he required. McIndoe promptly resigned his post at the Mayo and headed for London with his wife and young family. However, upon arrival in London in 1931, he discovered that Moynihan was unable to remember him. Furthermore, the Medical School at Hammersmith did not yet exist. At the suggestion of his mother, McIndoe consulted Gillies, who was a cousin of sorts, and he invited McIndoe to join his private practice. Like Gillies' partnership with Kilner, his professional association with McIndoe did not last. Hugh Johnson, who trained with McIndoe, wrote: "The two were really congenial but I can understand why the relationship wasn't lasting, for I've never known two such independent men. The loose partnership broke up before the war because, as Sir Harold put it 'The tail began wagging the dog'."[22]

18 For a full account of Pickerill's life and career, see Harvey Brown, *Pickerill: Pioneer in Plastic Surgery, Dental Education and Dental Research* (Dunedin: Otago University Press, 2007).

19 Janet Harding, personal communication.

20 R. Battle, 'Plastic surgery in the two World Wars and in the years between', *Journal of the Royal Society of Medicine*, 71:11 (1978), pp.844-848.

21 D.N. Matthews, 'Gillies: mastermind of modern plastic surgery', *British Journal of Plastic Surgery*, 32:1 (1979), pp.68-77.

22 H. Johnson, 'A brush with the golden decade of plastic surgery, 1949 to 1959', *Annals of Plastic Surgery*, 8:2 (1982), pp.166-178.

The Impact of the Second World War

It took the threat of war in 1938 to engender any serious effort to re-establish plastic surgery in England.[23] In 1932, the army began to develop a plan for plastic surgery organisation in the event of war and commissioned a report from a small committee including Gillies, William Kelsey Fry, and William Warwick James, the dental surgeon from the 3rd London General Hospital. The report contained an outline of the size and organisation recommended for a plastic surgery unit, along with an appendix which recorded the constituents of the liquid diet developed at Aldershot.[24] The conclusions of the report were based on the success of the Queen's Hospital and acknowledged its importance. The report lay dormant until 1938, when further discussions led to the conclusion that simply reopening Sidcup was impracticable as it lay under the projected route for bombers on their way to London, a prophesy which proved accurate during the war when the site at Frognal was twice damaged by enemy action.[25]

Rather than being concentrated in one location, the provision of facial reconstruction in the Second World War took place across a number of sites. Gillies' base was at Rooksdown House near Basingstoke, where Ivan Magill continued to anaesthetise his patients. Gillies looked after army and a smattering of RAF patients at Rooksdown, as well as civilian casualties, since civilians had become as likely to become the casualties of high-explosives as combatants thanks to bombing raids. Mowlem went to Mount Vernon and St Albans Hospitals, where he was joined as an artist by Dickie Orpen, daughter of the famous war artist Sir William. McIndoe set up base at the Queen Victoria Hospital, East Grinstead, where he was advised by Kelsey Fry. Kilner continued to work at Roehampton under the direction of the Ministry of Pensions, and later moved his base to Stoke Mandeville Hospital near Aylesbury. As none of the other Sidcup surgeons returned to work on the new influx of patients, a new raft of nascent plastic surgeons joined the various teams.

The rivalry between Gillies and McIndoe rumbled on during the Second World War as McIndoe's fame grew. McIndoe was an ebullient, even threatening personality, whose character was magnified by the particular glamour of his position. Being chief consultant to the RAF, his patients were drawn from the ranks of the RAF's fighter pilots. These men have become thought of as the pioneer subjects of plastic surgery, overshadowing the burns surgery undertaken on around 60 patients at Sidcup during the First World War.[26] Gillies and his family resented the manner in which McIndoe's media machine, with his establishment of the 'Guinea Pig' club which gained substantial publicity, consigned Gillies' own proto-guinea pigs to near oblivion. Yet McIndoe was the quicker – and perhaps better – surgeon of the two, whilst Mowlem was arguably a better surgeon than either of them.

Despite the arrival of new and inexperienced surgeons, record-keeping at Rooksdown was just as meticulous in the Second World War as it had been at Sidcup in the earlier conflict. Again, Gillies took advantage of modern technology. Operations and progress reports were typewritten onto proforma notes, and diagrams and photographs were made serially. Sellotape, rather than glue, was used to attach photographs to the case notes. Unfortunately, this material has not

23 P.J. Sykes and A.N. Bamji, 'Plastic surgery during the interwar years', *Annals of Plastic Surgery*, 65:4 (2010), pp.374-377.

24 *Report to the Army Council of the Army Advisory Standing Committee on Maxillo-facial injuries* (London: His/Her Majesty's Stationery Office, 1935).

25 In the first instance, a bomb landed in the courtyard of Frognal House. In the second, a V1 'Doodlebug' destroyed two wards in The Jungle in 1944.

26 Despite the glamour of the Spitfire and Hurricane, in fact most of McIndoe's patients were from Bomber Command. See Emily Mayhew, *The Reconstruction of Warriors: Archibald McIndoe, the Royal Air Force and the Guinea Pig Club* (London: Greenhill, 2004).

withstood the test of time, and as a result the case notes from Rooksdown are in a poorer condition than those from Sidcup. Instead of tasking artists with the production of watercolours, Gillies enlisted the help of Percy Hennell of the Metal Box Company. Hennell had discovered a three-lens camera invented by the Devin Colorgraph Company of New York, with which it was possible to reconstruct colour images by overlaying acetate monochrome negatives (See Colour Section, p.xxi). Hennell went on to produce a large number of photographs for the various units, a number of which survive in the collections of the RCS and BAPRAS.

The First World War had led to a brief and intense development in plastic surgery among British surgeons, followed by a largely dormant period. The effects of the Second World War on the specialty were profoundly different. While surgery for hare-lip and cleft palate had been performed prior to both wars it became apparent that the techniques applied to injured servicemen could be applied to other congenital deformities, and the number of surgeons who gained experience during the Second World War was sufficient to provide most general hospitals with at least a partial presence. In 1946, Gillies, Kilner, McIndoe and Mowlem, despite their professional differences, were instrumental in the establishment of the British Association of Plastic Surgeons, now BAPRAS. The British Association of Plastic Surgeons was a professional organisation for plastic surgeons that provided both a political presence and the opportunity to develop specialist education and research. The advent of the NHS in 1948, coupled with a change in attitudes towards cosmetic procedures, sustained a growth in the specialty upon which Gillies, Kilner, McIndoe and Mowlem's influence was undeniable. As late as 1978, one of the 'Big Four' had been responsible for the training of every consultant in plastic surgery in the United Kingdom.[27]

The many articles in the medical literature on Gillies express similar opinions: that he was brilliant, innovative, and difficult, this last feature perhaps not unusual among polymaths. He received a variety of honours, including a knighthood, honorary membership of overseas societies, a caricature in *Punch*, and even immortalisation as a golfer on a cigarette card. Gillies was content to push the boundaries of accepted practice, such as in 1946 when he became the first surgeon to perform a female to male gender reassignment procedure, on Laura Dillon.[28] Before he attempted the reverse procedure in the early 1950s on an ex-pilot named Robert Cowell, Gillies' conduct was highly questionable. He and two colleagues borrowed a corpse from a nearby hospital mortuary in order to do a practice run. The American plastic surgeon Jerome Webster suggested that Gillies' gender reassignment work was responsible for his being passed over for the Professorship of Plastic Surgery at Oxford, which was instead awarded to his old Sidcup colleague Tommy Kilner, yet Gillies' private practice, although highly lucrative on paper, did not bring him the riches he might have been expected to enjoy. In part, this was down to Gillies' somewhat cavalier attitude to money, which would later get him into trouble over unpaid income tax. Gillies' relaxed financial outlook was partly related to his generosity towards the less privileged. In cases where a young patient required work but the parents were in straitened circumstances, Gillies reduced or waived his fees, as in the case of Eric Wormleighton who was born with a cleft lip. Surgery at the Hammersmith Hospital had been unsuccessful, and Eric was seen by Gillies in 1933. Eric's father, a picture restorer whose business had been badly affected by the Great Depression, wrote that he was only earning £4 per week, and concluded "I must leave

---

27 Battle, 'Plastic surgery in the two World Wars'.
28 L. Hodgkinson, *Michael Nee Laura: The World's First Female to Male Transsexual* (London: Virgin Books, 1989); P. Kennedy, *The First Man-Made Man: The Story of Two Sex Changes, One Love Affair, and a Twentieth-Century Medical Revolution* (New York: Bloomsbury, 2007).

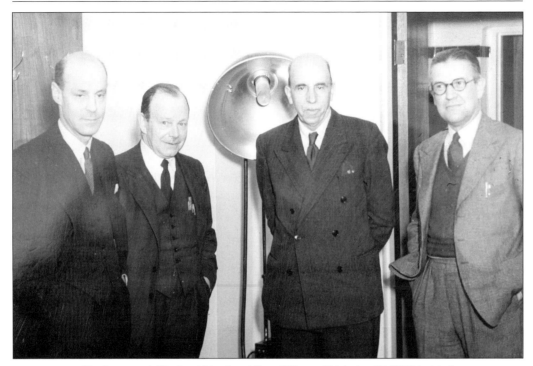

Plastic surgery's 'Big Four': Mowlem, Kilner, Gillies and McIndoe. (BAPRAS Archive)

myself in your good hands to charge me what you think fit."[29] A special rate, albeit at the quite substantial price of 30 guineas, was arranged, and Gillies also performed later operations at a vastly reduced rate. Bob Seymour, Gillie's secretary and ex-patient, appears to have had considerable discretion in financial matters, and Seymour's memory problems in the 1950s may have compounded the financial issues faced by the practice.

Beyond his surgical practice, Gillies was in great demand as a teacher. Despite mobility-limiting arterial disease, the result of a lifelong smoking habit, Gillies lectured, performed numerous demonstration operations, assisted at others, and developed many friendships overseas, particularly in India. He sustained correspondence with his students, and his personal papers contain many of the letters he wrote to compliment them on their technique in a way that must have brought great pride to their recipients. In 1957, alongside one of his trainees from Rooksdown, Ralph Millard, he authored a new and profusely illustrated two-volume textbook, *The Principles and Art of Plastic Surgery*. Although the light style of the work mirrored that of Gillies' correspondence, the lengthy exchange of letters between Gillies and Millard from 1952 onwards illustrates that Millard was actually responsible for writing the majority of the text whilst Gillies edited it.[30] However, between 1915 and 1957, Gillies had continually reflected upon the principles and the practice of plastic surgery, and the title of the book reflected its 40-year gestation. While much of the treatise was devoted to technique, the principles that underpin the specialty which were elaborated in Gillies' work hold true to this day.

Gillies also took up landscape painting, and had several successful exhibitions. However, although he could build faces, he could not draw them. He once painted a picture of the family

---

29 Correspondence kindly supplied by Mr Austin Wormleighton.
30 Correspondence from Gillies' files, courtesy of Ms Susie Winter.

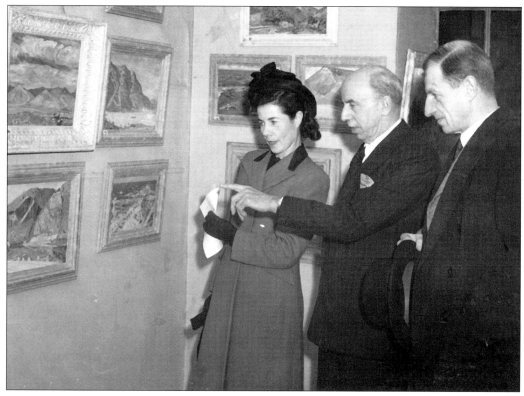

Sir Harold Gillies discussing his paintings at Foyles Art Gallery, 1948. (Author's collection)

dining room at Christmas which included the laid table, the mantelpiece, and the portrait of his grandmother that hung above it. His painting stopped at her shoulders, and the top of the frame was omitted.

Gillies was 12 years older than McIndoe, his erstwhile junior partner. However, Gillies outlived him, as McIndoe died suddenly in April 1960. The circumstances surrounding his death were mysterious. There was no mystery about his failing eyesight or his bid to become President of the RCS, yet his death, alone, just one day after he had been told that his Presidential bid had been unsuccessful, was not accompanied by a coroner's post-mortem, which was highly irregular. Some have suggested that the disappointment was too much, and that he took his own life. For all the tensions between them, Gillies wrote a fulsome tribute to his former colleague. However, at the end of it he added, as if to cement his own position as the king of plastic surgery: "The Prince is dead. Long live the Prince." The king's death followed just five months later, when Gillies succumbed to a stroke at the age of 78.

The Legacy of Sidcup

Under Gillies, modern facial surgery began at Sidcup. Yet the legacy of the Queen's Hospital is muddied by the specialty's failure to expand after the First World War, and the clear tensions between the various surgeons at Sidcup in subsequent years. The disagreement between Gillies and Aymard, the criticisms of Gillies' approach to the patients made by some of the staff, Pickerill's insularity and unwillingness to acknowledge the contributions of others, and the self-aggrandisement of some of the more senior figures in the military, such as Keogh and

Arbuthnot Lane, have combined to downplay the contributions of Gillies and the achievements of the Queen's Hospital. This pattern was evident even before the Queen's Hospital closed to patients.

In 1921, the *British Medical Journal* noted in a scathing editorial that none of the surgeons at Sidcup had been named in the first official report from the hospital:

> FACIAL SURGERY WITHOUT SURGEONS.
> We have received an exceedingly interesting publication … [from] the Queen's Hospital, Sidcup, for sailors and soldiers suffering from facial and jaw injuries … The report … gives an account of the last four years' working of the hospital, and states that the end of its labours is now happily in sight. The admiration which we had for the Queen's Hospital has, since reading this report, been greatly intensified, for it would appear … that the committee has achieved its thousands of brilliant results without the aid of any surgeons or dentists, except one honorary consulting surgeon and the presidents … It does mention, it is true, that at one time some overseas medical officers were at the hospital … but otherwise the entire work of the hospital was apparently carried on by the vice-presidents, general committee, commandant, matron, honorary secretary and treasurer, accountant, and auditor … absolutely no mention is made of the existence of any active surgical staff. A leaflet was enclosed in the report, printed in red ink, to which we turned eagerly as perhaps giving some explanation of this unusual method of staffing a hospital, but it merely expressed the regret of the honorary treasurer that, owing to an accidental omission, no mention had been made in the report of the Committee of the National Relief Fund. So the mystery – or the triumph – remains.[31]

This book has recognised the collective achievements of that surgical team, while emphasising the crucial personal contribution of Gillies himself. The seminal moment was Gillies' realisation that a single specialist hospital was advantageous because it would facilitate management of the increased workload brought about by the industrial nature of the war in France, and because surgeons engaged in the new discipline would learn more quickly if both patients and practitioners were concentrated within the same facility. Gillies also recognised the inadequacies of previous techniques and the need for immediate technical innovations, which respected the differences between hard and soft tissue. The need for the staff at Sidcup to adopt a multidisciplinary approach emerged from these ideas. Dentists, surgeons, anaesthetists, physicians, radiologists and their support staff all played different but important roles, and the surgeons' approach ensured the patient was part of the team.

Gillies was instrumental in ensuring that note-keeping at the Queen's Hospital was immaculate, and that illustrations formed a vital part of the medical records. Operative drawings, photographs, colour work and three-dimensional models augmented written notes which laid equal importance on the recording of successes and failures. Both were vital for further education and the continued development of the craft.

Alongside the physical treatment of the patients, Gillies also understood the importance of psychological rehabilitation. Disfigured men who made it to Sidcup usually survived, so the psychology of disfigurement had to be addressed. Whilst surgeons elsewhere operated on large numbers of patients, none benefited from viewing and discussing the results of their

---

31 'Facial surgery without surgeons', *British Medical Journal*, 2 (1921), p.859.

colleagues, and few on the continent seemed interested in the rehabilitation of their patients for life after the war. In this regard, the Queen's Hospital at Sidcup was unique.

After the Queen's Hospital closed to facial casualties in 1925, it was used to house patients with shellshock and tuberculosis. Following its sale to London County Council, it reopened as Queen Mary's Hospital in 1930. It became a so-called out-county hospital, and received patients from the whole of London. No records survive of the period between 1930 and 1948, except for the 'stand by' telegram received at the outbreak of the Second World War and a few photographs of the V1 rocket damage sustained in 1944. The establishment of the NHS led to a review of all hospitals in England which recommended Queen Mary's for closure, since its temporary buildings had outlived their expected shelf life. The plan was thwarted by the personal intervention of the local Member of Parliament, George Wallace, with the Health Minister Aneurin Bevan. As a result of Wallace's representations, Queen Mary's was transformed into a small general hospital. A new outpatient hall was completed in 1956 and, as maintenance of the old buildings became increasingly expensive, a phased development for a new hospital was agreed in 1960. Building began with a Maternity Unit and staff accommodation, and the huts of the old hospital were demolished once the new main block opened in 1974 (See Colour Section, p.xxii). Despite continued financial problems the hospital survived as a district general hospital until 2009, when it was subsumed into the South London Healthcare Trust. Within a year it had lost its identity, along with its Accident and Emergency and Maternity departments.

Frognal House was sold off in the early 1980s, and ultimately became a residential care home as part of the Sunrise Assisted Living group. The lawn upon which Gillies practised his golf swing remains intact, as does the iconic turkey oak depicted in Thomas Ireland's 1830 print. The site of the old hospital itself is now a wilderness, fenced off from public access following the discovery that the old asbestos huts had been ploughed under the ground after demolition rather than removed from the site as specified in the contract. The remains of the entrance driveway from Watery Lane are now all that can be seen of it.

The Post-War Lives of Sidcup's Patients

At the end of the First World War, those who had survived it returned to their homes. The accounts of numerous soldiers indicate that adjustment was not easy. Men had been exposed to dreadful conditions, and had to endure mud, shellfire, hand-to-hand combat and fear. These men had also experienced a lifestyle that was quite alien to their previous, mundane peacetime existences. The war had been both frightening and exciting. The environment of the Western Front was foreign in every sense of the word. Because their experiences were so profound, the men who returned from the war often felt restless. And because men felt that those who had not endured the same hardships would not understand them, many chose not to talk about their wartime experiences.

The Sidcup case notes allow an examination of the surgical results of the Queen's Hospital's patients beyond the examples charted in Harold Gillies' post-war textbooks. Gillies maintained contact with a handful of patients, but the brief descriptions which he recorded do not permit a full evaluation of the effects of facial injury and the wartime experience upon the men who were treated at Sidcup. What was the long-term impact of wartime facial injury on the victims? How did injuries and disfigurements affect their post-war lives? The reconstruction of many men's faces was remarkable, but the results were variable and the prospects for Sidcup patients were mixed. A few, like Albert Mears, died from surgical complications. Others succumbed to the Spanish Flu or tuberculosis, although this outcome was little different from the likely course of the disease in the uninjured. For some, their injury changed the course of their life or, as in David Howard's case, materially contributed to their death. Contemporary accounts in the press, as well as those written by nursing staff, outline the pity which many felt towards the wounded. Certainly, some men struggled with their disfigurements, became isolated and withdrawn from society, and formed awkward relationships with those who were horrified or revolted by their appearance. This chapter, however, argues that isolation and rejection was not the outcome for all of those who suffered from facial injuries. Hitherto unknown accounts of men are drawn upon here to demonstrate that many Sidcup men went on to lead relatively normal lives after the war.

During the period in which the Gillies Archives were housed at Queen Mary's Hospital, Sidcup, connections were established with many relatives of former patients of the Queen's Hospital, who shared reminiscences and personal accounts of how the lives of these patients unfolded after their treatment. In total, six essays written by Sidcup patients and nearly 100 family accounts have been collected, an unparalleled source of the long-term impact of the war on men who experienced facial injuries. Many of these accounts relate to patients who married and procreated after the war, so they tend to reflect more positive long-term outcomes. Nonetheless, collectively the accounts challenge previous assumptions that disfigurement invariably led to isolation and depression. In addition, photographs provided by the families allow us to track the reconstruction process beyond the walls of the Queen's Hospital and the pages of Gillies' books. The photographs of Sidcup men in their old age attest to the success of the facial surgery undertaken by Gillies and his surgical team during the First World War. Alongside the stories of those men's lives, they further emphasise the long-term effects of the strategies employed by British surgeons in response to facial injury, and the better outcomes in comparison with those on the continent.

Men who are disfigured or mutilated by war are often thought to experience PTSD. Men disfigured in the First World War were undoubtedly traumatised by their injuries. The effects of this trauma were complex and nuanced. Today, injury in the armed forces leads to discharge from service; thereafter there may be poor support. Uninjured men may also suffer. Simon Weston, the Falklands veteran severely burned on the *Sir Galahad*, has indicated that many of his fellow-soldiers with PTSD suffered because they had seen, acutely and in close-up, the injuries of their friends rather than suffered any physical injury themselves.[1] By the same token it has been reported that uninjured men sometimes felt guilt that they had not been injured, and there is evidence that PTSD sufferers without obvious physical injury have found it difficult to obtain closure. When demobilised men returned to a mundane life after an intense period of activity, they may have felt a profound sense of anti-climax. At the same time, their families had no conception of their experiences. Men's isolation, and inability to speak of what had happened to them, often worsened their condition. Whilst the wounded man's reluctance to discuss his wartime experiences is a common theme within the accounts from Sidcup patients, the vast majority of cases demonstrate that the men got on with their lives after the war. They encountered challenges and prejudice, but their children and grandchildren mostly report that they were well-adjusted and content. Where problems did occur, these issues were similar to those experienced by uninjured men, for whom there was an equally powerful draw towards the maintenance of silence over their experiences. The experience of war, rather than the experience of disfigurement, was the main factor which caused post-traumatic stress. At Sidcup, as at East Grinstead in the Second World War, there was a spectrum of adjustment to post-war life, from those who shrugged off their injuries with complete insouciance to those who were and would remain withdrawn from society. Little correlation can be found between the severity of injury and the ability of the individual to cope with their disability.

Stories of the Men

Returning Home to Pick Up where they Left Off

The Star and Garter Home in Richmond opened in January 1916, and provided a permanent home for men severely disabled in the war. It is a testimony to the success of the Queen's Hospital that only 12 Sidcup men entered the home, all between 1924 and 1929. The notes of just two of these men survive. Leslie Boorman, RAF, was injured in 1919. The circumstances of his injury are unknown, but he had severe facial burns and a deformity in one hand. Boorman left the home in 1929 to get married. Leo Hancox developed severe back pain, with rarefaction of the lumbar vertebrae, whilst a patient at Sidcup. The Sidcup notes hint at a slowly progressive malignancy, but it is impossible to determine the cause. He was admitted to the Star and Garter in 1925, and died there three years later.

The majority of Sidcup patients slowly returned to their homes after the war. Some returned to their old occupations or those for which they had been trained at Sidcup. Many of their lives were normal, contented, and unremarkable. Artilleryman Francis Grayer returned to the

---

1   Simon Weston, personal communication, 2016.

railways after the war, and retired after 40 years of service at Waterloo Station with his railway pension and presentation mantel clock. His grandson, born in 1956, wrote of the family Grayer produced after the war:

> I am a Chartered Surveyor and have developed numerous offices, factories and shopping centres over 30 years having worked for funds, property companies and the Millennium Commission. My Brother is an Architect. I live in Weybridge and he lives in Godalming. My mum lives in Guildford and my Aunt and cousin Kate live in Reigate and my Cousin Michael lives in Knightsbridge so we Grayers have all remained SW Londoners for over 100 years. One of my boys is at … Jesus College [Oxford] reading Chemistry, and one of my brother's boys is at St Andrews doing Geography. Amazing that all this family descends from a Gillies patient.[2]

Grayer died in 1958. He fell off his bicycle whilst cycling to his allotment, and hit his head on the kerb. It was a sudden end to a simple life, which seems to have been unimpaired by the burns he suffered in 1916 (See Colour Section, p.xxi).

Harold Chilvers, from Greenwich, already had an 11-month-old son before the war. A machine gunner, Chilvers was wounded at 3rd Ypres in August 1917 by a sniper who had already killed two members of his crew. After his return home, Chilvers had four further children and worked at the Greenwich gasworks where he helped with experiments to run motor cars on coal gas. He later moved to Dagenham, Essex, where he worked for the Ford motor company, before he became a maintenance man at a caravan site in Clacton-on-Sea. In 1972, Chilvers developed gangrene after cutting his toenails, and had to have both legs amputated. Despite this, he lived into his nineties and was described by his grandson-in-law, Alan Wright, as a jolly man. Wright also recalled that Chilvers had a "nasty scar" from his wartime injury, and that he could often be found perching a pipe on the one tooth which remained in his bottom jaw.[3]

One of the Sidcup men, Walter Yeo of HMS *Warspite*, even returned to active service after he left Sidcup. Yeo was discharged unfit in 1921 and, with the aid of a lump sum, he became landlord of the Western Hotel in his home town of Plymouth. He later worked in the naval stores at Devonport. As a legacy of his eyelid injuries, Yeo was treated for a corneal ulcer in 1938, but he lived to the age of 70 and died in 1960. His naval compatriot, Willie Vicarage of HMS *Malaya*, returned to his native Wales and had a successful career as a plumber, and later in the Swansea Borough Architect's department, despite the severe injuries to his hands. A 1970s photograph of Vicarage in a rowing boat with his granddaughter shows a disfigured but happy man.

James Dawson, from Keighley in West Yorkshire, also moved back home after the war. However, Dawson returned a married man, having met his wife-to-be in Sidcup whilst a patient at the Queen's. Dawson had been shot through the right cheek and had part of his skull plated behind the ear. His face was pulled up to the right after treatment, and his sight was impaired in the right eye. Nevertheless, he bought a house and gained work as a wood machinist. The family story, submitted by Dawson's grandson Keith Lloyd, was that Dawson's right eye had been impaired by his wartime injury, whilst his left eye was blinded by a sliver of wood which entered it whilst Dawson was chopping firewood on the doorstep. Despite his impediments, Dawson lived a happy and rewarding life, and died of a heart attack on 20 August 1952.[4]

---

2   John Grayer, personal communication.
3   Alan Wright, personal communication.
4   Keith Lloyd, personal communication.

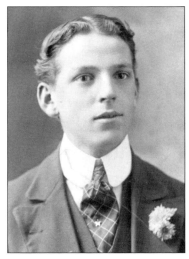

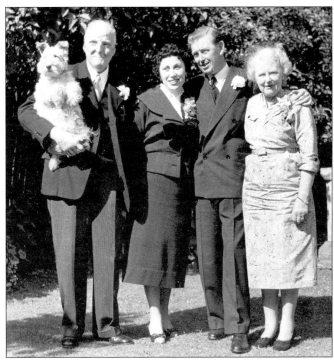

Francis Grayer before his injury (in 1915) and at a family wedding in the 1950s. (Courtesy of the Grayer family)

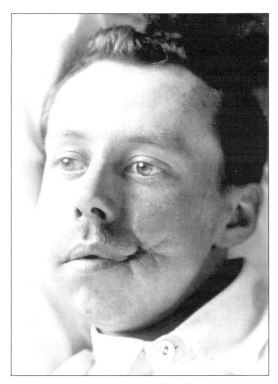

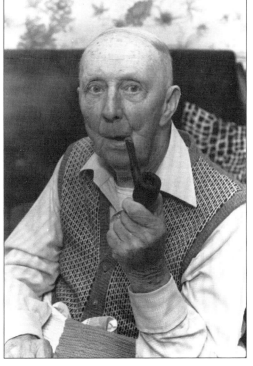

Harold Chilvers, Machine Gun Corps. Admission photograph, 18 March 1918; as an old man c.1960. (Courtesy of the RCS and the Chilvers family)

Stent and grafts were then placed into position and the edges of this portion of the flap sewn down again.

Progress: I Obvious pressure over "nasal" prominence necessitated removal of stitches

II Patient ran a temperature with a considerable amount of pus which did not clear up until the removal of the stent.

Eighteen days later the condition was considered sufficiently clean to undertake a Second stage Extensive suppuration occurred due to septic granulations of chest flap. Drainage was provided with tubes along the top incision near the Eyebrows & in the lateral nasal region. The condition has cleared up. Fomentations were applied. Sloughing occurred in one or two situations along the upper border of the flap above the Eyebrows and over the tip of the nose (a small portion) marked black in diagram

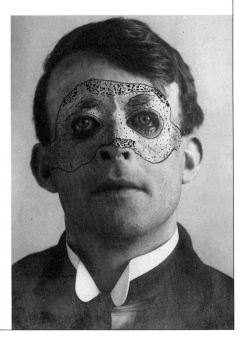

1st Stage after removal of stent.

pedicle Tubed →

← pedicle tubed

Central raised portion

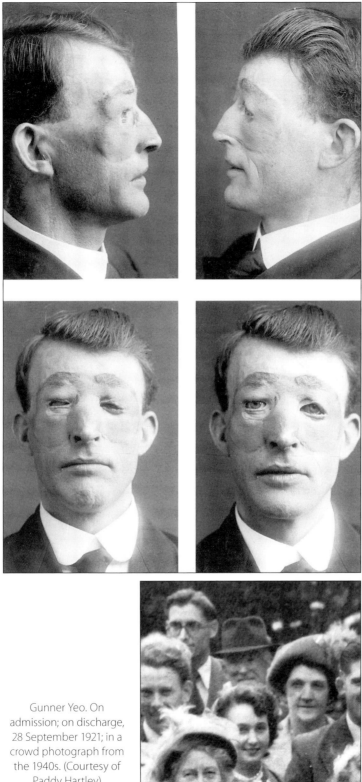

Gunner Yeo. On admission; on discharge, 28 September 1921; in a crowd photograph from the 1940s. (Courtesy of Paddy Hartley)

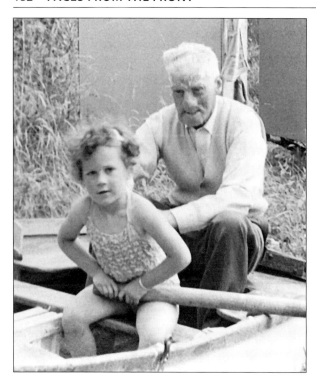

William Vicarage. Family photograph taken in the early 1970s. (Author's collection)

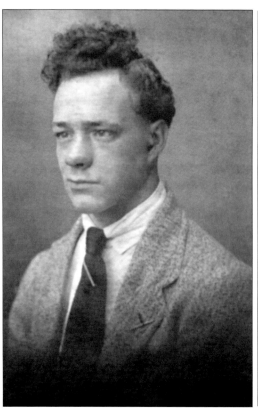

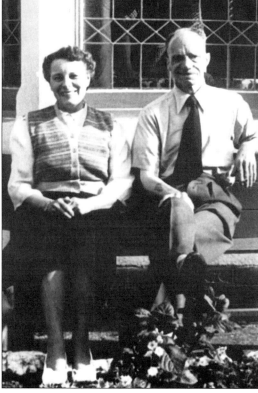

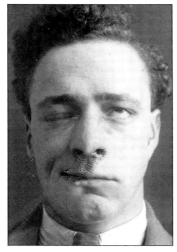 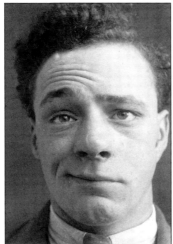 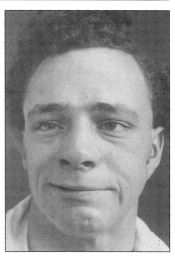

Bottom left, opposite and above: James Dawson. Family photographs from 1916 and the 1940s; admission photograph demonstrating the left-sided facial palsy caused by a bullet wound below the left ear, 12 May 1920. (Courtesy of the RCS and the Dawson family)

Henry Jones also lived a full and productive life after the war. Born out of wedlock in Shoreditch, East London, in 1883, Jones first enlisted in the army in 1900 and was awarded the South Africa Medal. He married Sarah Reeves in 1904 under his legal name of Monksfield, and the couple went on to have 13 children. After his discharge in 1906, Jones became a French polisher, but the outbreak of war in 1914 saw him among the first to enlist. Jones re-entered his old regiment on 1 September and was wounded at Neuve Chapelle the following spring. He was treated at Aldershot and discharged after his wounds had healed. He returned to his old life as a French polisher and seemingly lived a contented life until his death on Christmas Eve 1944. His daughter Betty remembered him as a slight, calm, unassuming man, who never showed anger and did not see his injuries as an impediment.[5]

Many of the Sidcup men appear to have been kind and gentle, and clearly enjoyed their post-war lives. Albert Roberts, born in Liverpool in 1894, provides a notable example. Roberts left school at the age of 14, when he became a solicitor's clerk in the family's home town of Nelson, Lancashire. In 1915, he joined the Royal Welch Fusiliers alongside his close friend Tommy Dearden. At Serre on 13 November 1916, in one of the last actions of the Battle of the Somme, Roberts was captured and Dearden killed in the same attack. Roberts spent the next two years in Germany as a POW, before he was repatriated to King George's Hospital Stamford Street, London and eventually referred to Sidcup. During his time at Sidcup, Roberts assisted the photographer as part of his occupational therapy, and an album of prints that he made has survived. After he was discharged, Roberts returned to his family and his previous employer in Nelson, where he continued as a clerk before later becoming an estate agent. He married Nellie Woodhouse in 1924, and four years later they had a son, Derek. In 1940, Roberts joined the Home Guard and, after the death of Nellie the following year, he married Maude Robinson in 1943.

---

5   John Basford, personal communication.

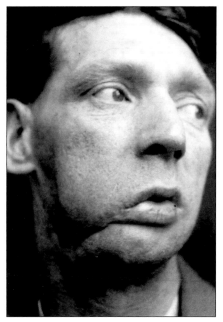

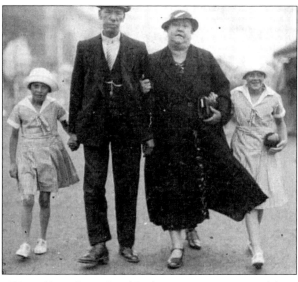

Private Henry Jones, Royal Fusiliers. 18 January 1921; with his family, c.1935. (Courtesy of the RCS and the Jones family)

The couple had one daughter, Betty, who remembered her father fondly:

> He was a quiet, friendly man, very generous and dearly loved by his family and friends. He liked nothing better than to have a few drinks and then recite limericks and other jokes until everyone was helpless with laughter. Despite his facial disfigurement he was never reclusive or aggressive but he did sometimes show signs of unfounded jealousy of his wife.[6]

Far from becoming a recluse, Roberts remained an active participant in the community. A keen snooker player, he won several tournaments at the local Conservative Club and was an ardent follower of Burnley Football Club. In the 1950s, Roberts completed a correspondence course to become a certified accountant, and took a job at Castle Castings in Clitheroe where he worked until he was 80. After his retirement, Roberts and his wife moved into British Legion Sheltered Accommodation in Wythenshawe, Manchester, where they lived happily until his death at the age of 90.

Not all men had a comfortable transition back into civilian life, however. Stanley Cohen lost his face to burns, and his fiancée deserted him because of his appearance. He lived alone, and moved from west London to Bickley, near Sidcup, in the 1950s. Despite this personal setback, he had a successful career after the war. In 1921, he was hired by Lord Northcliffe to run a motor insurance scheme sponsored by *The Times*, and later became secretary of the newspaper's pension funds. He did eventually marry, but the union only lasted for a year. His obituary, published after his death in 1972, referred to his erect bearing, high standards, and his predilection for sending sympathetic notes to sick staff.[7] According to John Clarke, a pupil at a Sunday school class which Cohen ran, 'Stan' was a prolific correspondent. Cohen used to send

---

6   Barbara Prater, personal communication.
7   *The Times*, 6 May 1972. I am grateful to John Taylor for this information.

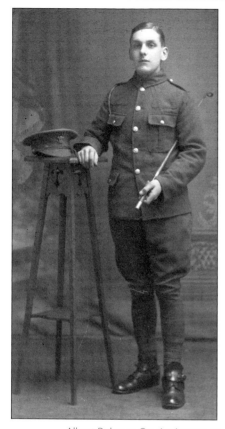
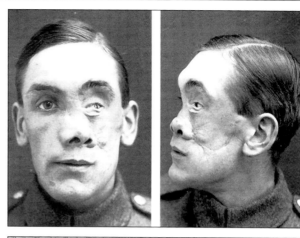
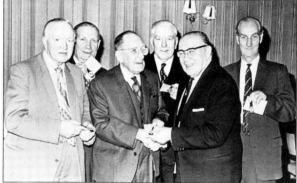

Albert Roberts. On signing up; on admission to Sidcup; in his eighties, upon retirement.
(Courtesy of the RCS and the Roberts family)

a postcard to each of his pupils whenever he went on holiday. He also intimated that he found it easier to face children than adults, because children responded to his deformity with curiosity rather than disgust or horror.

Walter Ashworth had a similar experience to Cohen. Ashworth had been engaged to a lady from Cheadle, Cheshire, before he joined the army. After he was wounded, according to Ashworth's granddaughter Diane Smith, his fiancée called off the engagement. One of the lady's friends was disgusted by this and began to write to Ashworth whilst he recovered in hospital. She also visited him, and the two became engaged, married, and produced a baby daughter. Ashworth returned to Bradford after the war to take up his old job as a tailor. According to Smith, his employers "had not expected him to have facial scars and so refused to let him work in front of shop."[8] Ashworth was relegated to a menial role in the back area, a demotion which "upset him so much that he gave his notice." Although his former employer later asked if Ashworth would be willing to return, as their customers had refused to deal with anyone else, Ashworth's confidence had been dented and he refused.

Ashworth was advised to live in a warmer climate to help him recover his strength after his operations, which led to his accepting a two-year position as a butler on a sheep station

---

8   Diane Smith, personal communication. Unless otherwise stated, all quotations in this passage are taken from this source.

in New South Wales. The work was not too demanding, and Ashworth benefited greatly from the warm weather and the good treatment he received from the family who owned the sheep station. Smith believes that the experience "built his confidence up greatly" after the rejections he had experienced during and immediately after the war. Ashworth was also reunited with his surgeon in Australia, as he met Gillies while the latter was on a teaching visit. Gillies reminded Ashworth that the two had unfinished business, and it appears that Ashworth had further surgery after his return to England. He was clearly one of Gillies' favourite patients, and appears next to him in a large group photograph taken at the Cambridge Military Hospital (see p.53).

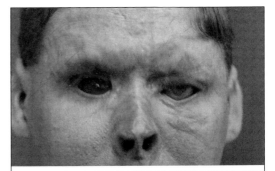
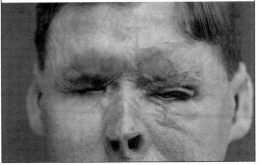

Final photograph of Lieutenant Stanley Cohen, Tank Corps. (RCS)

At the end of the two-year contract, Ashworth had earned enough money to buy a house in Blackpool. Once back in England, he returned to the profession of tailoring. His granddaughter recalled that "he was always employed and became quite successful in his trade." Ashworth's wounds remained a constant problem for him, however. Shrapnel was removed from his back as late as the 1950s, and he was unable to eat a number of foodstuffs. A family photograph of Ashworth as an old man shows him with a twinkle in his eye, and the same crooked smile from his injury that was evident in all the photographs he appeared in at Aldershot and Sidcup. His granddaughter remembers him as "an extremely popular man, very dapper … [He] always carried himself proudly and without embarrassment and socialised a great deal." His post-war tale was very much one of triumph over adversity.

Ashworth's antipodean encounter with Gillies was not the only example of men with a Sidcup connection meeting again in later life. In the case of surgeon Charles Smith, his father's treatment at the Queen's came in very handy. In 1947, Smith attended an interview at St Thomas' Hospital, accompanied by his father Cecil who, as Lieutenant Smith of the Royal West Kent Regiment, had been a Sidcup patient. Charles wrote:

> We arrived … and went to the Dean's office, sat around for a considerable length of time when I imagine I was fairly apprehensive as Thompson was known to be very irascible … In due course the door opened and a large man came bustling in, took one look at my father who … had 20 plastic surgical operations to restore some sort of normality without much success for the lower part of his face, and following that look said 'Good God, Smith of the Dirty Half-Hundred!'[9] I am not sure that I exchanged any words with him and I certainly was not interviewed, nor did he ask why I wanted

---

9   The 'Dirty Half-Hundred' was the Royal West Kent's nickname – obtained during the Peninsular War, where they were the 50th Regiment of Foot. As the black dye in their jackets had run, the soldiers had covered their faces with black streaks as they wiped away sweat with their sleeves.

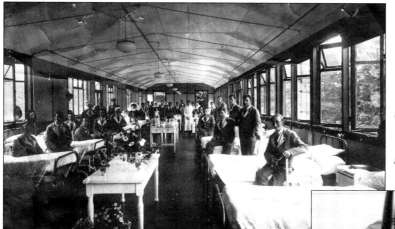

Walter Ashworth at the Queen's Hospital (far right) in 1918; Ashworth in the 1960s. (Courtesy of the author's collection and the Ashworth family)

to take up medicine or whether I wanted to take up medicine, but he disappeared into a little room with my father for twenty minutes. I eventually heard that I had been accepted.[10]

The Dean had been attached to Sidcup during the war.

The Smiths maintained a far more regular contact with Sidcup. They lived in Harrow, north-west London, where Cecil was a bank clerk. Their next-door neighbours were the Wimbushes. Norman, an engineer by profession, had also been a patient at Sidcup and his thespian aspirations had led him to produce the hospital's 1920 Christmas show. His wife Ida had attended the Royal Academy of Dramatic Art, and their daughter Mary went on to play Nigel Pargeter's mother in the long-running radio serial *The Archers*. Before he arrived at Sidcup, Wimbush had originally been treated by Hippolyte Morestin, who considered that he had finished the job. As Wimbush's admission photograph demonstrates, he arrived with a substantial disfigurement which underlines the inadequacy of surgical repair standards in France. Charles Smith records an anecdote from their time as neighbours. One day, a man walking down the road had approached Cecil Smith, who had been gardening, to ask for directions. Cecil did not recognise the destination, and called over the fence to see if Wimbush could assist. Cecil had noted the discomfited appearance of the traveller, and assumed he was uncomfortable with talking to a disfigured man. However, when Wimbush appeared, the traveller's look turned to horror and he disappeared as quickly as he could. The two former Sidcup men found the affair amusing rather than tragic, a response which seems to reflect the outlook of many of the men who left Sidcup behind after their treatment had been completed.

Some adults could be hurtful rather than horrified, however. Before the war, Sydney Twinn had driven a carrier's cart in the Cambridge area. He met his wife whilst at work, as he delivered

---

10 Charles Smith, personal communication.

hats from a milliners to the home of the economist John Maynard Keynes. Mary Russell's grandmother worked as a maid for the Keynes' at the time, and the Keynes family even paid for Twinn's wedding. However, as Russell wrote, Twinn's homecoming after the war was a difficult one:

> His two children didn't recognise him because of his injuries and hid under the table when he arrived home. My grandmother described her visit to the hospital in Sidcup was very traumatic. His injuries were very obvious and my mother told stories of people calling out unpleasant names as they walked down the street. My grandmother told how, when she had had another child, people crowded around the pram, expecting the baby to have inherited his father's deformities. However, he went on to have another five children, my mother being one of them.[11]

Twinn bought a shop with Russell's grandmother, and the pair ran a successful small business selling groceries and animal feed in Cambridge. Twinn lived into his eighties and, unlike many, he was keen to talk about life in the trenches. Although he told tales which were "quite disturbing" to his grandchildren, Russell's memories of a "kind and gentle man" echo those of many of the relatives of Sidcup men whose accounts are recorded here.

The men treated at Sidcup came from all over the British Empire. After the war, these men returned to their home countries and faced uncertain futures. In 1914, Bruce Fowler was a farm worker in New Zealand, but had lived for a time in London following the death of his mother. Taken to Britain by his father when he was three years old, Fowler had been cared for by an aunt and studied at the Central Polytechnic School. He enlisted as soon as war was declared, but missed the Gallipoli campaign after he developed jaundice. He was wounded in the elbow in France, but made a good recovery and returned to the front line after four months. He was wounded again in October 1918, and married a childhood friend in London in 1919 whilst he was a patient at the Queen's (See Colour Section, p.xxiii). The newlyweds established themselves in New Zealand, where Fowler was awarded land in central Otago in a ballot for returning soldiers. However, the farm was too small, and the weather unsuitable for dairy farming. After six years Fowler abandoned the farm and moved to Christchurch, where he established a general store and grocery business.

Fowler eventually moved to Wellington where he remained for the rest of his working life. He had always had an interest in radio, and whilst in London he had been offered an apprenticeship at Marconi. In Wellington, Fowler began work with a wireless company, became a shop manager, and ultimately bought his own premises and diversified into other electrical goods and repairs. His wife died in 1960, but Fowler married again in 1963. With his second wife, Fowler became a founder member of the local Samaritans and a hospital volunteer, and took charge of a Sunday school. Despite a series of strokes, he remained active and made baskets and tapestries. His daughter reflected that "he gave himself fully to his work, was staunch and unyielding in his faith, and totally loyal to his friends and family until his death at 93 years of age."[12]

The experience of another New Zealander was far less fortunate. Jasper Watkins, 1st New Zealand Rifle Brigade, was wounded at the Somme and arrived at Sidcup after initial treatment at the New Zealand Hospital at Mount Felix. He underwent a series of operations on his cheek and jaw, and made friends with one of the Sidcup nurses. However, he returned to New Zealand alone, where he met and married Maisie. It was a marriage of convenience; Maisie was

---

11   Mary Russell, personal communication.
12   Joan Markley, personal communication.

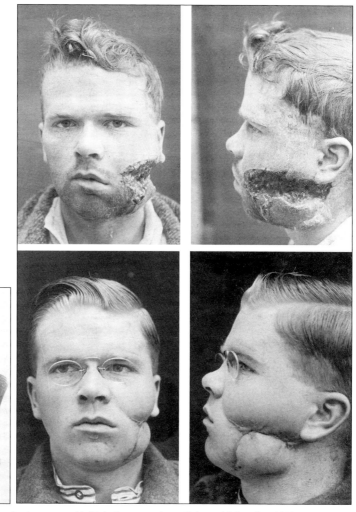

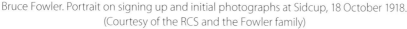

Bruce Fowler. Portrait on signing up and initial photographs at Sidcup, 18 October 1918.
(Courtesy of the RCS and the Fowler family)

pregnant by another man, and Jasper was disfigured. Neither of them, therefore, was thought to be particularly eligible. The illegitimate child was put up for adoption, and Jasper and Maisie went on to have five children, including two sets of twins, of their own. The family settled on a farm near Pukekohe, south of Auckland, before Maisie suddenly died from appendicitis in 1930. Unable to cope with the demands of raising five children, Jasper contacted his nurse friend from Sidcup and she migrated to New Zealand to help. Yet tragedy would strike the family again when Jasper was asked to help a friend break in a difficult horse. Jasper received a kick in the stomach from the horse, but declined the offer of a doctor and instead proceeded to walk home. He collapsed and, shortly after, died in hospital from what appears to have been a ruptured spleen. The Sidcup nurse, known as 'Auntie' by the family, could not cope with the children and they were dispersed among other family members. As a final misfortune for the Watkins family, Jasper's eldest son was killed near Arezzo during the Second World War.

The story of Norman Eric Wallace, the Canadian artillery observer with the RAF, contains elements of both tragedy and triumph. Unlike his New Zealand counterparts, Wallace did not return to his homeland after the war, but instead remained at Sidcup where he met a nurse from Grantham, Marguerite Baxter. The two married in her home parish church on 23 June 1920, and Eric gave his address as the hospital. Sadly, less than a year later, Marguerite died from an abdominal tumour. Eric was discharged from the hospital in November 1921 and promptly vanished from the records. Nothing is known of his whereabouts for the next four years, but thanks to Jeremy Stevenson we can piece together Wallace's life from 1925 onwards. In 1914, Stevenson's grandfather, Frank Lironi, had purchased the Lake Hotel in Llangammarch Wells, Powys. In 1925, Wallace checked in for a weekend. He stayed for the next 35 years, and became a "father figure" to the young Stevenson.[13] Wallace taught him to hunt, shoot, fish, and how to fly model aeroplanes, and encouraged Stevenson's love of tape recording. The two also enjoyed an annual week in London, where they spent "practically every night in the theatre." In 1939, Captain Wallace helped organise the Home Guard and, at some point during the Second World War he obtained a promotion to Major. He was issued a car by the Ministry of Defence, and Stevenson's mother told stories of Wallace driving it on the wrong side of the local roads. Stevenson left the Lake Hotel in 1960, when he and his mother went to live in a house opposite the hotel. There was a lot of land, and Major Wallace was able to have a chalet there in which he lived until his death in 1974. Although "he was a guest at the hotel ... on the other hand he was a close friend of the family as well." Stevenson and his family knew that Wallace had been married, but he never spoke of it to them or to James Hogg, another guest at the hotel in the early 1950s who remembered Wallace. Hogg's principal memory was of being taught to fish by Wallace, and his lasting impression was of Wallace's "dignity and gentleness, with a hint of sadness which only now do I fully understand."[14] While Wallace never did return to his native Canada, and endured heartache before his treatment at Sidcup was over, he nevertheless found peace in mid-Wales and lived an active and fulfilled life.

Remaining at Sidcup

Not all those who were treated at the Queen's Hospital chose to return to their pre-war homes. Some men preferred to leave their pre-war lives behind and stayed in Sidcup or nearby Bromley. While this may have reflected an unease at possible interactions with old friends and neighbours, in several cases it was the result of relationships which the men had established with local girls whilst in residence at the hospital. Bob Davidson was one such case, but also a man who demonstrates the subtle ways in which a disfigurement could modify a man's behaviour. Born in Dublin as one of 12 children, Davidson had enlisted in the RAMC in 1914 and was wounded on 28 April 1916 while bringing in a stretcher case (See Colour Section, p.xxiv). His injuries were extensive and, although a reasonable superficial reconstruction was achieved in 11 operations, he was left with a large defect in the hard palate. Henceforth, he was unable to eat without making a loud snuffling sound. Davidson was one of the patients who took advantage of the offer of a photograph set which documented his treatment, and obtained a set of glass negatives of himself.[15] As part of his rehabilitation, Davidson was sent into Sidcup with the hospital mail. The girl behind the post office counter subsequently became his wife. Their wedding photograph was heavily retouched. They had two daughters, one of whom recalled Davidson's self-consciousness over his palatal defect. Due to the difficulties he had with eating,

---

13   Jeremy Stevenson, personal communication. Unless otherwise stated, all quotations in this passage are taken from this source.
14   James Hogg, personal communication.
15   The quarter-plate negatives were donated to the author by Davidson's daughter, and now reside in the Antony Wallace Archive, BAPRAS.

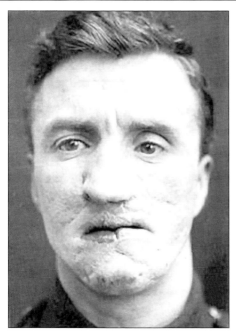

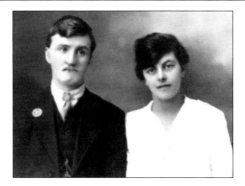

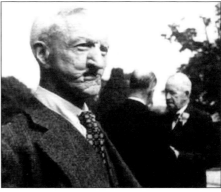

Bob Davidson, RAMC following surgery; on his marriage; in 1958. (RCS and the author's collection)

when people went to lunch Davidson would eat alone in the kitchen.[16] Davidson remained attached to the hospital, and appeared in the 1927 hospital staff photograph. He was still there in the 1950s, and the last photograph of him is at a meeting of old patients outside Frognal House in 1958.

Bill Hollins also married a local girl and continued to work at Sidcup until his retirement, as did his friend Jocky Anderson. James Best, who was sent to Sidcup after the war following unsuccessful surgery, married one of the nurses and established himself as a barber in the local area. Barbering the disfigured men was a difficult task, as barbers shaved as well as cut hair, and it is likely that Best learned his trade at Sidcup. His deformity was not severe, but he had a facial palsy which affected his speech. Sadly, his wife died in 1928, although he did re-marry and lived happily until 1978. Frank Heaton, known to his family as Steve, stayed on as a porter and then trained as a nurse, working at the hospital until the 1950s. These men do not appear to have allowed their appearance to affect their lives. However, one patient who remained at Sidcup was very self-conscious of his burned face. As a result, he would only work night shifts. Two of the nurses from the 1950s were saddened by his apparent isolation, and when they discovered it was his birthday they duly made him a cake. It was, he said, the first birthday cake he had ever had.[17]

Edward Albert Palmer, who was actually Herbert Arthur Palmer,[18] had no such insecurities. Despite the fact that his face collapsed twice and required revision, Palmer was a fearless player of both football and cricket after the war. Much to the concern of his family he would

16 Shelagh Davidson, personal communication.
17 Sheila Anstall, personal communication.
18 Herbert had borrowed the birth certificate of his dead infant brother, three years his senior, in order to enlist in 1914.

head a football with no thought for the condition of his face. Palmer married his childhood sweetheart, Rose, in 1919, and she successfully talked him out of his desire to emigrate to Australia and lose himself in the outback. Palmer first became a gas lamp lighter and then a lorry driver for Bromley Borough Council, a job which required many trips to Coventry to pick up new council vehicles from the Dennis Company factory. In the Second World War, Palmer joined the Air Raid Precautions Heavy Rescue Group. In the early 1970s, Palmer and his wife met Gillies' daughter and son-in-law by chance in a pub in Chelsfield, a small village about five miles from Sidcup. Palmer's son Roy records that "there were hugs and kisses between her and Father and [the] drinks flowed freely." Sadly, Palmer developed dementia before he died at the age of 81. Nevertheless, he was "sadly missed but always remembered and loved." His eldest son Albert wrote with great pride about his father, and noted that "he has been gone 2 years yet I still yearn for him."[19] Like Stanley Cohen, Palmer was subjected to a great deal of persecution from the general public. However, whilst Cohen found adults more difficult to deal with, Palmer had to cope with the taunts of the local children.

Although many of the men who remained at Sidcup did so because of an attachment to the hospital or a local girl, two men became attached to Gillies instead. The first, Bob Seymour, one of the men from the first day of the Somme offensive, took over the role of Gillies' secretary from another Sidcup patient named Greenaway. He remained in post until the mid-1950s. At that stage, age had caught up with Seymour and he began to make errors in Gillies' accounts. In combination with Gillies' own lackadaisical approach to finances, Gillies' tax bills went unpaid. Seymour was quietly pensioned off. The second, Sidney Beldam, became Gillies' chauffeur and went on to build a large and happy family (See Colour Section, p.xxiv).

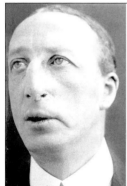
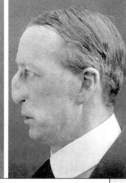
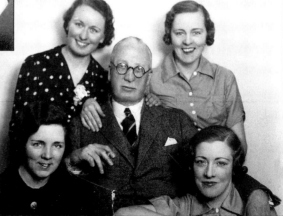

Bob Seymour following reconstruction; in the 1950s. (RCS and the author's collection)

---

19   The details in this passage were gratefully received from Roy and Albert Palmer, and Lynne Judge.

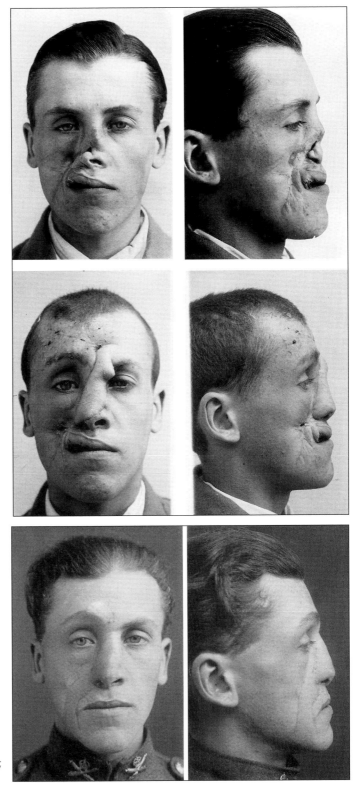

Sidney Beldam on admission;
post reconstruction. (RCS)

Retraining at Sidcup

Two of the most compelling post-war stories belong to men whose injuries resulted in a complete dislocation of career and life. Malcolm Shirlaw, known as Micky, was brought up in Lanarkshire. He was a miner when war broke out and, perhaps with a desire to soar above the ground rather than toil beneath it, he volunteered for the RFC. However, his eyesight was not good enough, and he ultimately enlisted in the Gordon Highlanders. He was wounded in the jaw on 26 August 1917, during the regiment's assault on Gallipoli Farm near Ypres. It took him almost two years to reach Sidcup, and he was transferred from Brook Street Hospital in May 1919. A football enthusiast from his youth, not even surgery could deter Shirlaw from joining the football team alongside his friend Bill Hollins. But his future career plans were also foremost in his mind during his time at the Queen's, and Shirlaw took a great interest in the dental techniques which were being used to treat his wound. He retained his own dental splint as a memento of his treatment at Sidcup, though after his death it disappeared in the house clearance. Shirlaw was ultimately taken on and trained by Archie Lane, before he found a job of his own in Tunbridge Wells. He was a speedy and meticulous worker, and his daughter recalls the kitchen table of the family home being a mass of teeth and dentures.[20]

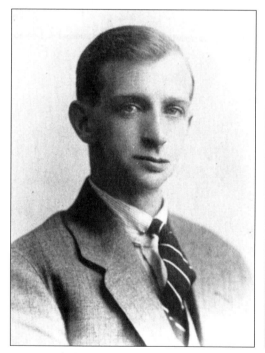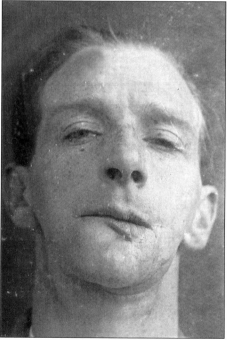

Malcolm Shirlaw. Pre-war; at Sidcup in 1919. (Courtesy of the RCS and the Shirlaw family)

Shirlaw's professional leap from the mines of Motherwell to dental technician in Tunbridge Wells was a significant one, but the transformation of Walter Bowen was perhaps even more remarkable. Known to all as Mike, Bowen began his working life as a railway clerk in South Africa. He enlisted in the militia, and went to Europe with the 2nd Regiment, South African Infantry. He was promoted to Sergeant, but severely wounded at Ypres on 18 September 1917 by

---

20 Pauline Pratt, personal communication.

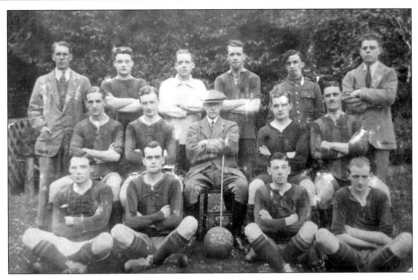

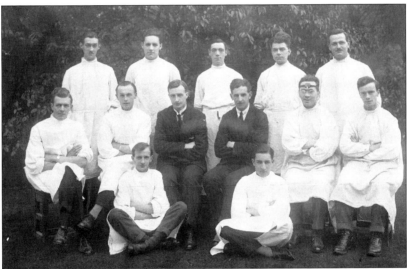

Shirlaw (left) in the hospital football team, 1919-1920, where he is seated bottom right; and (right) in his new role as a dental technician, seated bottom left. Archie Lane is on the far right of the back row. (Author's collection)

a shell fragment which blinded him and took away his nasal bridge. A rhinoplasty attempted at the 2nd London General Hospital was unsuccessful, and Bowen was sent to St Dunstan's Lodge in Regent's Park. Although discharged with a full disability pension, Bowen was determined to overcome his blindness. He rapidly learned braille and, encouraged by St Dunstan's, decided to become a lawyer. He gained a place at Caius College, Cambridge, in 1918, and graduated three years later. While in Cambridge, Bowen fell in love with Eleanor Gillies, Harold's sister, and the pair married early in 1919. Unsurprisingly, as a new member of the Gillies family, Bowen was admitted to Sidcup in May 1919 for the repair of a persistent hole in the upper part of his nose. The procedure was ultimately unsuccessful, but he was under treatment periodically for the next two years.

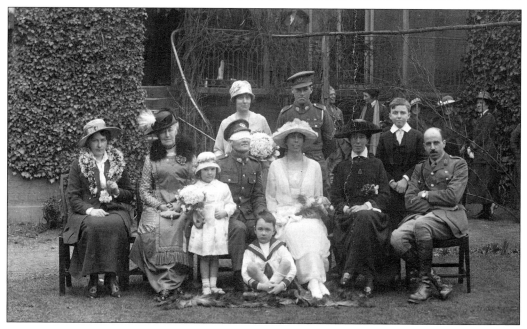

Sergeant Bowen, South African Infantry. Wedding photograph with his wife Eleanor. Gillies is seated on the far right. (BAPRAS Archive)

Bowen was called to the bar in 1922 and returned to South Africa where he became a successful lawyer. In 1924, he became a member of the Cape Province Legislative Assembly. Five years later, Bowen was elected as Member of Parliament for the Cape Town (Central) constituency, where he played a major role in the establishment of the South African National Council for the Blind and helped to found the Athlone School for the Blind which still exists today. Hilary Marlow, the son of its Headmaster, recalled a meeting with Bowen:

> Memories came back to me of a young boy being introduced to this man, puzzled as to why a man would want to have his eyes covered by a white mask. Introducing me, my father said, 'This is Mr Bowen and, because he is blind, like the children in the school, he would like to feel your face.' The big man bent down and his fingers traced the outlines of my face to create a mental picture in his mind of my appearance. I cannot recall anything more of the meeting but his face remained fixed in my memory.[21]

Bowen's untimely death in 1948 was a great shock to all who knew him. "Blindness," he wrote, "should not be viewed as a calamity but rather as an incentive to unleash energies hitherto thought impractical." Arthur Pearson, the proprietor of the *Daily Mirror* who himself suffered blindness at the age of 47 as a result of glaucoma, had established the St Dunstan's rehabilitation service which an ethos that he would not be "a" blind man, but "the" blind man. The energy, determination, and success of Mike Bowen epitomised that sentiment.

Although he did not scale the same heights as Mike Bowen, or leave his pre-war home and career behind to the same extent as Micky Shirlaw, Joseph Pickard also retrained after the war.

---

21 Hilary Marlow, 'The legal career of R.W. Bowen', *Winston Churchill Memorial Trust Fellowship Report*, 2006. Unless otherwise stated, all quotations in this passage are taken from this source.

He was also the only Sidcup patient whose experiences are contained within the IWM's extensive sound archive of interviews with veterans of the First World War. Pickard spent a number of months at Sidcup, and after the war he trained as a watchmaker in a government-sponsored "instructional factory." He went on to successfully pursue watchmaking as a career in his home town of Alnwick, but continued to visit Tommy Kilner in Harley Street, Roehampton, and Oxford. His new nose had held up well; his only minor complaint was that one nostril had closed up because he had become lazy with his silver dilators. David Hiscocks has argued that what was said in these interviews may have been influenced by the interviewee's perception of who would listen to the result, and that they therefore have the potential to skew our own perception of the wartime experience. However, Pickard's tone and demeanour throughout the interview are impressive.[22] His laconic black humour infuses the recording, and makes it evident that he was a happy, well-adjusted man.

Disfigurement, not Disability

The accounts above demonstrate the variety of post-war circumstances that the former patients of Sidcup experienced. Some led happy and rich lives, others were less fortunate. From the majority of accounts, it is clear that disfigurement was not considered analogous to disability. Yet self-consciousness was a difficulty with which a number of the patients struggled to cope after the war. Some men declined to be photographed after their injury, whilst others would turn their heads to conceal their deformities from the camera. Reginald Fellowes' granddaughter, Carol Claxton, notes that there are very few surviving photographs of her grandfather, and those in the family's possession were taken at a distance with Fellowes in the background.[23] Fellowes' war had been a short one. He had landed at Suvla Bay with the 5th Norfolks on 10 August 1915, and was wounded just two days later. According to Claxton, Fellowes had been a handsome man, and had attempted to cut ties with her grandmother as a result of his disfigurement, "but she would have none of it and they were married in 1919." Alongside concealing his disfigurement from family photographs as best he could, Fellowes also spoke little of his time as a soldier and a patient to his relatives. However, Claxton does recall that whenever Fellowes encountered anyone begging or selling matches on the streets and purporting to be blind, he could adjudge whether they were telling the truth purely by their reaction to his face.

Some men were, in the accounts offered by their families, profoundly different after the war. William Spreckley, who had lost his nose but received a reasonable reconstruction, was an unhappy man (See Colour Section, p.xxiv). Although he superficially dealt well with his disfigurement, he began to drink and gamble, and things became difficult for his children as a result of marital arguments. However, with his grandchildren he was a loving and kind grandfather, and he went on to serve in the Home Guard during the Second World War. Like Spreckley, Harold Cullimore was kind and patient with his grandchildren. However, he abused his wife and locked his children in a cupboard under the stairs for hours at a time over trivial misdemeanours. His granddaughter believed that his treatment of her was the result of an attempt to make up for the way in which he had brought up his own family. Cullimore had been a hot-tempered man before the war, and there is nothing to suggest that his disfigurement exacerbated the aggressive tendencies he had previously displayed. His treatment of his wife and children may well have occurred without the intervention of injury.

---

22 D. Hiscocks, 'Keeping the individual in focus: making use of interviews with Great War veterans from the IWM sound archive', *Stand To!*, 105 (2016), pp.24-26.
23 Carol Claxton, personal communication.

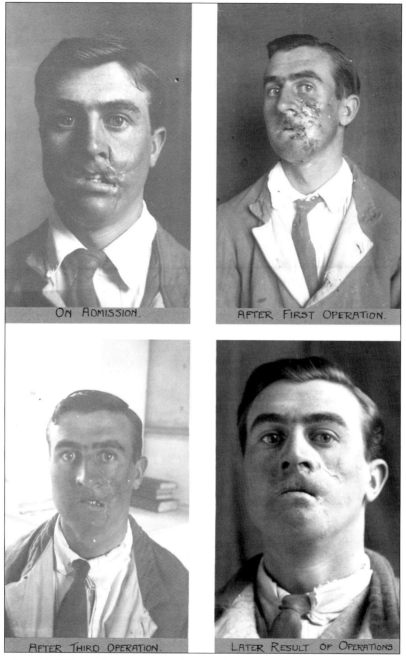

Reginald Fellowes. Demonstration photographs prepared for a lecture tour. (RCS)

Whilst injury may not have been the determining factor in the post-war difficulties experienced by former patients, we do have evidence that the horrors of the war were a major factor in the life of one of the men in particular. Although Stanley Cohen's face had deterred his fiancée, he remained haunted for the rest of his life by images of the machine gunners that his tank had run over on his orders. After his account of the event his narrative contains a lengthy religious reflection. His thoughts, worries, and regrets were of the war, not his disfigurement.

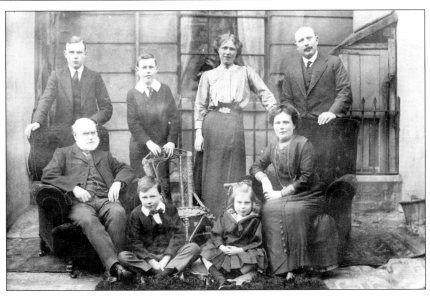

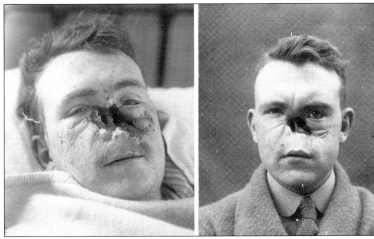

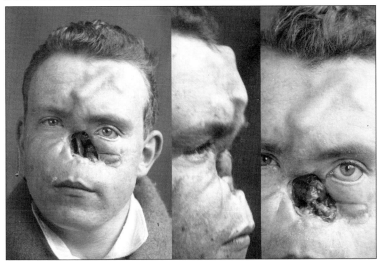

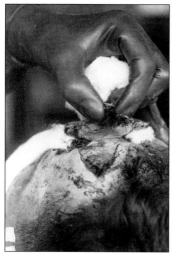
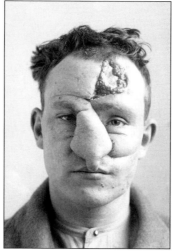
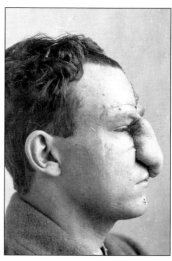

William Spreckley before the war; initial photograph; during the surgical process; post-war. (Courtesy of the RCS and the Spreckley family)

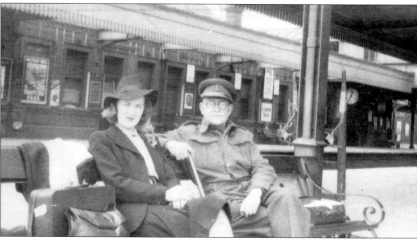

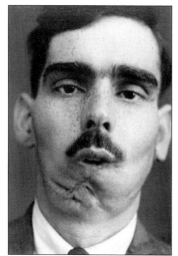
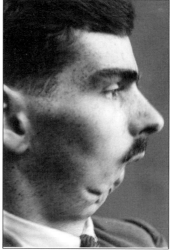
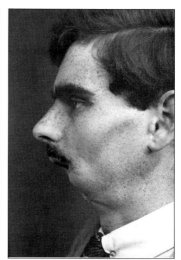

Harold Cullimore. Before surgery, 2 November 1920. (RCS)

Conclusion

Family accounts show that not all wounded men were pitiable, miserable wrecks, embittered and destroyed by the First World War. Many of those who served in the First World War enlisted at the very outset and were not thrown into battle against their will. Despite their dreadful injuries, their enthusiasm persisted. The essays produced by men in the literacy class at Sidcup merit reconsideration here:

> To summarise my whole experience in the Army, I must confess that I enjoyed soldering [sic] which was a very clean life to those who adapted it in the proper manner. When I look back and think things over which has happened in my service I feel proud, I also feel proud to think I was wounded fighting in such a famous regiment as 'The Black Watch'.[24]

In addition to regimental pride, the men displayed a patriotic attitude to the country in the service of which they had been wounded. As Private McGowan wrote: "I like my country, and if I can earn a respectable living in it I shall never have anything to say against it."[25]

The army had given men a life they would otherwise have been unable to experience. It had expanded their horizons and revealed qualities within them that they were unaware existed. As Private Murray expressed:

> I cannot say I am sorry I joined the army as it has broadened my outlook on life, and given me many friends, whom I otherwise would never have known. So after all I lost little, and gained much, through The Great War.[26]
>
> Looking back over the last five or six years of my life, I find that the time spent in the army has not been in vain. Apart from the physical well being [sic] I enjoyed while serving with the colours, it has given me a broader outlook on life, and brought out qualities hitherto unsuspected in me. In closing I cannot speak too highly of the splendid work done by women in the Great War. In hospitals this was especially noticeable, but whether in hospitals or any other branch of the service, they entered into their work so zealously that we are indebted to them as much as anything else, for the peace we now enjoy.[27]

Joseph Pickard reflected that the First World War had made him a man: "I was determined to go; I was glad I went; I've never complained about being in the war. I was standing on my feet when I was fifteen and a half, amongst men."[28]

These are not the words of men who wrote or said what they hoped their audience wanted to read or hear. Their sense of patriotism and duty were real. For all its horrors, the war made men of them, gave them new experiences, and changed many of them for the better. And the medical services treated them well. The war produced casualties on a scale hitherto unseen,

---

24 BLSC: LIDDLE/WW1/GA/WOU34, My Personal Experiences of the Great War, Private McGowan, Black Watch, Essay in Lady Gough's class, January 1922.

25 BLSC: LIDDLE/WW1/GA/WOU34, My Personal Experiences of the Great War, Private Murray, North Staffs Regt, Essay in Lady Gough's class, January 1922.

26 BLSC: LIDDLE/WW1/GA/WOU34, My Personal Experiences of the Great War, Private Best, 2nd Royal Scots Fusiliers, Essay in Lady Gough's class, 27 January 1922.

27 BLSC: LIDDLE/WW1/GA/WOU34, My Personal Experiences of the Great War, Private Faragher, Lancashire Fusiliers, Essay in Lady Gough's class, January 1922.

28 IWM: 8946, Joseph Pickard (IWM interview).

and created injuries whose resolution had never before been attempted. It took time for lessons to be learned, from triage through the management of surgical shock and sepsis, to the development of surgical method and rehabilitation. Sidcup's patients were experimental subjects, and although losses may have been avoided with hindsight, what was done with the resources available was nothing short of remarkable.

Finally, as the accounts discussed here testify, many of the former patients of the Queen's Hospital went on to lead normal lives and raised families. In some cases, the men were able to access opportunities which substantially improved their lives, and which may not have been available to them had they not been wounded. Many men, some 10 percent of the surviving accounts, met their wives at the Queen's Hospital.[29] The hospital had life-changing effects upon its patients. The final word goes to one of those descendants, Joan Markley, whose father Bruce Fowler's story has been discussed above:

> As a family we give thanks for those at Sidcup who enabled our father to live such a full and active life.[30]

---

29 These men included Thomas Bearpark, Peter Brady, Bob Davidson, George Florence, Maurice Herne, Bert Hollins and Norman Wallace.
30 Joan Markley, personal communication.

Bibliography

Unpublished Material

Australian War Memorial, Canberra
AWM11 1506/8/43, [Australian Imperial Force Administrative Headquarters registry, 'A' (Adjutant-General's Branch) medical (subject) files:] The Queen's Hospital, Frognal [Minutes of Meetings of General Committee] (October 1917 – August 1918), Queen's Hospital Minute Book.

Bexley Local Studies and Archives Centre, London
Papers of Doctor Andrew Bamji.

British Association of Plastic, Reconstructive and Aesthetic Surgeons Archive, London
Report on the work of the Queen's Hospital, 1917-1929, c.1930.

Brotherton Library, Leeds
Bamji Collection, QUE, The Queen's Hospital, 1917-1929: The Queen Mary's Hospital, 1929-1967: Sidcup: Kent.
Liddle Collection, LIDDLE/WW1/GA/WOU/34, 6 Mss essays by patients with facial injuries in Sidcup Hospital.
Liddle Collection, LIDDLE/WW1/WF/REC/01/B43, Budd, JGH.

Glasgow University Library, Glasgow
Papers of Donald Sutherland MacColl.

Imperial War Museum, London
1697-2, Private Papers of Captain A.D. Chater.
8946, Joseph Pickard (IWM interview).
12007, Private Papers of Captain, J.K. Wilson.

London Metropolitan Archives, London
H02/QM, Queen Mary's Roehampton Trust.
H02/QM/Y/01/005, The Queen's Hospital, Sidcup, Kent: newspaper cuttings.

The National Archives of Australia, Canberra
B2455, First Australian Imperial Force Personnel Dossiers, 1914-1920.

The National Archives of the United Kingdom, London
WO 363/W644, Army Service Record File for George Eliot Webster.

Privately held personal papers
Papers of George Brooks.
Papers of Reginald Evans.
Papers of Stanley Cohen.

Royal Archives, Windsor
Diary of Queen Mary.

Royal College of Surgeons, London
Case files of the British section of the Queen's Hospital.

Wellcome Library, London
CMAC RAMC/760, 2 albums of photographs of plastic surgery cases at the King George Military Hospital, (later Red Cross Hospital), Stamford Street, London, taken by Dr. Albert Norman, Honorary Scientific Photographer.

Unpublished theses
Pickerill, H.P., 'Facial Surgery' (unpublished Masters Dissertation, University of Birmingham, 1923).

Published Material

Books
Albee, F.H., *A Surgeon's Fight to Rebuild Men* (London: Robert Hale, 1950).
Anon., *A Train Errant: Being the Experiences of a Voluntary Unit in France and an Anthology from their Magazine, 1915-1919* (London: Simson & Co., 1919).
Anon. (K.E. Luard), *Diary of a Nursing Sister on the Western Front* (London: William Blackwood & Sons, 1915).
Barker, Pat, *Life Class* (London: Hamish Hamilton, 2007).
——, *Regeneration* (London: Viking Press, 1991).
——, *Toby's Room* (London: Hamish Hamilton, 2012).
Bengston, B.P. and Kuz, J. (eds.), *Photographic Atlas of Civil War Injuries: Photographs of Surgical Cases and Specimens* (Grand Rapids, MI: Medical Staff Press, 1996).
Blackham, R.J., *Scalpel, Sword and Stretcher* (London: Sampson, Low, Martin & Co., 1931).
Blair, J.S.G., *Centenary History of the Royal Army Medical Corps, 1898-1998* (Edinburgh: Scottish Academic Press, 1998).
Braam, Conny, *The Cocaine Salesman*, trans. by Jonathan Reeder (London: Haus, 2011).
Breitner, B. (ed.), *Ärtzte und ihre Helfer im Weltkriege 1914-1918* (Vienna: Verlag Amon Franz Goeth, 1936).
Brenton, Howard, *Doctor Scroggy's War* (London: Nick Hern, 2014).
Brown, Harvey, *Pickerill: Pioneer in Plastic Surgery, Dental Education and Dental Research* (Dunedin: Otago University Press, 2007).
Bruhn, C., *Die Gegenwärtigen Behandlungswege der Kieferschussverletzungen. Ergebnisse aus dem Düsseldorfer Lazarett für Kieferverletzte (Kgl Reservelazarett)* (Wiesbaden: Verlag von J.F. Bergmann, 1915-1917).
Cohen, D., *The War Come Home. Disabled Veterans in Britain and Germany, 1914-1939* (Berkeley, CA: University of California Press, 2001).

Crumplin, M.K.H. and Starling, P., *A Surgical Artist at War: The Paintings and Sketches of Sir Charles Bell, 1809-1815* (Edinburgh: Royal College of Surgeons of Edinburgh, 2005).

Cushing, H., *From A Surgeon's Journal* (London: Constable & Co., 1935).

Delaporte, Sophie, *Les Gueules Cassées: Les Blessés de la Face de la Grande Guerre* (Paris: Nöesis, 1996).

Deranian, H.M., *Miracle Man of the Western Front: Dr Varaztad H. Kazanjian, Pioneer Plastic Surgeon* (Worcester, MA: Chandler House, 2007).

Dolby, R.A., *A Regimental Surgeon in War and Prison* (London: John Murray, 1917).

Dowd, J.H., *The Doings of Donovan in and out of Hospital* (London: Country Life, 1918).

Dugain, M., *La Chambre des Officiers* (Paris: Éditions Jean-Claude Lattès, 1998).

Gibbs, P., *Now It Can Be Told* (New York: Garden City, 1920).

Gillies, H.D., *Plastic Surgery of the Face: Based on Selected Cases of War Injuries of the Face Including Burns* (London: Hodder & Stoughton, 1920).

Gillies, H.D. and Millard, R., *The Principles and Art of Plastic Surgery* (London: Butterworth & Co., 1957).

Glubb, J.B., *Into Battle* (London: Cassell, 1978).

Gordon, A., *The Rules of the Game: Jutland and British Naval Command* (London: John Murray, 1996).

von Graefe, C.F., *Rhinoplastik* (Berlin: Realschulbuchhandlung, 1818).

Guillebaud, P., *From Bats to Beds to Books. The First Eastern General Hospital (Territorial Force) in Cambridge – And What Came Before and After It* (Cambridge: Fern House, 2012).

Gurner, Ronald, *Pass Guard at Ypres* (London: J.M. Dent & Sons, 1930).

Haeseker, B., *Dr. J.F.S. Esser and his influence on the development of plastic and reconstructive surgery* (Rotterdam: Erasmus Universiteit, 1983).

Harrison, Mark, *The Medical War: British Military Medicine in the First World War* (Oxford: Oxford University Press, 2010).

Hay, M.V., *Wounded and a Prisoner of War. By an Exchanged Officer* (Edinburgh: Blackwood, 1916).

Hodgkinson, L., *Michael Nee Laura: The World's First Female to Male Transsexual* (London: Virgin Books, 1989).

Hone, J., *The Life of Henry Tonks* (London: Heinemann, 1939).

Ivy, Robert, *A Link with the Past* (Baltimore, MD: Waverly Press, 1962).

Judd, J.R., *With the American Ambulance in France* (Honolulu, HI: Star-Bulletin Press, 1919).

Keegan, D.F., *Rhinoplastic Operations with a Description of Recent Improvements in the Indian Method* (London: Baillière, Tindall & Cox, 1900).

Kennedy, P., *The First Man-Made Man: The Story of Two Sex Changes, One Love Affair, and a Twentieth-Century Medical Revolution* (New York: Bloomsbury, 2007).

Klein, F., *Diary of a French Army Chaplain* (London: Andrew Melrose, 1915).

Layton, T.B., *Sir William Arbuthnot Lane, Bt.* (Edinburgh: E. & S. Livingstone, 1956).

Lindemann, A., *Leitfaden der Chirurgie und Orthopädie des Mundes und der Kiefer* (Leipzig: Verlag von Hermann Meusser, 1939).

MacCurdy, J.T., *War Neuroses* (Cambridge: Cambridge University Press, 1918).

McDowell, F., *The Source Book of Plastic Surgery* (Baltimore, MD: Williams & Wilkins, 1977).

Macpherson, W.G., Bowlby, A.A., Wallace, C. and English, C. (eds.), *Official History of the Great War: Medical Services; Surgery of the War*, volume 2 (London: His/Her Majesty's Stationery Office, 1922).

Martin, C., *De La Prothèse Immédiate, Appliquée à la Résection des Maxillaires: Rhinoplastie sur Appareil Prothétique Permanent; Restauration de la Face, Lèvres, Nez, Langue, Voute et Voile du Palais* (Paris: G. Masson, 1889).

Martinier, P. and Lemerle, G., *Injuries of the Face and Jaw and their Repair; and the Treatment of Fractured Jaws*, trans. by G. Lawson Whale (London: Baillière, Tindall & Cox, 1917).

Mayhew, Emily, *The Reconstruction of Warriors: Archibald McIndoe, the Royal Air Force and the Guinea Pig Club* (London: Greenhill, 2004).

Meikle, Murray C. with Bamji, Andrew, Marchant, Bob and Morgan, Brian, *Reconstructing Faces: The Art and Wartime Surgery of Gillies, Pickerill, McIndoe and Mowlem* (Dunedin: Otago University Press, 2013).

Mitchell, T.J. and Smith, G.M., *History of the Great War Based on Official Documents: Medical Services, Casualties and Medical Statistics* (London: His/Her Majesty's Stationery Office, 1931).

Muir, W., *Observations of an Orderly* (London: Simpkin, Marshall, Hamilton & Kent, 1917).

——, *The Happy Hospital* (London: Simpkin, Marshall, Hamilton & Kent, 1918).

Mütter, Thomas Dent, *Cases of Deformity from Burns: Successfully Treated by Plastic Operations* (Philadelphia, PA: Merrihew & Thompson, 1843).

Natvig, P., *Jacques Joseph: Surgical Sculptor* (Philadelphia, PA: W.B. Saunders, 1982).

Nélaton, C. and Ombrédanne, L., *La Rhinoplastie* (Paris: Steinheil, 1904).

——, *Les Autoplasties* (Levres: Joues Oreilles Tronc Membres, 1907).

Nichols, Alan, *Sons of Victory: 1914-1918* (privately printed, N.D.).

Nicolson, Juliet, *The Great Silence: Britain from the Shadow of the First World War to the Dawn of the Jazz Age* (London: John Murray, 2009).

Nobbs, G., *English Kamerad! Right of the British Line* (London: Heinemann, 1918).

Pickerill, H.P., *Facial Surgery* (Edinburgh: E. & S. Livingstone, 1924).

Pound, R., *Gillies. Surgeon Extraordinary* (London: Michael Joseph, 1964).

Reid, G. (ed.), *Poor Bloody Murder: Personal Memoirs of the First World War* (Oakville, ON: Mosaic Press, 1980).

Rémi, H., *Hommes sans Visage* (Lausanne: Editions Spès, 1942).

Report by the Joint War Committee and the Joint War Finance Committee of the British Red Cross Society and the Order of St. John of Jerusalem in England on voluntary aid rendered to the sick and wounded at home and abroad and to British prisoners of war, 1914-1919 (London: His/Her Majesty's Stationery Office, 1921).

Report of the Joint War Committee of the British Red Cross and Order of St John on Voluntary Aid rendered to the Sick and Wounded at Home and Abroad and to British Prisoners of War, 1914-1919 (London: His/Her Majesty's Stationery Office, 1921).

Report to the Army Council of the Army Advisory Standing Committee on Maxillo-facial injuries (London: His/Her Majesty's Stationery Office, 1935).

Riaud, Xavier, *Pionniers de la Chirurgie Maxillo-Faciale* (Paris: L'Harmettan, 2008).

Sassoon, S., *Sherston's Progress* (London: Faber & Faber, 1936).

Schama, S., *The Face of Britain: The Nation through its Portraits* (London: Penguin/Viking, 2015).

Schulte am Esch, J. and Goerig, M. (eds.), *Proceedings of the Fourth International Symposium on the History of Anaesthesia* (Lübeck: Verlag Dräger Druck, 1999).

Scotland, T. and Heys, S. (eds.), *War Surgery 1914-18* (Solihull: Helion & Company, 2012).

Scott, K., *Self-Portrait of an Artist, from the Diaries and Memoirs of Lady Kennet* (London: John Murray, 1949).

Shah, T.M., *Rhinoplasty: A Short Description of One Hundred Cases* (Soruth: Junagadh Sakari, 1889).

Staige Davis, J., *Plastic Surgery: Its Principles and Practice* (Philadelphia, PA: P. Blackiston's Son & Co., 1919).

Stallworthy, J. (ed.), *The Complete Poems and Fragments of Wilfred Owen* (London: Chatto & Windus, 1983).

Steel, Nigel and Hart, Peter, *Jutland, 1916: Death in the Grey Wastes* (London: Cassell, 2003).

Tagliacozzi, Gaspare, *De Curtorum Chirurgia per Insitionem* (Venezia, 1597).

Tait Mackenzie, R., *Reclaiming the Maimed: A Handbook of Physical Therapy* (London: Macmillan, 1918).

Tatham, M. and Miles, J.E., *The Friends' Ambulance Unit, 1914-1919: A Record* (London: Swarthmore Press, 1920).

Tennant, N.A., *A Saturday Night Soldier's War, 1913-1918* (Waddesdon: Kylin Press, 1983).

Thomson, J., *Report of Observations made in British Military Hospitals in Belgium after the Battle of Waterloo with some remarks on Amputation* (London: T. Cadell & W. Davies, 1816).

Vansittart, P. (ed.), *John Masefield's Letters from the Front, 1915-1917* (London: Constable & Co, 1984).

Vidler, D., *Rye Golf Club: The First 90 Years* (Rye: Rye Golf Club, 1984).

Warwick James, W. and Fickling, B.W., *Injuries of the Jaws and Face* (London: John Bale & Staples, 1940).

Whitehead, Ian, *Doctors in the Great War* (Barnsley: Pen & Sword, 1999).

Winter, J. and Baggett, B., *1914-1918: The Great War and the Shaping of the 20th Century* (London: Penguin, 1996).

Wise, S.F., *Canadian Airmen and the First World War* (Toronto: University of Toronto Press, 1980).

Yealland, L.R., *Hysterical Disorder of Warfare* (London: Macmillan, 1918).

Young, Louisa, *My Dear, I Wanted To Tell You* (London: HarperCollins, 2011).

——, *The Heroes' Welcome* (London: HarperCollins, 2014).

Articles

Anon., 'Facial surgery without surgeons', *British Medical Journal*, 2 (1921), p.859.

Bamji, A.N., 'The Macalister Archive: records from the Queen's Hospital, Sidcup, 1917-1921', *The Journal of Audiovisual Media in Medicine*, 16:2 (1993), pp.76-84.

Battle, R., 'Plastic surgery in the two World Wars and in the years between', *Journal of the Royal Society of Medicine*, 71:11 (1978), pp.844-848.

Bennett, John, 'Henry Tonks and plastic surgery', *British Journal of Plastic Surgery*, 39:1 (1986), pp.1-34.

Burkett, Robert, England, Andrew and Rayner, Richard, 'Private Harold Page: a Norfolk man', *Stand To!*, 106 (2016), pp.117-124.

Clarke, R.C., 'Evolution of a casualty clearing station on the Western Front', *British Medico-Chirugical Journal*, 54 (1937), pp.1-20.

Cole, P.P., 'Plastic repair in war injuries to the jaw and face', *The Lancet*, 189:4881 (1917), pp.415-418.

Colyer, J.F., 'A note on the treatment of gunshot injuries of the mandible', *The British Medical Journal*, 2:1 (1917), pp.1-3.

Converse, J.M., 'Plastic surgery, the twentieth century, the period of growth (1914-1939)', *Surgical Clinics of North America*, 47:2 (1967), pp.261-278.

Dorrance, G.M., 'Observations on the work at Queen's Hospital in England', *The Dental Summary*, 39 (1919), pp.865-867.

Dunham, T., 'Method for obtaining a skin-flap from the scalp and a permanent buried vascular pedicle for covering defects of the face', *Annals of Surgery*, 17:6 (1893), pp.677-679.

Esser, J.F.S., 'General rules in simple plastic work on Austrian war wounded soldiers', *Surgery, Gynaecology and Obstetrics*, 24 (1917), pp.737-748.

Filatov, V., 'Plastic procedure using a round pedicle', *Vestnik Ofalmol*, 34:4 (1917), pp.149-158.

Freshwater, M.F., 'A critical comparison of Davis' principles of plastic surgery with Gillies' plastic surgery of the face', *Journal of Plastic, Reconstructive and Aesthetic Surgery*, 64:1 (2011), pp.17-26.

——, 'Denis F. Keegan: forgotten pioneer of plastic surgery', *Journal of Plastic, Reconstructive & Aesthetic Surgery*, 65:8 (2012), pp.1,131-1,136.

——, 'Joseph Constantine Carpue and the bicentennial of the birth of modern plastic surgery', *Aesthetic Surgery Journal*, 35:6 (2015), pp.748-758.

Freshwater, M.F., Su, C.D. and Hoopes, J.E., 'Joseph Constantine Carpue – first military plastic surgeon', *Military Medicine*, 142:8 (1977), pp.603-606.

Hiscocks, D., 'Keeping the individual in focus: making use of interviews with Great War veterans from the IWM sound archive', *Stand To!*, 105 (2016), pp.24-26.

Ivy, R.H., 'The mysterious A.C. Valadier', *Plastic and Reconstructive Surgery*, 47:4 (1971), pp.365-370.

Johnson, H., 'A brush with the golden decade of plastic surgery, 1949 to 1959', *Annals of Plastic Surgery*, 8:2 (1982), pp.166-178.

Kaufman, M.H., McTavish, J. and Mitchell, R., 'The gunner with the silver mask: observations on the management of severe maxillo-facial lesions over the last 160 years', *Journal of the Royal College of Surgeons of Edinburgh*, 42:6 (1997), pp.367-375.

Keegan, D.F., 'Rhinoplasty', *The Lancet*, 137:3521 (1891), pp.419-422.

Lalardrie, J.P., 'Hippolyte Morestin, 1869-1918', *British Journal of Plastic Surgery*, 25 (1972), pp.39-41.

Lindsay, D., 'Five men', *Medical Journal of Australia*, 18 January 1958.

McAuley, J.E., 'Charles Valadier: a forgotten pioneer in the treatment of jaw injuries', *Proceedings of the Royal Society of Medicine*, 67:8 (1974), pp.785-789.

McGee, R.P., 'The maxillofacial surgeon in a mobile hospital', *Journal of the American Medical Association*, 73:15 (1919), pp.1,114-1,118.

Marlow, Hilary, 'The legal career of R.W. Bowen', *Winston Churchill Memorial Trust Fellowship Report*, 2006.

Matthews, D.N., 'Gillies: mastermind of modern plastic surgery', *British Journal of Plastic Surgery*, 32:1 (1979), pp.68-77.

Munby, W.M., Forty, A.A. and Shefford, A.D., 'Notes on the principles and results of treatment in 200 cases of injuries to the face and jaws', *British Journal of Surgery*, 6:21 (1918), pp.86-91.

Penfold, E.A., 'A battleship in action', *The Journal of the Royal Naval Medical Service*, 3:1 (1917), pp.44-56.

Pickerill, H.P., 'Intraoral skin grafting: the establishment of the buccal sulcus', *Proceeding of the Royal Society of Medicine, Section of Odontology*, 12 (1919), pp.17-22.

Remensnyder, J.P., Bigelow, M.E. and Goldwyn, R.M., 'Justinian II and Carmagnola: a Byzantine rhinoplasty?', *Plastic & Reconstructive Surgery*, 63:1 (1979), pp.19-25.

Ryu, J., Horkayne-Szakaly, I., Xu, L., Pletnikova, O., Leri, F., Eberhart, C., Troncoso, J.C. and Koliatsos, V.E., 'The problem of axonal injury in the brains of veterans with histories of blast exposure', *Acta Neuropathologica Communications*, 2:153 (2014), <http://actaneurocomms.biomedcentral.com/articles/10.1186/s40478-014-0153-3> (accessed 26 January 2016).

Staige Davis, J., 'Plastic surgery in World War I and in World War II', *Annals of Surgery*, 123:4 (1946), pp.610-621.

Sykes, P.J. and Bamji, A.N., 'Plastic surgery during the interwar years', *Annals of Plastic Surgery*, 65:4 (2010), pp.374-377.

Valadier, A.C., 'A few suggestions for the treatment of fractured jaws', *British Journal of Surgery*, 4:13 (1916), pp.64-73.

Wakeley, C.P.G., 'Skin grafting in the treatment of war burns', *The Lancet*, 191:4943 (1918), pp.736-737.

——, 'The treatment of burns in naval warfare', *American Journal of Surgery*, 33:3 (1919), pp.61-63.

——, 'The treatment of war burns', *Journal of the Royal Naval Medical Service*, (1917), pp.156-162.

Wallace, A.F., 'The development of plastic surgery for war', *Journal of the Royal Army Medical Corps*, 131:1 (1985), pp.28-37.

Newspapers and periodicals

Daily Sketch
The Lancet
Liverpool College Magazine
National Review
The Times

Websites

Bamji, A.N., *The Gillies Archives from Queen Mary's Hospital, Sidcup*, <http://www.gilliesarchives.org.uk/> (accessed 15 June 2016).

Royal College of Surgeons, 'Cole, Percival Pasley (1878-1948)', *Plarr's Lives of the Fellows Online*, <http://livesonline.rcseng.ac.uk/biogs/E003978b.htm> (accessed 10 January 2016).

Index

Africa xiii, 18, 26, 32, 74, 183, 194, 196

Albee, Fred H. 42, 73, 137

Aldershot i, vii-x, xvi, 19, 41, 49-53, 59, 61, 66-68, 71, 73, 77, 87, 89, 93, 95, 101, 107, 120, 123, 130-131, 140, 142, 148, 168, 170, 183, 186

American Civil War xi-xii, 123, 159

Amiens 18, 103, 112

Arbuthnot Lane, Sir William ix, 48-49, 52, 59-62, 68, 116, 163-165, 174

Ashworth, Walter 73, 185, 187

Auckland vii, 130, 151, 189

Australia i, ix, 62, 106, 122, 146, 161, 168, 186, 192

Australian Imperial Force x, 26, 106, 122

Aymard, Captain John Law ix, 49, 95, 169, 173

Barker, Pat vii, x, 123, 140, 157

Beldam, Sergeant Sidney 89-90, 192-193

Birmingham viii, 63, 68, 78, 90, 136, 167

Blair, Vilray xii-xiii, 63, 116, 168

Boer War xiii, 26, 122

Boston vii-viii, x, 116

Boulogne 34, 39, 44, 48-49, 105, 130, 164

Bowlby, Sir Anthony 26, 31, 113, 129

Bromley viii, 190, 192

Brooks, George 26, 37, 146-149

Budd, Captain J.G.H. 29-30, 34, 37, 145, 148, 152-153

Cambridge i, ix, 36, 47-49, 52, 123, 148, 157, 186-188, 195

Canada i, vii, ix, 67, 113, 168, 190

Chubb, Gilbert 61, 73, 167-168

Cohen, Lieutenant Stanley vii-viii, 21-22, 103-104, 119, 145, 184-186, 192, 198

Cole, Herbert xiv, 46, 122-123, 138, 140

Collins, Albert viii, 151, 155

Colyer, Sir Frank 67, 163, 167

Crimean War xiii, 26, 35

Croydon 67, 163, 167

Cullimore, Harold 158-159, 197, 200

Davidson, Bob viii, 190-191, 202

Delaporte, Sophie vi, x, 92, 112-113

Derwent Wood viii, 45, 128, 151, 166

Dorrance, George M. 63, 68, 104, 116, 162, 168

Dublin 18, 44, 190

Dunedin vii-viii, x, xiv, 63, 110, 129, 140, 168-169

Edinburgh xi-xiii, 32, 38-39, 68, 94-96, 164, 167

Ellerman, Sir John 29, 125, 145

Esser, Dr Johannes F.S. 42-43, 95, 101, 116-117

Evans, Sergeant Reginald vii, 49, 52

France ii, vi, x-xi, 20, 27, 29, 34, 41-45, 47-48, 50, 62, 66, 70, 112-113, 116, 118, 122, 137, 144, 153, 162, 164, 168, 174, 187-188

Frognal x, 53-54, 57, 59, 66, 149, 155, 166, 170, 175, 191

Fry, Captain William Kelsey viii-ix, 60-61, 65, 91, 107, 137, 170

Gallipoli 18, 188, 194

George V, King viii, x, 46-47

Germany xi, 38, 48, 77, 87, 101, 112, 116, 118-119, 129, 145, 183

Gillies, Major Harold D. i, iii, viii-x, xiii-xv, 19, 24, 40-41, 47-54, 57, 59-62, 65-71, 73-75, 77-78, 81-82, 84, 86-92, 94-95, 97-98, 100-101, 103-104, 107-110, 112, 116-121, 123, 128-132, 134-138, 140-146, 148-149, 152-153, 155, 159, 161-162, 164, 167-178, 186, 192, 195-196

Glubb, John Bagot 30, 32, 35-37, 148-149

Gough, Lady viii, 59, 158-159, 201

Grayer, Gunner Cecil 95, 101, 177-179

Green, Private Percy vi, 47, 88, 103, 136

Hampshire i, 52, 54, 70, 100, 123

Harris, Private John 22, 54, 95

Hollins, Bill 154, 191, 194

Hornswick, Sidney 121-123, 132-133

India 26, 50, 172

Jones, Private Henry 48-49, 103, 183-184
Jones, Sir Robert 48-49, 103, 183-184
Jutland, Battle of 22-23, 94, 96, 167

Kazanjian, Dr Varastad viii, x, 42, 113, 115-116,
    168
Kenderdine, Sir Charles 53-54, 58-59, 130,
    165-166
Keogh, Sir Alfred ix, xiii, 49, 164, 173
Kilner, Dr Thomas 76, 161, 169-172, 197

Lancashire 101, 183, 201
Lane, Archie viii-ix, 48-49, 52, 59-62, 68, 72,
    74-75, 90, 93, 110, 116, 128-129, 143, 146,
    163-165, 174-175, 194-195
Leeds vii-viii, xvi, 46, 67, 167, 169
Lindsay, Daryl viii, xiv, 62, 81, 105, 120, 122-123,
    128, 132, 134, 138-140, 161
London i-ii, vii-viii, x-xi, xiv-xv, 17, 19, 22, 29-30,
    32-35, 37-40, 42, 45-48, 50-54, 58, 60-61,
    67-68, 74, 81, 84, 90-91, 93, 101, 103, 106,
    109, 112, 115, 122-123, 125, 129-131, 139-140,
    142-145, 147, 149-151, 154-155, 157-158, 162,
    164-167, 169-171, 175, 183-184, 187-188, 190,
    195
Lumley, Lieutenant Ralph 24-25, 97-98, 104,
    138

Machine Gun Corps 89-90, 123, 146, 179
Manchester viii, 113, 149, 167, 184
McIndoe, Archibald vii, x, 169-173
Mears, Private Arthur Albert 104-106, 123, 126,
    176
Melbourne viii, xv, 62-63, 75, 139-140, 168
Millard, Dr Ralph vi, xv, 19, 48-50, 53, 61, 65, 68,
    70-71, 74, 91, 101, 108-109, 119, 131, 162, 172
Morestin, Dr Hippolyte xii, 41-43, 48-49, 101,
    112-113, 187
Muir, Ward 91, 93, 128, 143, 150

Nélaton, Charles xi-xii, 50, 77, 123
Neuilly 28, 42, 48, 73, 101, 114-115, 137
Neuve Chapelle 44, 52, 183
New Zealand i-ii, vii, ix-x, xiv-xv, 47, 63-64,
    67-69, 80, 122, 129, 140, 151, 155, 163, 168,
    188-189
Newland, Colonel Henry 62-63, 116, 122, 161,
    168
Norfolk Regiment 20, 31, 89
North Sea xiii, 38, 97

Oxford 25, 68, 171, 178, 197

Paris viii, x-xii, 41-42, 44, 48, 50, 61, 76, 92-93,
    101, 112-114, 164-165
Parkwood 59, 61, 65
Philadelphia 44, 68, 94, 116, 167
Pickard, Joseph 75-77, 196-197, 201
Pickerill, Henry Percy viii, x, xiv, 63, 68-69, 73,
    78, 86-89, 92, 110, 136, 138, 168-169, 173
Pound, Reginald 47-48, 50, 52, 60, 81-82, 84,
    142-144, 149

Red Cross viii, 46-48, 52-53, 58, 153, 164
Richmond 145, 165, 177
Rifle Brigade 19, 73, 158, 188
Risdon, Dr Fulton xv, 61-62, 168
Roberts, 'Bobs' C.W. 48, 50, 168, 183-185
Roehampton viii, xv, 48, 53, 159, 163, 165, 167,
    169-170, 197
Royal Field Artillery 21, 80, 98-99, 101, 133
Royal Naval Division 77-78, 131-132

Second World War 17, 94, 110, 131-132, 159,
    170-171, 175, 177, 189-190, 192, 197
Serre 19, 73, 183
Sewell, Trooper Horace 81, 84, 142-143
Seymour, Private Robert 19, 77, 172, 192
Sidcup i-iii, v-vii, ix-x, xiii-xvi, 18-19, 21, 24-26,
    38, 41, 51, 53-54, 58-63, 65-69, 71, 73-75, 77-78,
    81, 87-90, 92-93, 95-98, 100-114, 116-117,
    120-125, 128-131, 134, 136-140, 142-149,
    153-156, 158, 160-171, 173-178, 183-192,
    194-195, 197, 201-202
Smith, Ferris viii, 17, 20, 63, 104-105, 116, 124,
    168, 185-187
Somme, Battle of i, 18, 21, 27, 31-33, 41, 52, 70, 73,
    77, 87, 89, 183, 188, 192
South Africa xiii, 26, 32, 183, 194, 196
Spreckley, Lieutenant William 77, 79, 121, 138,
    197, 200

Thomas, Private William 49, 81-82, 94, 164, 169,
    175, 186, 202
Tonks, Henry viii, 50-52, 61, 73-74, 87, 90-91, 101,
    120-123, 125, 128, 130, 132, 135, 137-140
Toronto viii, xiv, 25, 61
Tringham, Private Leonard 78, 81, 88, 136

United States ii, 42, 63, 94, 100, 115, 129, 164,
    168

Valadier, Dr Charles Auguste 44-45, 48, 61, 113,
    130, 135, 164-165
Vicarage, William 95-97, 178, 182

Wade, Captain Rubens 50, 57, 107-108
Wakeley, Cecil P.G. 94, 96, 167
Waldron, Dr Carl viii, 61-62, 168
Wales 60, 90, 146, 178, 186, 190
Wallace, Major Norman Eric vii, 98-100, 133,
    189-190, 202
Wandsworth 37-38, 45-46, 91, 128, 143
Waterloo xi, 149, 178

Whipp, Private Frank 87-88, 146, 151-152
Williams, Private vii, 74-75, 116, 148
Wimbush, Lieutenant Norman 101-102, 149, 187
Wimereux 44-45, 61, 156, 164

Yeo, Gunner Walter 96-97, 178, 181
Yorkshire 73, 91, 154, 178
Ypres vii, 18, 21, 40, 101, 178, 194